TECHNIQUES IN NONINVASIVE VASCULAR DIAGNOSIS

An Encyclopedia of Vascular Testing

Third Edition-Revision 3

ROBERT J. DAIGLE, JR. BA, RVT, FSVU

Published by Summer Publishing

Summer Publishing, LLC.
4572 Christensen Circle
Littleton, CO 80123

303-734-1789
fax- 1-866-519-0674
email address: Sales@SummerPublishing.com
website: www.summerpublishing.com

Book illustrations by Rodney Summer
Cover design by Pam McKinnie, Concepts Unlimited
Thanks to Nancy Chouinard for proof reading and editing.

ISBN 978-0-9720653-6-8

FOREWORD

Having both been in the field of vascular diagnosis for over 30 years, we have been part of the effort which has seen Doppler Ultrasound, in particular, progress from initially being a curiosity, to be one of the major non-invasive techniques used in vascular diagnosis. During this time, several textbooks have appeared which have tried to explain the technology and application for all who are interested in diseases of blood vessels. Most of them have their merits but there has not been, in our opinion, a book which explains how to carry out the examinations, indicated clinically, how to interpret the results of these investigations, and which also explain the basic technologies involved in a simple but rigorous way.

This present text, we have found, to be direct and to the point, and is not burdened with too much theoretical background. It contains very good technical explanations of basic Doppler ultrasound methods, Duplex and Colour Flow systems. It is also equally as good in the area of physiological testing. The book contains explanatory diagrams and emphasizes the pitfalls which can lead to misdiagnosis. It is easy to assimilate and is an excellent, practical guide and handbook.

We would recommend this book to Vascular Technologists, Clinical Applications Specialists in industry, and anybody who wishes to learn about the practicalities of vascular examinations.

J. P. Woodcock BSc, PhD, FInstP
Professor of Medical Physics and Bioengineering,
University of Wales College of Medicine, Cardiff, UK

R Skidmore BSc, PhD, MIEE, FinstP, FRSA
Managing Director, Scimed Ltd, UK

ACKNOWLEDGMENTS

Many friends and colleagues have influenced the content and style of this book and for their help I am very grateful. A special thanks goes to Dr. Richard Kempczinski for teaching me the fundamentals and laying the groundwork for a career in vascular diagnosis. He taught me the courage to say I don't know when I lacked the knowledge, and encouraged me to investigate, learn and teach. I'd like to thank Rod Summer for his excellent drawings and sketches included in this book.

This book is dedicated to my wife Sandy, who has essentially been without a husband while I've written this third edition, and to my children Kelly and Kristin.

PREFACE

Noninvasive vascular technology is a growing field with an increasing number of practitioners from radiology, ultrasound, echocardiography, cardiopulmonary, physician assistant and nursing backgrounds. A question often posed by people entering the field to those currently practicing the art is "what's a good textbook for vascular technology?" Although there are many excellent textbooks available, the focus of existing books is varied; many are directed exclusively towards the novice, others are designed to aid in passing the vascular registry exam, and others contain information on obsolete tests. Currently, there is no single book with sufficient information to cover this diversity of educational and clinical needs. This book is no exception.

This book will broaden the knowledge of the reader, assist in registry preparation, and provide a basic understanding of a wide range of vascular tests, however, it is not intended to be comprehensive preparatory text for the vascular registry examination. Other publications are better suited for this task. The focus of this textbook is exam protocol and interpretation: what exam to use for specific clinical indications, how to perform the exam(s), and how to interpret the results.

There are very few "standard" protocols within the field of vascular technology. A few testing methods have remained unchanged for 20 years, as they've proved to be effective, cost efficient and accurate, and there have been no good replacements. Most protocols, however, have changed as we find better ways, and because technological advances mandate new test methods. The protocols explained in this book are a mixture of traditional methods and new techniques that as of this writing are "state of the art" and are used by leading vascular laboratories.

There is one rule, or fact of vascular life, which has not changed in 30 years, and one that perhaps distinguishes vascular technology from other technical fields. *The accuracy of the noninvasive examination is almost exclusively dependent on the skill and the experience of the operator.* No matter how knowledgeable the interpreter, if the technologist misses the disease during the scan, it is unlikely that it will be detected. This places a unique responsibility on the technologist or operator, and they must strive to gain the knowledge and competency required. Protocols are merely a guideline for applying knowledge and experience in obtaining a technically good result.

The protocols in this book generally subscribe to the standards recommended by the Intersocietal Commission for the Accreditation of Vascular Laboratories (ICAVL).

Learn as much as you can and enjoy this unique profession. RJD

TABLE OF CONTENTS

CHAPTER 1: PRINCIPLES OF DOPPLER ULTRASOUND

THE DOPPLER SHIFT - HISTORY

In 1842, Christian Andreas Doppler presented his hypothesis "On the coloured light of the double stars and certain other stars of the heavens". He postulated that light emitted from stars moving away from the earth (or towards) was shifted in its wavelength and color. The stars moving away were "red-shifted", and those moving towards us were "blue-shifted" in the light spectrum.

He stated that color perceived by the eye is dependent upon the frequency of the pulsation that stimulates it. Anything that changes the interval between the pulsations changes the perceived color. If the light source and the observer are both at rest, then the observed frequency and emitted frequency are the same.

His ideas were met with great skepticism and in 1845, Christoph Hendrik Diedriek Buys Ballott attempted an experiment to disprove Doppler's theory. It was impossible at the time to challenge the theory with light waves, so Ballott used sound waves in his experiment.

The fastest vehicle at that time was a train capable of 40 MPH that operated between Utrecht and Amsterdam. Ballott positioned a horn player on the train and musicians along the track. As the train approached, all musicians played the same note in an attempt to detect (or not detect) a change in the pitch of the note. The experiment was hampered by adverse winter conditions, so the experiment was postponed until summer. At that time Buys Ballot had arranged a more sophisticated experiment involving teams of musicians. Musical conductors were placed at the train station along with one team of horn players, while the other team rode on a flatbed car of the train. As the trained passed the station at 40 mph, the frequency of the note played by horn players on the train was perceived to increase by a 1/2 note as the train approached and decrease by a 1/2 note as the train sped away. This confirmed part of Doppler's theory of frequency shift related to motion, at least with sound. It was not until the 20th century that it was confirmed with light waves.

In 1846 Doppler said "I still hold the trust, indeed stronger than ever before, that in the course of time this theory will serve astronomers as a welcome help to probe the happenings of the universe". [1]

THE DOPPLER SHIFT - BASIC PRINCIPLES

Echo Doppler is the principle we use to detect blood flow.

As the red blood cells do not emit sound, we rely on our instruments to send sound and receive the echo from moving reflectors. The difference in the transmitted frequency and the reflected and changed frequency from moving blood is called the Doppler shift, or Δ f (delta f).

Piezoelectric crystals

Elements (groups of elements) in the ultrasound transducer are stimulated with electricity to oscillate and produce a high frequency sound signal.

*   The frequency of the transmitted signal depends on the size of the elements: the small the elements, the higher the frequency.

*   Frequency is expressed in hertz , 1 sound wave or cycle per second = 1 hertz.

*   For diagnostic ultrasound, Doppler frequency is between 2.0 - 10 MHz.

*   Piezoelectric elements are similar in function to sound speakers; they both convert electrical energy into the mechanical energy (the moving speaker baffle).

*   Returning ultrasound echoes mechanically stimulate the crystals and the mechanical motion is converted into electrical current.

The returning signal is demodulated and processed and the resulting frequency shift happens to be within our range of hearing. <u>The transmitted frequencies are, in a fashion, compared and subtracted from the reflected frequencies</u> by quadrature signal processing so that the Doppler shifted frequency is expressed as a positive or negative value, depending on the direction of blood flow relative to the Doppler beam direction.

$\Delta f = f_r - f_t$

Δf is the Doppler frequency shift

f_r is the returning frequency

f_t is the transmitted frequency

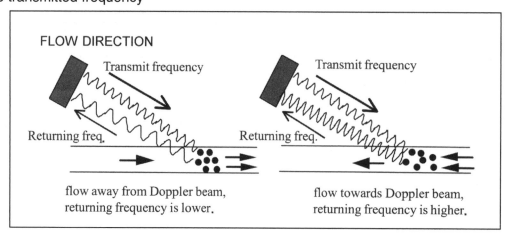

FLOW DIRECTION

Transmit frequency   Transmit frequency

Returning freq.   Returning freq.

flow away from Doppler beam,   flow towards Doppler beam,
returning frequency is lower.   returning frequency is higher.

- If the returning frequency is lower than the transmitted frequency, the Doppler shift is considered a NEGATIVE (-) shift.

- If the returning frequency is higher, the Doppler shift is POSITIVE (+).

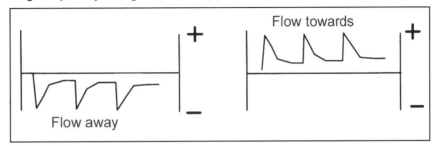

- Generally, negative shift (flow away) is displayed below spectral baseline, unless "spectral INVERT" is enabled. Positive shifts are displayed above baseline. Look for the negative sign on the side of the spectral display (or the "invert" indication).

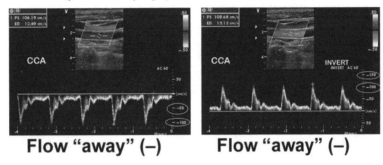

Flow "away" (–)   **Flow "away" (–)**

- If the returning frequency is the same as the transmit frequency, there is theoretically no Doppler shift.

- Some new Doppler systems will automatically "flip-flop" the directional sign when the Doppler beam is changed in the opposite steer direction. Waveforms will stay above baseline and the negative sign will invert. (Unfortunately, most manufacturers don't provide a POSITIVE sign, only a NEGATIVE sign.

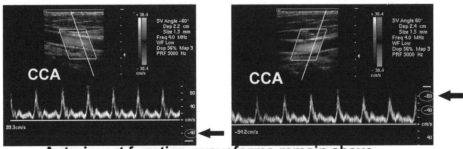

**Auto-invert function: waveforms remain above
baseline, but scale with negative signs flips.**

- Hewlett-Packard, now Philips Ultrasound, uses the "intelligent Doppler" feature on some of their ultrasound systems. The Doppler angle adjustment cursor contains an arrow. The arrow should be adjusted to point in the direction that flow is supposed to going, whether arterial or venous flow. The spectral invert function should be left off. Normal antegrade flow will be above baseline, regardless of steering direction. Retrograde, abnormal flow will be below baseline.

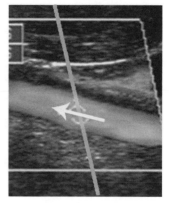

FREQUENCY SHIFT is what we hear and see on the spectral display. It is affected by:

1. <u>The transmitted Doppler frequency:</u> the higher the transmitted frequency, the higher the frequency shift for any given velocity.

2. <u>The Doppler beam "angle to flow"</u> or "angle of incidence": the lower the angle (numerically), the higher the frequency shift. A zero degree angle (Doppler beam parallel to flow) results in the maximum frequency shift, whereas a 90 degree angle results in the lowest frequency shift for any given velocity.

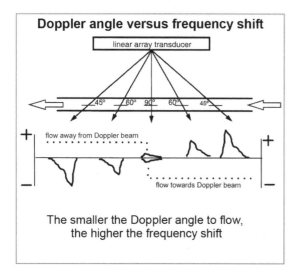

Doppler angle versus frequency shift

The smaller the Doppler angle to flow, the higher the frequency shift

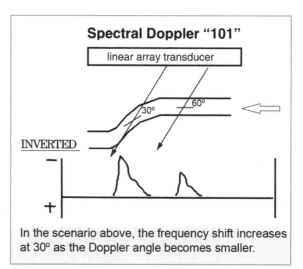

Spectral Doppler "101"

In the scenario above, the frequency shift increases at 30° as the Doppler angle becomes smaller.

3. <u>The velocity</u> of red blood cells: the faster the velocity, the greater the frequency shift.

The Doppler equation expresses the relationship between these factors:

$$\mathbf{\Delta}f = \frac{2\,f_t\,V\,\cos\,\theta}{C} \quad \text{or} \quad V = \frac{C\,\mathbf{\Delta}f}{2\,f_t\,\cos\,\theta}$$

C = average speed of sound in tissue (1540 m/s); this is programmed into the duplex systems.
f_t = transmitted Doppler frequency; this is also programmed into the ultrasound system.
Δf = (delta f); this is the frequency shift.

cos θ = cosine of theta; this is the cosine value of the Doppler angle of incidence. In order to correctly calculate velocity, this angle must be set by the user with the angle correction cursor.

V = estimated velocity.

Doppler Steering

- Beam steering in linear array transducers is accomplished by a signal phasing process that allows the Doppler beam to be steered to the left or to the right. If the beam is not phased (un-steered), it appears straight down and perpendicular to the face of the transducer.

- The amount of steering (phasing), whether 10, 15, 20 or 30 degrees is dependent on transducer design, the element spacing (pitch), the number of elements, the number of channels and the transducer frequency.

- Many Doppler systems allow steering to only 20°. In a horizontal vessel, parallel to the transducer face, this will result in a Doppler angle of incidence of 70°.

- It is important to understand the difference between Doppler beam angle, and angle of insonation to the vessel.

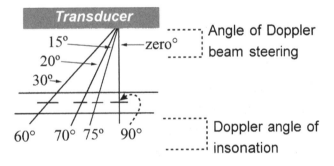

- Velocity estimates become less accurate when the Doppler angle exceeds 70°. It is recommended that the Doppler angle of insonation be 60 degrees or less for accurate velocity measurements.

- If the vessel is horizontal and the Doppler steering angle is 20° or less, the operator must "heel and toe" the transducer to achieve a lower Doppler angle of incidence.

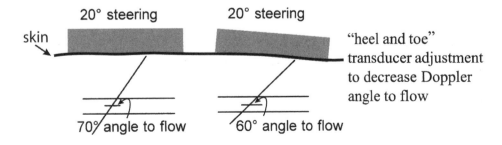

- If the vessel is not horizontal, steer the Doppler in a fashion that will lower the angle of incidence. *see below*

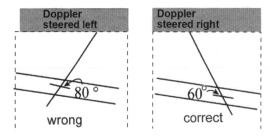

NOTE: A common mistake made by "newts..." is to place the Doppler beam into a vessel and adjust the angle correction cursor, not to the axis of the vessel, but to the numerical value of 60 °. THIS IS NOT THE DOPPLER ANGLE OF INSONATION, and this scenario will result in a false velocity calculation. See Below.

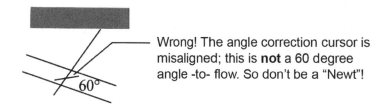

- At low Doppler angles, small errors in cursor alignment have a minimal effect on the velocity estimation. As Doppler angle increases, however, small misalignment can have greater effect. The diagram below illustrates the effect on the velocity estimation of a 5° misalignment of angle cursor at 40, 60 and 80 degree Doppler angles on the velocity estimation. A 5° misalignment at an 80 degree angle will result in nearly 100% overestimation of the actual velocity.

- Doppler angles of >60° can be used as long as velocity measurements are not essential. As previously stated, angles of 60° or less are required for accurate velocity estimation.

Angle cursor misalignment

<u>Actual velocity = 100 cm/sec.</u>

<u>Velocity read-out with errors:</u>

5° error at 40° angle = 108 cm/s

5° error at 60° angle = 118 cm/s

5 ° error at 80° angle = 195 cm/s

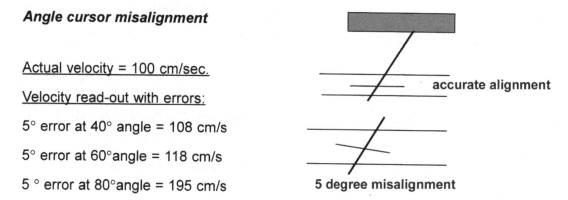

CONTINUOUS WAVE (CW) DOPPLER

CW Doppler uses two piezoelectric elements; one constantly transmitting and the other constantly receiving.

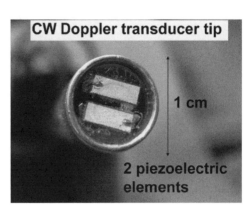

CW Doppler transducer tip

1 cm

2 piezoelectric elements

Advantages of CW Doppler:

* It is not specific for depth, and it will detect flow in any and all vessels in the beam path.

* It is useful and convenient for obtaining systolic blood pressures in lower arterial exams.

* There is no aliasing artifact.

Disadvantages of CW Doppler:

* It is not specific for depth, and it's difficult to isolate specific vessels along the beam path.

PULSED WAVE (PW) DOPPLER

* In PW Doppler, the same piezoelectric elements are used for transmission and reception.

* PW Dopplers may consist of a single crystal or an array of elements. In linear array transducers, multiple elements are used together for Doppler.

* The pulse sequence is as follows:

    * A pulse is transmitted from the piezo elements; then the elements "turn off".

    * At a specific time interval, WHICH IS DETERMINED BY THE DEPTH OF THE SAMPLE GATE, elements are "turned on" in the receive mode for a brief period.

    * The frequency content of the returning pulse from a specific depth is then compared to the transmitted signal for frequency content.

    * The transmit - receive cycle is then repeated.

> REMINDER: The transmit pulse length is set by the sample volume length. A long sample gate results in a prolonged "ring time" of the elements and pulse length is long. Conversely, a small sample volume length results in a short transmitted pulse.

Range-Gating in Pulsed Wave Doppler

The range gate or sample volume, positioned within a vessel and at a specific depth, sets the time interval of the pulsed wave Doppler. A deep range-gate requires a greater time interval between pulse transmissions, as the system must wait for the returning echo before the next pulse transmission. Conversely, a shallow range-gate requires a shorter time interval.
The rate of this pulse-echo cycle is known as the **pulse repetition frequency or PRF.**

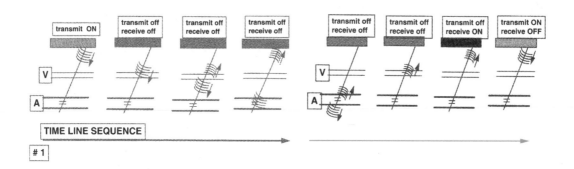

Pulse Repetition Frequency

* PRF is the number of pulse-echo cycles occurring in one second.

* PRF ranges from several hundred to many thousands of times per second.

* PRF is expressed as hertz (Hz), 1000 pulse-echo cycles in one second = 1000 Hz. (PRF "hertz" is not the same as one sine wave cycle per second in transmitted sound frequency.)

* The PRF on most systems is linked to the SCALE control in spectral and color Doppler.

Aliasing

* Aliasing will occur when the Doppler frequency shift exceeds one half of the PRF. This is known as the <u>Nyquist limit.</u>

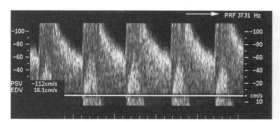

Typical appearance of aliased spectra with peaks coming up from the bottom. PRF is at 3731 Hz.

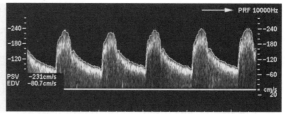

PRF increased to eliminate aliasing. PRF is now at 10,000 Hz.

To eliminate or reduce aliasing:

* Increase the PRF (practical solution).

* Drop or reposition the baseline (practical solution).

* Eliminate the time-sharing features like "triplex" Doppler, where color, image and spectra are all happening simultaneously (practical solution).

* Use a higher Doppler angle to decrease the frequency shift (theoretical solution).

* Decrease the Doppler transmit frequency (theoretical solution).

* Decrease the sample volume depth (not always possible) (theoretical solution).

Note: System PRF is not related to the transmitted frequency of the transducer.

DISPLAYING THE DOPPLER SIGNAL

Fast Fourier Transform (FFT)

⇒ FFT processes thousands of Doppler shifts each second and subdivides the frequency shifts into "bins".

⇒ Frequency shift is displayed in the vertical axis on the spectral display.

⇒ Time is displayed on the horizontal axis of the spectral display.

⇒ Amplitude, or Power, is displayed as brightness of each pixel in the FFT spectral display. The higher the density of reflectors, the higher the number of frequency shifts in each "bin". The higher the "bin" density, the brighter the pixel on the display screen.

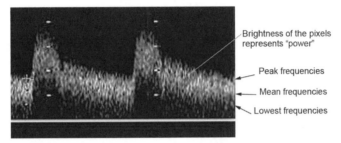

Brightness of the pixels represents "power"

Peak frequencies

Mean frequencies

Lowest frequencies

Other Doppler parameter adjustments.

Wall Filters

• Spectral and color Doppler have wall filters, also called "thump", or high-pass filters.

• Wall filters are often linked to the PRF scale. As the scale increases, so does the wall filter level.

• Wall filters should be set to less than 100 Hz for venous flow detection.

• Filters should be set low for the detection of low velocities in a near total occlusion of an ICA.

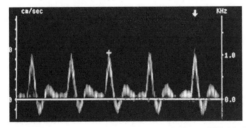
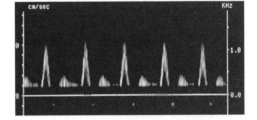

Popliteal artery with low wall filter (55 Hz)   Popliteal art. with high wall filter (200 Hz)

Sample volume

The sample volume (aka, range-gate) length is adjustable. Increasing the size increases the "ring time" of the Doppler elements during a pulse, i.e., it increases the spatial pulse length. Decreasing the SV size has the opposite effect. A large SV increases spectral broadening as there are more "lanes of traffic" being sampled. A small SV samples a more discrete area of flow.

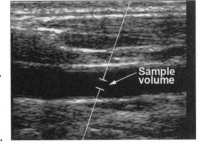

Sample volume

COLOR DOPPLER

• Color Doppler uses multiple scan lines contained within the color box or region of interest (ROI) to create a real-time image of frequency shifts related to movement. This process must occur relatively fast to be perceived as "real-time". If the range gate method were used similar to spectral Doppler, it would take too long to generate a color scan line, let alone a single color frame.

• Color information obtained from one sweep of all scan lines equals one frame. Most color images are displayed at a rate of 8 frames per second or greater.

• Frequency shifts detected within sample sites along the scan lines are processed with autocorrelation.

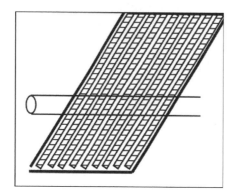

Autocorrelation

• Most color Doppler systems use <u>autocorrelation</u> to generate a color image. In this mathematical technique, multiple pulses sent along a single scan line are analyzed for frequency shift at various depths. On a color Doppler display, there are typically hundreds of Doppler sample sites per scan line.

• An initial pulse is transmitted down a scan line into the tissue. The non-Doppler-shifted information is processed for gray-scale content, while the Doppler-shifted echoes from the multiple sample sites along the scan line are stored in memory. The echoes are converted to voltages for each echo.

• Subsequent pulse echoes are obtained, stored and then compared to the initial pulse echo.

• Shifted echoes (voltages), related to motion within the sample locations, are detected by the comparison.

Autocorrelation provides the following information: [2]

1) direction (sign, negative or positive)
2) average or mean frequency shift
3) power or amplitude
4) variance (frequency spread).

Autocorrelation requires at least 3 pulses per line, but typically manufacturers use between 6 and 20. A high number of pulses per line (often called High Resolution Mode) results in a more robust color image, but at the expense of frame rate. A lower number of pulses per line compromises color quality, but allows faster color frame rate.

Pulses per scan line

The number of pulses per line is known by the following terms:

⟹ Packet size

⟹ Ensemble length

⟹ Color sensitivity

⟹ Color quality

Color quality is also affected by axial resolution. Increased axial resolution (using a higher transmit frequency) makes pixels smaller in the vertical plane. Conversely, decreasing axial resolution increases pixel vertical length.

Scan Line Density

High scan line density	**Low scan line density**
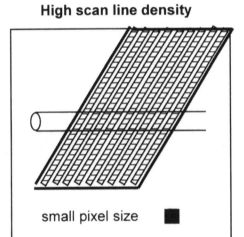	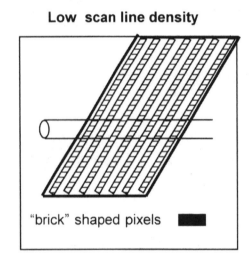
small pixel size ■	"brick" shaped pixels ▬

- The density or number of scan lines affects the color image and the frame rate; the higher the line density, (high number of scan lines within the color box), the better the color resolution.

- High scan line density requires more time to generate an image, so frame rate is slower. Conversely, higher frame rates result when scan line density is lower. The line density control is often referred to as Color Resolution.

- Instruments that offer a high "RES" mode increase the scan line density.

- Most color duplex systems use line averaging to compensate for reduced scan line density.

- The information between the scanlines is interpolated and filled in. This is performed to maintain higher frame rates.

- The color frame rate usually can be improved by decreasing the width of the color box. This decreases the number of functioning color scan lines.

Color Coding and Direction

Adjust and optimize color parameters including gain and PRF scale controls.
See Color plate #1: A-F.

Color angles game "101".

The typical color-coding assignment for direction is "Blue Away, Red Towards, or **BART**. Color can be <u>inverted</u> to allow blood away to be red. The examples below attempt to illustrate that color coding is based on flow relative to the transducer color beam.

Figure pg.12:1-4   Transducer, color unsteered

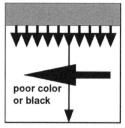 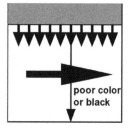 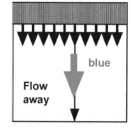 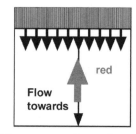

Flow at 90° to Doppler, flow neither towards nor away, poor color coding.   Flow <u>away,</u> blue.   Flow <u>towards</u>, red.

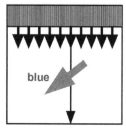 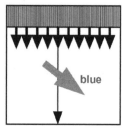 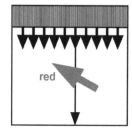 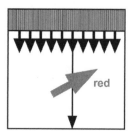

Flow from right to left and <u>away.</u>   Flow from left to right and <u>away.</u>   Flow from right to left and <u>towards.</u>   Flow from left to right and <u>towards</u>.

See Color Plate #2: A-E.

Color directional coding is related to flow either towards or away from the Doppler beam direction, and not necessarily based on whether flow direction is left or right on the ultrasound image.

Figure pg.13:1

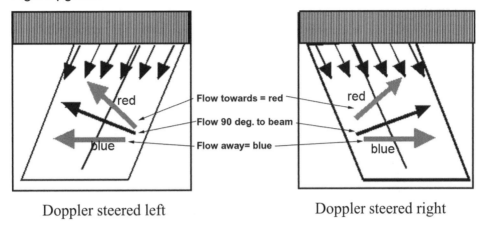

Doppler steered left   Doppler steered right

See Color Plate #2: E.

Frame rate

Color frame rate is slower than B-mode ultrasound due to the necessity of several pulse transmissions per scan line.

<u>Color Frame rate variables:</u>

⇒ Packet size.

⇒ Density of scanlines.

⇒ PRF.

⇒ Color box width.

⇒ Color box depth.

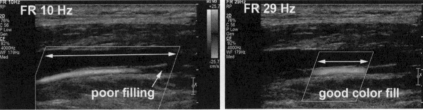

Figure pg.13:2 *See Color Plate #2: G-H.*

POWER DOPPLER

Traditional color Doppler methods assign blue or red color for flow direction, and hue or saturation for variation in frequency shift. As with spectral Doppler, color flow is angle dependent. Higher angles result in lower frequency shift and darker color hues, and vice versa. At a 90° angle, Doppler sensitivity is poor, and color coding ambiguous.

Power Doppler (PD) color method encodes the amplitude or "power" of the blood cells. In FFT spectral Doppler, pixels within the spectral display are assigned a brightness dependent upon the density of frequency shifts within the "bin". That is, the higher the number of blood cells traveling at the same speed (amplitude/power), the brighter the pixel in the spectral display. Power Doppler uses a similar method; the color brightness is based on the density or distribution and number of blood cells, and not on their velocity. Although some ultrasound systems encode for direction, all use various color intensities to colorize the "power" of blood cell density along the color scan lines.

Advantages of Power Doppler:

⇒   No aliasing.

⇒   Less angle dependency, color encoding and good filling at 90 degrees.

⇒   Improved noise filtering.

⇒   Improved sensitivity.

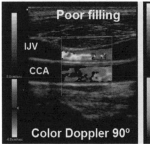 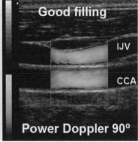

Figure pg. 14:1, 2

Renal perfusion with Power Doppler

See Color Plate #1: G-H.

These advantages allow improved flow detection in organs, tumors, and in low velocity situations. Power Doppler is often useful in detecting the carotid "string sign".

Disadvantages of Power Doppler:

⇒ High persistence.

⇒ Lack of aliasing.

⇒ No velocity encoding.

⇒ Absence of direction encoding (exceptions exist).

⇒ Not able to demonstrate flow turbulence.

The high persistence inherent in many systems causes the color to bleed over vessel walls into surrounding tissue. Although this appears to be "improved flow detection", often it's merely color overwriting onto adjacent tissue. This is exacerbated when the tissue or vessel is pulsating strongly.

Power Doppler removes hemodynamic information; it does not show frequency/velocity increase, nor post stenotic turbulence. For these reasons it is currently not a good tool for evaluating arterial stenosis, except in situations of near total occlusion where "trickle flow" may exist.

Power Doppler at this time does not replace color Doppler for peripheral vascular diagnosis, although it may be used as an adjunct to color Doppler. The advent of directional Power Doppler has improved its utility. The clinical utility of power Doppler is unfolding, but at present it appears to find its best utility in organ perfusion and tumor flow detection. The use of Power Doppler with 3-D rendering and contrast agents is a promising tool.

ARTIFACTS OF DOPPLER ULTRASOUND

B-mode ultrasound is designed to provide images that <u>represent</u> actual tissue lying in the path of the transmitted sound wave. This representation is based on the strength of the reflected echo from tissue interfaces and impedance differences. Color and Spectral Doppler supplement this information by detecting frequency shifts from moving objects (red blood cells and tissue). Artifacts occur that alter the representative image of blood and tissue. It is important for the sonographer, technologist and physician to recognize common "ghosts" of ultrasound.

The Mirror-Image Artifact

*   This color duplex artifact is commonly seen in the left supraclavicular region when imaging the proximal subclavian artery or vein. [3]

*   A second artery or vein appears deep to the actual vessel. This phantom artery or vein can be seen in gray scale image, color Doppler and spectral Doppler.

*   The Doppler signals are usually weaker than those generated by the actual vessels which lies closer to the transducer surface.

*   Occasionally, this artifact can be seen below the common carotid artery.

*   This artifact has been referred to as a "ghost" artery.[4]

Figure pg.15:1

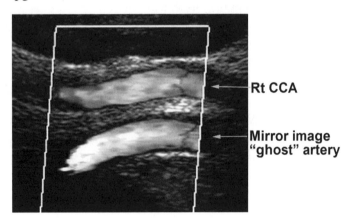

Rt CCA

Mirror image "ghost" artery

Common carotid artery "ghost" artifact. ***See Color Plate #3: A.***

The mirror imaging artifact is often confused with a aberration of normal anatomy. In the neck (image above), it may be confused with an ECA and ICA originating from the innominate artery. In the supraclavicular region, it is mistakenly thought to be a dual subclavian artery.

The diagrams below illustrates how the reflection phenomenon occurs.

In the <u>image on the right</u>, the ultrasound beam (A) strikes the "object" and most of the signal is scattered away from the transducer.

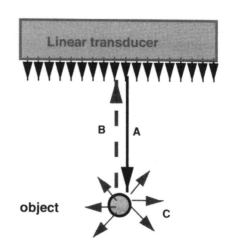

Some of the signal (B), however, is reflected back to the transducer where it is received and processed.

Based on the <u>transit time</u> of the signal down and back, and the known speed of sound in tissue, the system can estimate the distance of the reflector, in this case the target object. It will be displayed in the image at the appropriate depth.

In the next diagram on the transmitted sound from the left side of the transducer depicts the object in its correct time/ depth orientation.

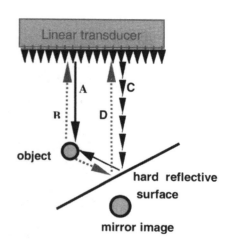

The transmitted beam (C) from the right side however, strikes the hard, reflective surface (caused by the impedance difference between air and tissue) of the pleura /lung interface.

Some of the signal deflects towards the object, strikes it, and reflects back to the lung surface, and back to the transducer (D).

Because the time of flight is longer on the right (C & D), the system interprets this as a reflection from a great depth, and it displays the object at a greater depth in the field of view.
So two objects will be displayed, the more superficial one is the actual object, and the deeper one (below the pleural- lung interface) is the artifact. The reflective object can be tissue or red blood cells.

This type of "goblin" can appear below any "hard" reflective surface and is often seen below calcified arteries, atherosclerotic plaque, and in abdominal ultrasound, near the diaphragm. It's also common see the region of the left subclavian artery from a supraclavicular scan approach.

See Color Plate #3: B.

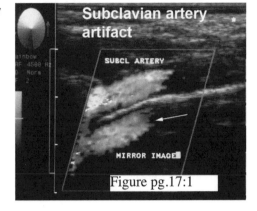

Figure pg.17:1

Elevation Plane Focus Artifacts.

There are 3 focal planes in ultrasound that affect image resolution:

⇒ Lateral

⇒ Axial

⇒ Elevation plane; this is the slice thickness of the beam (sometimes referred to as the "Z" axis)

Remember: a linear array transducer displays a two dimensional image of a three-dimensional object.

The lateral resolution depends on beam forming and focusing characteristics. Good lateral resolution can separate and distinguish objects that are beside each other. Multiple focal zones increase the <u>lateral</u> resolution along the vertical axis (depth)..

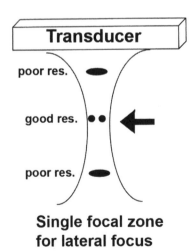

**Single focal zone
for lateral focus**

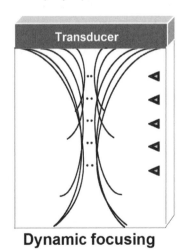

Dynamic focusing

Axial resolution is determined by the axial pulse length, which in turn is dictated by the transmit frequency. The higher the frequency, the better the axial resolution. Axial resolution is the ability to distinguish small adjacent objects along the axis of the ultrasound beam.

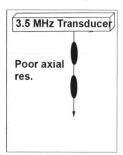

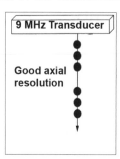

There is a <u>third dimension</u> of the ultrasound beam and it's called the <u>elevation plane</u>.

From Scanlon KA. Sonographic Artifacts and their Origins. 5

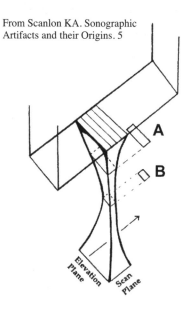

The focal zone of the elevation plane is fixed and is not affected by the adjustment of lateral focal zones. This plane is sometimes called the "slice thickness", but this term implies a uniform thickness to the slice and this is not the case with most current ultrasound systems.

The elevation plane focal area is set at a specific depth and varies by transducer design and frequency.

The resolution of an object depends on where the object lies in the beam path. A small object at point B will be seen with good resolution, whereas a small object at point A will be adversely affected by the slice thickness.

The slice thickness in this diagram has been exaggerated for effect.

With this vessel in <u>longitudinal view</u>, the image displayed will be only two dimensions. The thickness between the arrows will be displayed as one flat plane, as in a photograph. However, the flat plane image will be a composite of the vessel and the tissue on each side that is within the thickness of the beam. It will appear as though the tissue is inside the vessel. (See next figure).

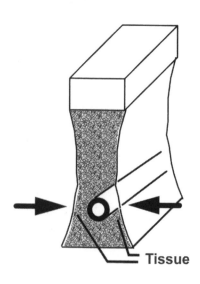

- When surrounding tissue becomes "averaged" with the main object of interest, the image becomes a composite.

- This is also referred to as the "partial volume effect".

- The erroneous depiction of tissue or echoes within an otherwise anechoic object can cause cystic structures to look solid.

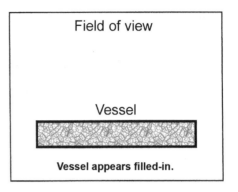

Field of view

Vessel

Vessel appears filled-in.

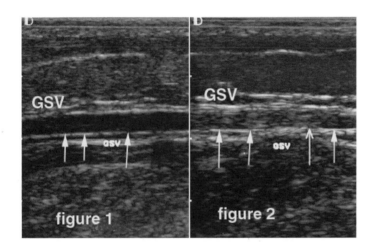

figure 1   figure 2

Figure 1 was obtained with a 10 MHz transducer with a short (shallow) elevation plane focus. This superficial great saphenous vein lies within the narrow segment of the slice thickness.

Figure 2 was obtained with a 5 MHz transducer with an deeper elevation plane focus. The vessel appears filled-in due to a wide beam at this superficial depth.

Some manufacturers have developed transducers that focus more uniformly in the elevation plane. This allows better resolution over a greater depth and improves the B-mode image by reducing the "partial volume" effect. These vessels will appear free of tissue. These transducers are sometimes called matrix array or 2-D transducers.

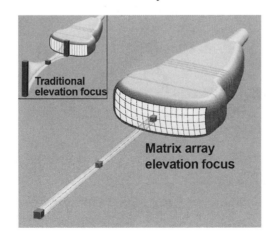

Traditional elevation focus

Matrix array elevation focus

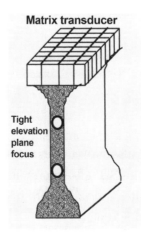

Matrix transducer

Tight elevation plane focus

Intrinsic Spectral Broadening[6]

- Spectral broadening, or increased bandwidth within the FFT spectral display, has traditionally been associated with an increase in the "spread" of velocities of red bloods cells (RBCs) within the sample volume caused by disturbed, non-laminar blood flow.

- Modern linear array transducers employ relatively large Doppler apertures to allow beam steering (phasing) and good depth penetration.

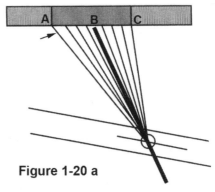

Figure 1-20 a

- These large apertures cause a spectral spread, or broadening, that is unrelated to blood cell distribution or flow patterns.

- This phenomenon, called Intrinsic Spectral Broadening (ISB), occurs to a greater or lesser extent on all linear array transducers.

- ISB artificially increases the peak frequency on the spectral display and can cause velocity overestimation.

- The larger the aperture, or number of elements used for Doppler, the greater the spectral broadening.

- In a typical Doppler ultrasound display, a single Doppler cursor is shown along with the sample or range gate. This Doppler line represents the center of the Doppler beam. There are, however, multiple elements on either side of the Doppler line that form the Doppler beam. Frequency information from all elements, A-C above in Figure 1-20a, are displayed in the spectra, and the result is intrinsic spectral broadening. The highest frequency shifts come from the end elements (A, above), while angle correction occurs with the center elements (B).

- There are additional issues at play that effect the ISB, but these are beyond the scope of this text.

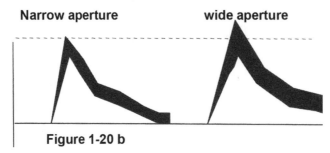

Figure 1-20 b

- The spectral waveform on the left above in Figure 1-20b, (produced with a small aperture), has minimal ISB, and improved peak velocity estimation. The waveform on the right demonstrates increased broadening resulting in an increase in peak frequency/velocity measurement values.

- Intrinsic spectral broadening is minimal at low Doppler angles, but increases in a non-linear fashion as the Doppler angle increases. Above 65 or 70 degrees, ISB can cause a significant overestimation in the velocity calculation and this can adversely affect disease categorization.

- Some clinicians have suggested using a fixed Doppler angle to standardize the overestimation brought on by ISB. Unfortunately, ISB appears to be <u>related to Doppler beam steering</u>, as well as angle Θ.

Some systems produce different frequency shifts for the exact same Doppler angle depending on the Doppler beam being unsteered (straight down), or steered to the side (30 degrees of beam steer). When the beam is fired straight down (zero degrees of steering), maximum "effective aperture" is used for that depth, and depth penetration is optimized.   However, maximum ISB occurs when the full aperture is used. When the beam is steered to one side or the other, *effective Doppler aperture is reduced,* as is intrinsic spectral broadening. As discussed above, the size of the "effective" aperture affects ISB and the appearance of the spectral waveform. The amount of steering, the size of the aperture, and other Doppler configurations vary considerably from manufacturer to manufacturer.

WHAT TO DO ABOUT THIS ARTIFACT?

⇒ When an accurate measurement is essential for disease classification, use Doppler angles of 60 degrees or less; if possible keep the Doppler angle between 50 and 60 degrees.

⇒ Lower Doppler angles result in less intrinsic broadening and more accurate velocity estimations.

⇒ During disease follow-up exams, use the Doppler angle employed in the previous exam and, if possible, use the same beam steering configuration, i.e., Doppler unsteered, left or right.

Doppler Range-gate depth ambiguity [7]

<u>Normal pulse repetition frequency (PRF)</u>

- When one sets the Doppler sample volume or range gate at a specific depth in the ultrasound field of view, the operator is actually setting a time interval between transmission and receive mode in the pulsed Doppler system.

- The system sends a Doppler pulse, waits for a specific length of time, and then turns on the piezo elements to receive and process the returning echo.

- The Doppler system rejects all returning echoes except those from the specific depth (time) of the sample gate.

- Because the propagation speed of sound in tissue is known, time and depth are synonymous.

- Normally, the system will not transmit another pulse until the previous pulse has been received, so the system knows the returning pulse has come from the sample volume and not from another vessel that might lie in the path of the Doppler beam.

High PRF

- This technique is used by some manufacturers to increase the rate at which this pulse-echo cycle, or pulse repetition frequency (PRF), can occur.

- The system will transmit a pulse at twice the normal interval, which means a second pulse is sent before the original pulse returns.

- The PRF is doubled in this method and aliasing is usually eliminated.

A problem can develop with high PRF if other vessels lie in the beam path. The system is not exactly sure of the depth from which the returning echo was reflected. It might have come from the sample volume, or from one of the other vessels. If there are no other vessels in the beam path, except the one specifically being examined, or if the secondary vessel does not lie at half or twice the sample volume depth, there's not problem. When in high PRF mode, manufacturers will often indicate the regions of potential secondary sample gates.

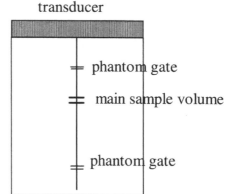

If the multiple or "phantom" sample gates lie in or near a vessel, the Doppler system will not be able to differentiate signals from the main sample volume from those of the phantom gates. **This is known as range gate ambiguity.** If this situation should occur, reposition the scan plane to keep the phantom gates out of more superficial or deeper vessels.

REFERENCES - ADDITIONAL READING

1. Alec Eden, Christian Doppler -Thinker and Benefactor. Druckerei Roser, Salburg-Publisher 1988

2. Kremkau FW. Diagnostic Ultrasound: Principles and Instruments. 7th Ed. Saunders-Elsevier 2006

3. Reading CC, Charboneau JW, Allison JW, Cooperberg PL. Color and Spectral Doppler Mirror Image Artifact of the Subclavian Artery. Radiology 1990;174:41-42

4. Middleton WD, Melson GL. The Carotid Ghost: A Color Doppler Ultrasound Duplication Artifact. J Med 9:487-493.1990

5. Scanlon KA. Sonographic Artifacts and their Origins. AJR 156:1267-1272 June 1991

6. Daigle RJ, Stavros AT, Lee RM. Overestimation of Velocity and Frequency Values by Multi-element Linear Array Dopplers: J Vasc Technol, 14(5):206-213,1990

7. Mitchell DG. Color Doppler Imaging: Principles, Limitations, and Artifacts. Radiology 1990: 177:1-10

CHAPTER 2: CAROTID COLOR DUPLEX SCANNING

CEREBROVASCULAR SYMPTOMS

1. Cerebrovascular accident (CVA)- completed brain stroke.

Causes:

- Embolism
- Thrombosis
- Hemorrhage

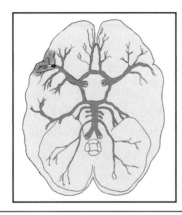

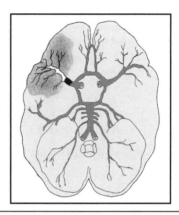

| If a thromboembolus is small, it will travel distally along a cerebral vessel (in this case the MCA) until it lodges in a small branch. A small area of brain tissue is affected and the ischemia may be transient (TIA). | If the embolus is large, it may occlude the proximal portion of a cerebral artery (in this case the MCA) and a much larger region of brain tissue is affected. Stroke and death are more likely consequences of large emboli. |

2. Transient Ischemic Attack (TIA) - symptoms resolve within 24 hours.

3. Reversible Ischemic Neurologic Deficit (RIND) — Symptoms resolve, but not within 24 hours.

4. Death is also a possible consequence of stoke.

Common Hemispheric symptoms and associated hemisphere:

- Aphasia - inability to speak or express oneself - dominant hemisphere, usually left.

- Dysphasia - impairment of speech, lack of coordination and failure to arrange words in proper order- dominant hemisphere.

- Dysarthria - imperfect articulation of speech due to disturbances of muscle control, slurring, etc. dysfunction of any number of brain centers.

- Lateralized paresthesia - tingling and numbness - contralateral hemisphere.

- Hemiparesis - lateralized weakness- contralateral hemisphere.

- Hemiplegia - lateralized paralysis - contralateral hemisphere.

- Amaurosis fugax (AF), AKA, transient monocular blindness (TMB), related to ipsilateral artery.

- Ataxia- gross incoordination of muscle movements, clumsiness of limb - contralateral hemisphere.

Vertebral - Basilar symptoms:

⇒ Diplopia-double vision   ⇒ Dizziness

⇒ Vertigo   ⇒ Drop attacks

⇒ Syncope   ⇒ Binocular blindness

Miscellaneous symptoms:

- Headaches, neck pain, death.

CAROTID ANATOMY

The distal vertebral arteries form the basilar artery. The basilar artery supplies blood to the posterior hemispheres of the brain via the posterior cerebral arteries.

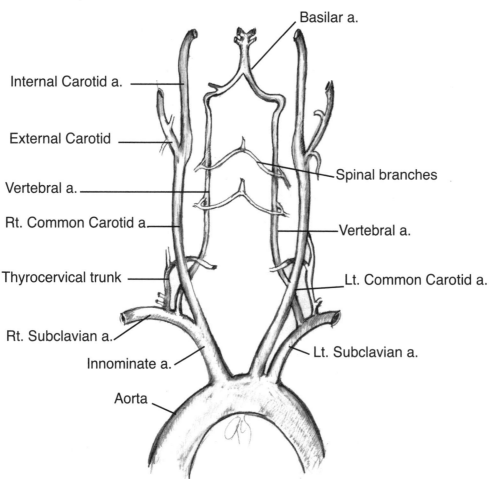

The innominate artery is also known as the brachiocephalic artery.

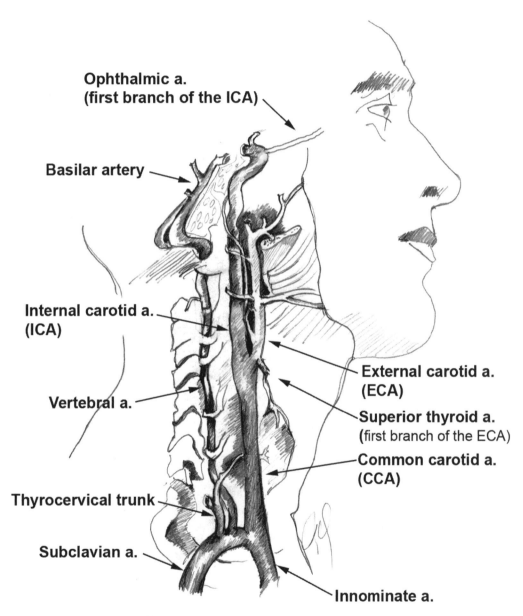

**Ophthalmic a.
(first branch of the ICA)**

Basilar artery

**Internal carotid a.
(ICA)**

Vertebral a.

Thyrocervical trunk

Subclavian a.

**External carotid a.
(ECA)**

Superior thyroid a.
(first branch of the ECA)

**Common carotid a.
(CCA)**

Innominate a.

Right Carotid Anatomy Diagram

PATIENT PREPARATION

Introduce yourself to the patient and to family members if present.

The duplex exam is begun after a pertinent clinical history has been obtained from the patient. History should include:

- Type of neurologic symptom(s), when they occurred and the duration.
- Myocardial infarction (MI).
- Hypertension (HT).
- Diabetes (DM).
- Smoking.
- Vascular operations.

⇒ To make the patient feel at ease, explain how long the exam will take and the nature of the test.

⇒ The patient is positioned supine on a comfortable exam gurney or bed (we use an extra 3-inch thick, full length foam pad on top of the exam table mattress) with a thin pillow placed under head and shoulders.

SCAN POSITIONS

⇒ The exam is performed with the operator sitting and positioned at the head of the exam table: use a table, gurney, pram etc., that will allow operators legs and knees to fit underneath.

⇒ Place a towel or tissue inside the patient's collar, and apply acoustic gel to the neck along the course of the carotid artery. Use plenty of gel.

⇒ Rest your right arm on the pillow and hold the transducer close to the "business end"; See below.

This is a good scan position for the right carotid. The ultrasound system is on the left side, controls are operated with the left hand.

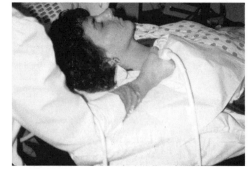

Although different scan positions are possible, all the sonographers that I consider to be "the Pros" scan from the head of the bed. Reasons include comfort, the ability to scan from posterior -lateral scan plane, and the ability to hold the transducer steady without drifting. The latter is particularly important when trying to hold a small Doppler sample volume in a tight (< 1 mm residual lumen) carotid stenosis to obtain several waveforms.

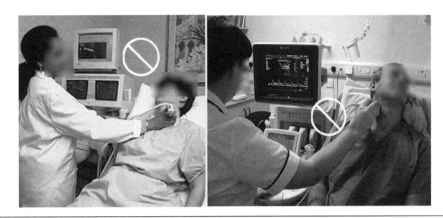

From the internet, these pictures demonstrate the worst possible scan positions: standing, no arm support, and transducer held in an anterior scan position. ***Don't do this!***

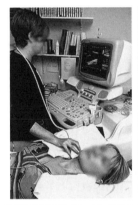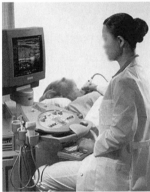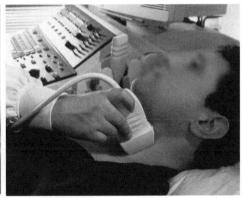

These scan positions, although inevitable when the head of the bed cannot be accessed, promote an anterior scan approach; OK for the ECA, but not the ICA If you use these (suboptimal) positions, you must be able to position the transducer posterolateral along the course of the ICA. Many sonographers who image from this position do not utilize the aforementioned optimum acoustic window.

More on appropriate scan positions later in the chapter.

There are a number of methods to scan the patient's left side. Many sonographers find it helpful to learn to scan with both right and left hands. The sonographer in this picture is scanning the left carotid with her left hand. The controls are operated with the right hand. This method will work only if the ultrasound control keyboard can be positioned very close to the operator; otherwise, it's a poor ergonomic position.

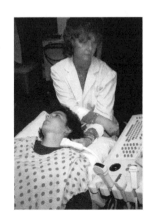

Scanning the left carotid

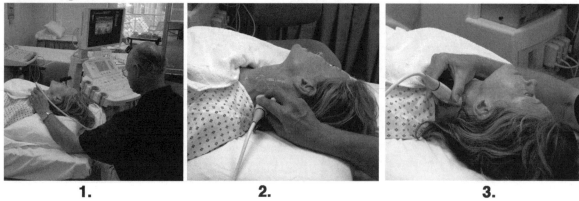

1.   **2.**   **3.**

1. US system moved to the right side, patient scanned with the left hand. Good method.

2. US system remains on left side: Sonographer shifts position to the left and scans with right hand. System is controlled with left hand.

3. US system remains on the left side: Sonographer scans left side with right hand with arm over top of patient. OK if posterolateral position can be achieved without choking the patient!

IMAGE SCAN PROTOCOL

Image orientation

Standard radiographic image orientation is used. In transverse (cross-sectional) plane, you're looking up through the body from the feet. The patient's right side is displayed on the left side of the screen and the patient's left side is on your right (see figure) below.

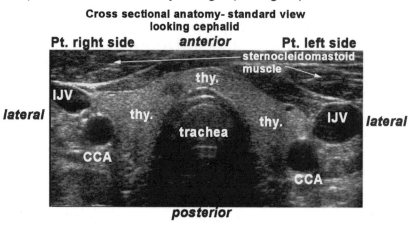

Cross sectional anatomy- standard view looking cephalid

In longitudinal view cephalad (towards the top of the head) is displayed to the left of the monitor, and caudal (towards the feet) to the right side of the monitor.

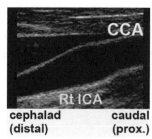

cephalad (distal)   caudal (prox.)

Transverse image

- Imaging is begun in a transverse plane with the patient's head slightly rotated away from the side to be examined. The transducer should be positioned with the "notch" downward for right side scanning.

- The common carotid artery (CCA) is identified at mid neck with an anterolateral transducer position and the image is oriented to the correct anatomical view. The thyroid should be to the right of the CCA on the image when scanning the right side; on the patient's left side, the thyroid should be on the left side of the CCA in the field of view.

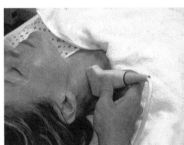

- Scan proximally, then distally to the bulb or bifurcation region. Identify, record, and note regions of disease.

- To optimize the image, try to keep the transducer perpendicular to the artery.

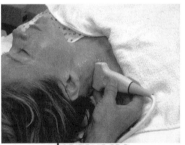

- Image the bifurcation, ICA and ECA from all three "windows" or scan planes illustrated below. Use the best acoustic window to clearly image the artery segment. <u>The best "acoustic window" for the ICA is usually from the posterolateral approach. The best window for the ECA is usually with the transducer anterolateral.</u>

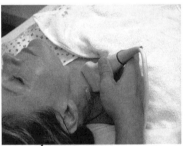

transverse,
anterolateral

transverse,
lateral

transverse,
posterolateral

- Differentiate the ICA/ECA and identify the ICA by its more posterior position in the neck. The ICA lies posterior in the neck 95% of the time, so in a lateral scan position, posterior direction is to the side of the field of view away from the thyroid. In the transverse images above, and to the right, posterior is indicated by a grey bar on the left of the field of view.

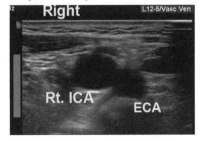

- If you've set up the image orientation correctly in transverse, the ICA will appear on the left side of the screen when scanning the patient's right side; ICA will appear on the right side of the screen when scanning the patient's left side.

Differentiation of ICA and ECA from transverse image

Cross-sectional view of the low neck in standard orientation. Anterior is where the chin is located, posterior is where the spine lies. If we scanned from an anterior to posterior direction, posterior would be in the far field, but we scan from the lateral aspect of the neck. Thyroid appears to the right of the CCA on the patient's right side, and to the left of the CCA on the patient's left side.

This mid-neck view, cephalad to the thyroid gland, demonstrates the ICA-ECA bifurcation. As diagrammed here, the ICA lies <u>posterior</u> in the neck. This occurs in about 95% of patients. Transducer position is anterolateral on the neck. Orientation is similar with transducer in lateral and posterior-lateral scan position.

Although the transducer is positioned on the side of the neck, the onscreen ultrasound image is displayed so that the transducer is at the top of the image.

In the B-mode image with the transducer in a lateral neck position, the right ICA bifurcates to the left of the screen, and the left ICA bifurcates to the right side in the field of view. The ECA position varies and may be lateral or medial (near field or far-field respectively).

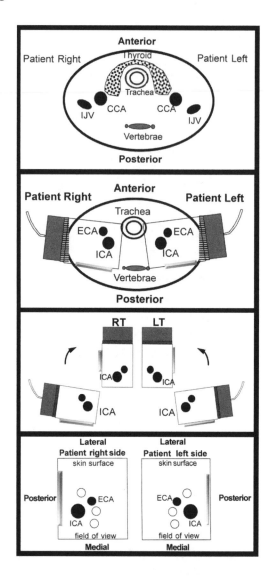

- A general rule of thumb in the transverse view is that the ECA will bifurcate towards the side where the thyroid was seen. The ICA may appear in the near field or the far field, as in the drawing above.

- In longitudinal view, the same relationship will exist, if scanned from the same approach, i.e., if the ICA lies in the near-field in transverse, it will be in the near-field in the long view (same for the ECA). If the ICA and ECA are in alignment vertically, other methods of differentiation may be used.

- In transverse, if the ICA and ECA splay apart abruptly, and the gap continues to widen, the patient has a tortuous ICA, and this information should be useful for aligning the transducer in the longitudinal view.

Anatomy tips:

⇒ The most common mistake in carotid imaging is the incorrect differentiation of the ICA and ECA in diseased bifurcations.

⇒ The ECA is usually smaller than the ICA, but not always. It has branches; this identification helps to differentiate it from the ICA. ICA and ECA differentiation is easy in normals but can become very difficult in the presence of extensive disease at the bifurcation.

⇒ Doppler waveform patterns and characteristic sounds are also used to distinguish the ECA from the ICA. This will be discussed later in this chapter.

Help hint on image orientation:

If the transducer is not oriented on the neck correctly, the image orientation will be "flipped" or

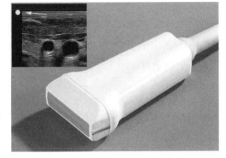

backwards. Most ultrasound transducers have a notch, an indentation or a bump on the casing that corresponds to a dot or mark on the ultrasound field of view. Many novice and some experienced sonographers rely on the "notch" to place transducer correctly. However, it's also easy to just simply slide the transducer on the skin and watch for the appropriate area to come into view in the correct location. For example, in longitudinal plane on the carotid artery, if you move the transducer distally (up the neck), you should see more tissue revealed on the left side of the screen. If more tissue is revealed on the right side of the display, you need to flip the transducer 180 degrees for correct orientation.

> **Orientation demo:** As you're looking at this page make a "lens" with your thumb and index finger similar to an OK sign. Put 👌 the "lens" to your eye and look through it to a section on this page. Move your "lens" and your head to the right; you should see the desk or vision field to the right (similar to moving your transducer and observing image "direction"). If you move to your right and you see page 30, the previous page through the "lens", your orientation is backwards (and you're in big neurological trouble)! If this happens when imaging, rotate the transducer 180° for correct orientation.

Longitudinal Image

• The CCA, ICA, and ECA are next viewed in longitudinal plane.

• Identify the CCA in mid neck from an anterolateral position, and scan proximally, then distally to the bulb or bifurcation region. Identify, record, or note regions of disease. Image the proximal, mid, and distal ICA from all three "windows" or scan planes.

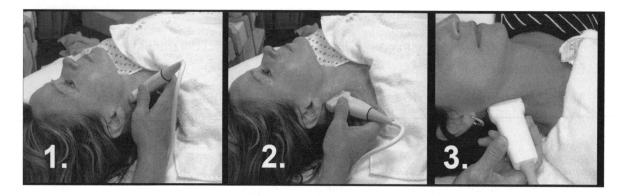

1. Anterolateral approach: good for the CCA and ECA.

2. At the bulb region, slide the transducer towards posterior (the back of the neck) and angle slightly upwards for a good view of the ICA.

3. This posterolateral approach allows the operator to scan distally along the course of the ICA. Note that the transducer is inferior to the angle of the mandible. <u>This is usually the best approach for the ICA</u>. The internal jugular vein provides an excellent "acoustic window" due to reduced US attenuation.

-   Record images of the ICA origin.

-   If plaque is present, optimize the image and demonstrate it clearly in the field of view and record it. For plaque characterization, record the view that demonstrates maximum plaque exposure, even though this view may exaggerate percent stenosis.

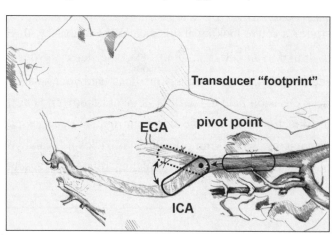

Transducer rotation for ICA and ECA. In longitudinal view, follow the course of the CCA to the bulb. Keep the proximal end of the transducer over the bulb and pivot the distal end slightly towards the chin (anterior) to locate the ECA, and towards the back of the neck (posterior) for the ICA Keep the proximal end of the transducer "fixed" as the pivot point.

In longitudinal plane usually only one vessel, either the ICA or the ECA is within the field of view. In a small percent of the patients, the "wishbone" bifurcation is observed, i.e., both the ICA and the ECA are imaged in the same plane; see below.

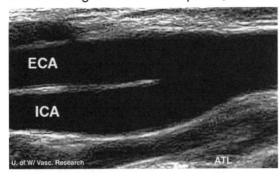

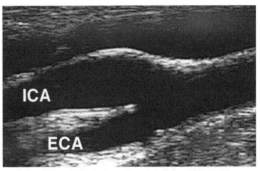

Pt. #1: ECA is in near field.   Pt. #2: ICA is in near field.

> Anatomic helpful hint: the "wishbone" or tuning fork bifurcation, as seen above, is only found in approximately 15-20% of patients. The ICA or the ECA may lie in the near-field (lateral). Remember, posterior is not "far-field" on the screen if you're imaging from the side of the neck.

Other methods of differentiating ICA and ECA:

⇒ The ECA has extracranial branches; the ICA does not.

⇒ The ICA has a lower resistance flow pattern than the ECA.

⇒ The ICA is usually larger in diameter that the ECA, although this can be misleading as the ICA can appear smaller if there is disease.

⇒ The "Temporal Tap" is an aid or tool for differentiating the ICA from the ECA when all else fails. The ipsilateral superficial temporal artery is palpated and "tapped" while the Doppler sample volume is in the vessel assumed to be the ECA. If the vessel being "sampled" is indeed the ECA, this will cause an oscillation in the Doppler waveform. This technique is fallible; if the temporal region is tapped too aggressively, the oscillation can appear in the ICA waveform as well. There is no need to perform this procedure on every patient, as the techniques previously mentioned should be the principal methods for ECA

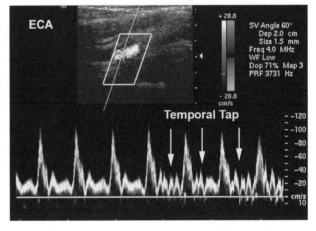

differentiation. But in situations where you are confused about the ECA and ICA, this technique can aid in the differentiation.

Plaque Characterization

In addition to the percent diameter reduction of carotid stenosis, investigators have attempted to identify plaque characteristics that may pose a greater risk for stoke or TIA. Various parameters of plaque morphology, including echodensity and surface characteristic have been correlated, in some reports with a higher rate of cerebrovascular events.

Terminology-definitions

ANECHOIC - Describes the property of being echo-free or without echoes (e.g., a fluid-filled cyst).

SONOLUCENT - Same as anechoic.

ECHOLUCENT - Same as anechoic.

ECHOGENIC - The ability to create an ultrasound echo.

HYPERECHOIC - Producing echoes of higher amplitude than normal for the surrounding medium.

HYPOECHOIC - Producing echoes of lower amplitude than normal for the surrounding medium.

ISOECHOIC - Areas which have similar echogenicity to each other. An isoechoic "property" makes it more difficult to see the desired tissue structure.

HETEROGENEOUS - mixed echoic pattern within plaque- areas of sonolucence and echogenicity.

HOMOGENEOUS - uniform plaque texture.

Assess for <u>plaque surface contour,</u> i.e., smooth versus irregular, and plaque texture, (echodensity) in longitudinal view.

More detail on plaque characterization can be found in the carotid interpretation chapter.

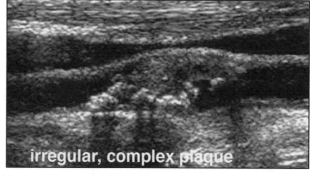

This is a complex, heterogeneous plaque, predominanately echogenic, with areas of sonolucence and calcification (note acoustic shadows).

irregular, complex plaque

Image measurements

⇒   Calculation of percent diameter reduction may be obtained by measuring the true vessel diameter (TD) and the residual lumen (RL) in transverse plane. Alternatively, the plaque diameter can be measured. The resulting percent diameter reduction is a rough estimate of the degree of stenosis, and may be used to quantitate plaque into various percentage groups.

Percent diameter stenosis
% D = PD ÷ TD x 100

Where:
PD: plaque diameter (true vessel diameter – residual lumen)
TD: true diameter of the artery

This is a 50% diameter stenosis

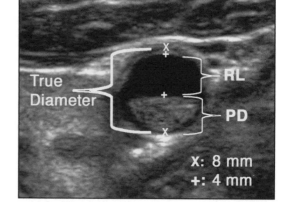

True Diameter

RL

PD

X: 8 mm
+: 4 mm

⇒ Diameter measurements provide a "ball park" estimate of degree of stenosis but are considerably less reliable in stenoses exceeding 60%. At this level the residual lumen becomes progressively more difficult to discern.

⇒ Area reduction can be measured from the transverse image, but must not be confused with diameter stenosis, as they are not the same. Report diameter, not area reduction. A math conversion between A and D is only valid if the plaque is purely circumferential (rare).

⇒ Diameter measurements in longitudinal view may grossly miscalculate percent stenosis, as the plaque can be made to appear more or less stenotic depending on the scan plane.

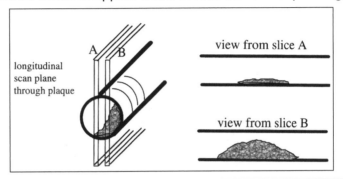

This stenotic plaque (approximately 30% stenosis on this diagram) can be made to appear differently in longitudinal view depending on the plane of the ultrasound beam.

To summarize, transverse and longitudinal B-mode imaging provides information on:

⇒ Anatomy and course of vessels.

⇒ Normalcy or disease.

⇒ Plaque characterization.

⇒ Stenosis estimation.

COLOR DOPPLER ASSESSMENT

General considerations:

Color Doppler is used to locate a region of stenosis or flow disturbance and allow placement of the pulsed Doppler sample gate. It is an essential tool for determining whether flow is present or absent, and is helpful in following the course of a tortuous vessel. Color Doppler has been shown to improve accuracy in differentiating very high grade ICA stenosis (>95%) from total occlusion. By illuminating branches of the ECA, color Doppler is also valuable in differentiating the ICA from the ECA.

Although color Doppler can identify the flow changes associated with a "hemodynamically significant" stenosis i.e., a stenosis of 60% D or greater, it cannot quantitate the stenosis. During the color Doppler exam, the following controls are frequently adjusted:

♦ Color velocity scale, or PRF.

♦ Color gain: to maximize sensitivity.

♦ Beam steering direction: for appropriate angle to vessel.

♦ Color invert: (if your ultrasound system does not have auto-invert).

<u>The following are general guidelines for optimizing color Doppler:</u>

1. **Beam steering**

   The color Doppler beam should be steered in a direction that provides the smallest angle of incidence to the blood flow. The bottom of the color box should point in the direction that the vessel dives.

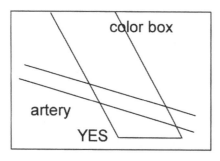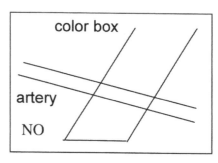

   Figure pg. 36:1-2   *See Color Plate #3: C-D.*

2. **Color scale, or pulse repetition frequency (PRF)**

   For high velocity flows, PRF must be increased to avoid or minimize ALIASING. For lower velocities, PRF scale must be reduced to improve sensitivity. Lower PRF until aliasing occurs, then increase one or two steps to allow good color filling without aliasing.

3. **Color gain**

   To insure appropriate color gain, increase the gain until "speckling" occurs in the image, or until color blooms over the artery wall, then reduce gain slightly, until speckling disappears or is minimized. This ensures that you are not "undergained".

4. **Width of the color region of interest (color box)**

   Frame rate is related to the width of the color box. A wide area of color insonation will reduce frame rate. If a higher color frame rate is desired, use a small color box.

5. **Color assignment**

   Flow away from the color Doppler beam is usually encoded blue (remember BART: <u>b</u>lue <u>a</u>way, <u>r</u>ed <u>t</u>owards), use invert controls to color code arteries red, veins blue if desired.

6. **Color steering**

   Some CDI systems lose color sensitivity when electronically steered. If depth penetration is an issue, turn off beam steering to fire the color beam straight down and angle the transducer (heel and toe) to achieve an appropriate Doppler angle. (See below).

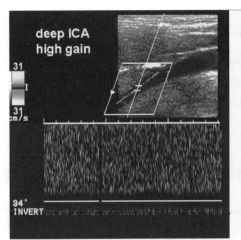 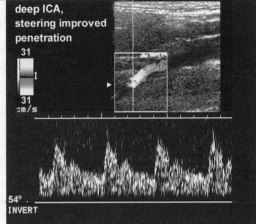

Color and Doppler steered left.   **Color and Doppler "unsteered".**

Other controls that are less frequently adjusted include:

⇒   Packet size (# of pulses per color scan line).

⇒   Scan line density.

⇒   Color maps.

⇒   Filters.

⇒   Color/write priority.

Color Doppler Protocol

⇒   The entire CCA is first evaluated with color Doppler.

⇒   The bulb and proximal ICA are next assessed with color. In the bulb, an area of flow separation, or "eddy flow" is often seen. Absence of local color filling may be due to plaque, low velocity flow, or poor local Doppler angle.

⇒   The mid and distal ICA segments are imaged with color.

⇒   The ECA is located and branches observed to confirm identity.

⇒   Any regions of flow disturbance, that is, increased frequency followed by a "mottled" color pattern, should be recorded and noted.

⇒   If total occlusion of an ICA is suspected, the artery should be interrogated with both low PRF for trickle flow, and with high PRF for stenosis. In the event the ICA is not occluded, color Doppler is idea for following the course of the distal ICA.

⇒   **Power Doppler** can be used if low velocity, trickle flow is suspected, or if the ICA is tortuous. Power Doppler is inherently more sensitive than color Doppler at high Doppler angles (close to 90°).

SPECTRAL DOPPLER ASSESSMENT

Spectral Doppler analysis: General considerations

1. For this text, percent diameter reduction refers to the diameter of the residual lumen at maximum stenosis compared to the true lumen diameter at that same location. This differs from the method now commonly used to measure angiogram, i.e., the residual lumen diameter compared to the true lumen of a disease-free portion of the vessel distally.

2. Velocity acceleration occurs when a stenosis reaches 60% in diameter reduction (some consider 50% the threshold).

3. Velocities do not significantly increase through lesser degrees of stenosis in the carotid arteries.

4. Most stenoses of 60% or greater cause significant turbulence distal to the plaque. The identification of this "post stenotic" turbulence is important confirmation for the presence of stenosis.

5. A focal velocity acceleration over the plaque followed by turbulence is an essential finding for a 50-60% stenosis or greater.

6. Doppler transmit frequency should be less that 5.0 MHz for optimum vascular performance. Frequencies of 5 MHz or greater may not allow adequate penetration on many patients.

The spectral Doppler exam complements the sonographic assessment and is used to determine the presence, location and severity of flow restrictive lesions, i.e., 60% diameter reduction or greater. If stenosis is less than 60%, generally there is no significant velocity increase over the stenotic region. The figures below demonstrate that this 50% stenosis does not increase the velocity over the plaque. The PSV in the CCA is 111 cm/s, and PSV over plaque is 86 cm/s.

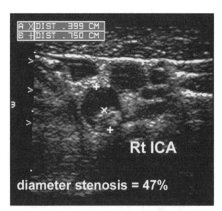

Figure pg. 38:1, 2   *See Color Plate #3: E-F.*

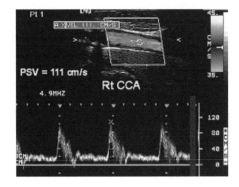

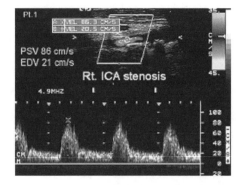

Flow characteristics in the cerebrovascular system

Obtain Doppler waveforms, from longitudinal plane, from the following locations as part of a normal examination.

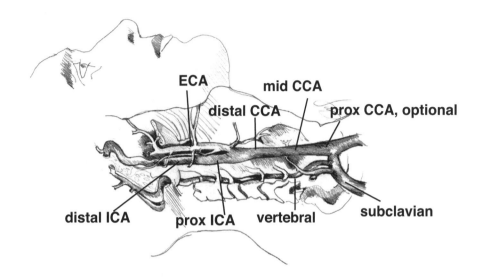

⇒ Mid and distal CCA: (proximal CCA may be obtained if any flow disturbance is seen with color Doppler in that region). Flow in the CCA is usually low resistance with flow throughout the cardiac cycle. The waveform pattern appears as a combination of the ECA and ICA waveforms. The proximal CCA waveform will appear more "pulsatile" (higher systolic velocity, lower diastolic velocity).

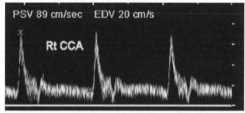

⇒ Proximal ICA (bulb): The CCA widens just before the bifurcation and this dilation extends into the proximal ICA (bulb) . There is a flow separation and often a helical flow pattern occurring in this region. This is normal, and should not be confused with post-stenotic turbulent flow.

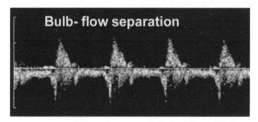

⇒ Proximal ICA, distal to bulb: flow should be "low resistance" as cerebral vessels are vasodilated. There should be forward flow throughout the cardiac cycle. Flow becomes laminar and spectral broadening decreased as one scans distal to the bulb region. Blood velocity may increase in the distal ICA as the artery tapers to a smaller diameter.

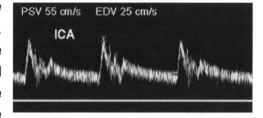

⇒ Proximal ECA: Doppler waveforms should demonstrate higher resistance than the CCA and ICA. Often a prominent dicrotic notch is present in early diastole. If orifice stenosis is suspected (if velocity appears high), sample more distally and look for post-stenotic turbulence to confirm stenosis.

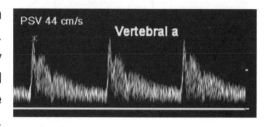

⇒ Vertebral arteries: normal flow should be in an antegrade direction and demonstrate low resistance. Often patients have a dominate vertebral artery with higher velocity on one side. If vertebral spectral waveform is abnormal or retrograde, evaluate the proximal subclavian artery for stenosis or occlusion.

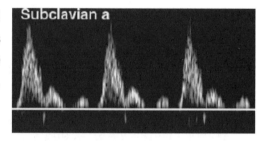

If retrograde flow is suspected, compare to the flow direction in the ipsilateral CCA. See chapter on Vertebral-Subclavian assessment.

⇒ Subclavian arteries: Obtain in mid to distal segments, as the proximal subclavian (on the left) is very deep. Doppler waveforms should demonstrate a high resistance pattern. If turbulence is found, scan more proximally.

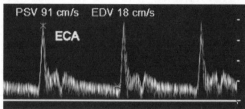

NOTE: Some labs record bilateral arm pressures, and if normal, do not scan the subclavian arteries. Other labs evaluate subclavian arteries only if indicated by abnormality in the vertebral waveform, or if symptomatic. However, ICAVL accreditation recommends that waveforms be obtained from subclavians bilaterally.

Doppler Measurements

Obtain these Doppler measurements from the following vessels:

* CCA: peak systolic velocity (PSV) and peak end-diastolic velocity (EDV).

* ICA: peak systolic velocity and peak end-diastolic velocity.

* ECA: peak systolic velocity.

* Vertebral and subclavian: peak systolic velocity.

* Maximum stenosis: peak systolic velocity and peak end-diastolic velocity.

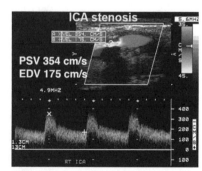

PSV and EDV at maximum stenosis in the ICA.

The following are general guidelines for optimizing spectral Doppler:

- The Doppler beam should be steered in a fashion that provides an appropriate angle, (see color steering above). If Doppler sensitivity is low due to a deep vessel and/or inappropriate Doppler frequency, steer the Doppler straight in, without steering. This provides maximum sensitivity, but Doppler angle may exceed 60 degrees unless the operator uses the "heel and toe" maneuver with the transducer to reduce angle.

- The frequency of the Doppler should be known to the operator. Absence of flow in a deep vessel may be due to inadequate penetration of a high frequency Doppler rather than an occluded vessel.

- Sample volume size is set in a range of 1.0 - 3.0 mm, but may be increased in stenosis.

- Spectral scale (PRF) and / or baseline is adjusted to accommodate the spectral waveform, don't use a large scale with a small waveform. Spectral waveform should be 1/2 - 2/3 of the scale in a normal exam.

- Doppler gain should be set appropriately, and not too high.

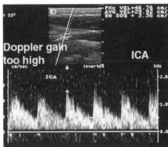

Spectral Doppler gain is too high, spectral broadening could mimic turbulence flow.

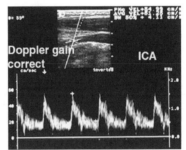

Spectral Doppler gain is adjusted correctly.

Doppler angle (angle theta)

Important information:

For improved velocity estimation, Doppler angles should not exceed 70 degrees. For carotid assessment, ideally, angles of 60 degrees or less should be used. Although Doppler may in some instances be used at angles exceeding 60 degrees, velocity measures will be somewhat overestimated. At 70 degrees or higher, velocities should not be recorded as the values are probably erroneously high, and unreliable.

There is evidence that velocity measurement variability exists between some ultrasound systems.[1] Additionally, some ultrasound systems, but not all, record different velocities at different Doppler angles. This limitation is not clinically important in normal, or minimally diseased patients. It does become an issue when obtaining measurements within a moderate to severe stenosis. If feasible, Doppler angles between 50-60 degrees should be used within stenosis.

Doppler Method for Stenosis

If plaque is seen or flow disturbance noted with color Doppler in the carotid or vertebral arteries, "map" the stenosis in the following fashion:

- Move the Doppler sample volume through the region. Look and listen for focal frequency/velocity increase, followed distally by post-stenotic turbulence.

- It is important for grading the degree of stenosis that velocity be obtained at maximum stenosis.

- The angle adjustment cursor should be carefully aligned to the axis of the vessel.

- Record the velocity proximal to the lesion, at maximum stenosis and distal to the stenosis, noting turbulence and a decrease in velocity.

- Measure the peak systolic velocity and end-diastolic velocity.

> NOTE: In a hemodynamically significant ICA stenosis, obtain at least 3 spectral waveform samples at maximum stenosis. These values should all be within the parameters for a category of disease. See criteria in carotid interpretation chapter.

Vertebral Artery Assessment

Obtain Doppler waveforms from both vertebral arteries and measure PSV. Check carefully for flow direction. See the chapter on Vertebral and Subclavian Artery Imaging for more detail.

A word about carotid ultrasound protocols.

Lab protocols are often based on obtaining, recording and measuring Doppler waveforms from multiple, predetermined sites. The primary purpose of carotid imaging often gets lost in accomplishing the requirements of the protocol. The primary goal of the carotid/vertebral ultrasound exam should be to identify stenosis (or occlusion) and quantify it based on Doppler velocity measurements. This concept should be the foremost principle in your protocol. On one occasion I witnessed a technologist perform a carotid exam according to "protocol" that included sampling in the proximal and distal ICA, but apparently did not include sampling at the point of maximum stenosis, or anywhere within a stenosis! The 60% plus mid ICA stenosis was completely missed (until I made a fuss)! So don't let "protocols" get in the way of identifying disease.

Mapping a carotid stenosis.

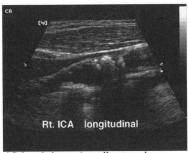

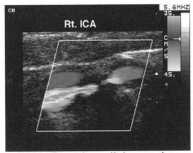

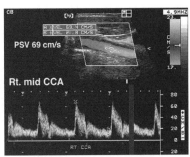

ICA origin not well seen in trans. due to calcified plaque.

Color Doppler: alising and flow disturbance at ICA origin

Mid CCA, PSV 69 cm/s

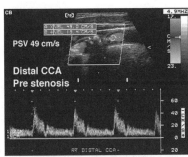

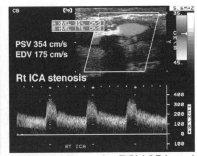

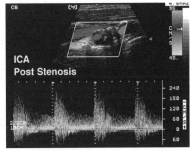

Pre-stenotic velocity PSV 49 cm/s in distal CCA.

ICA max stenosis, PSV 354 cm/s EDV 175 cm/s.

Post stenotic turbulence in ICA

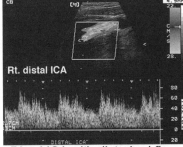

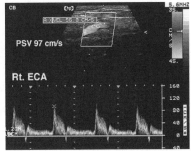

Distal ICA with disturbed flow.

Normal ECA flow.

Figure pg. 43:1-8   *See Color Plate #4: A-F, and Color Plate #5: A-B.*

Internal Carotid Occlusion

The correct diagnosis of carotid occlusion versus a high-grade stenosis is very important for subsequent patient management. If the internal carotid artery occludes, it becomes thrombosed intracranially as well as extracranially, and surgical intervention is usually not possible. Near-total occlusions are amenable to surgery, but the ability of duplex ultrasound to diagnosis this condition is hampered by a number of physiologic and technical factors. "Trickle flow" in a nearly occluded ICA may not be detected with Doppler or color Doppler if the velocity scale (PRF) is set too high.

To identify and characterize the ICA as being totally occluded:

♦ Use color Doppler (and power Doppler if available) at normal and low PRF.

♦ Establish that there is no flow in the ICA by sampling in multiples sites with spectral Doppler.

♦ Observe the course of the ICA in transverse plane to discern tortuosity that might make the ICA difficult to locate in longitudinal plane.

♦ Observe the ICA for thrombus: you must be able to see some length of the thrombosed ICA.

♦ The ICA may be contracted in appearance.

♦ Rule out potential technical problems.

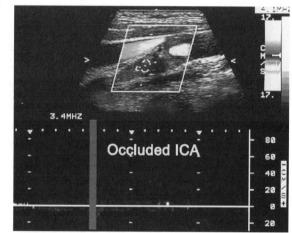

✳ Don't sample under calcified plaque, which may block the Doppler signal.

✳ Use an appropriate Doppler scale (PRF).

✳ Avoid a 90° angle with spectral or color Doppler.

✳ Use sufficient Doppler gain, but don't overgain.

✳ Do not mistake the ECA for the ICA. Occasionally, the ECA waveform may look like the ICA. This is a very common mistake among "Newts".

✳ Don't mistake an ECA branch for the ECA and the ECA itself as the ICA.

♦ The diastolic flow situation in the CCA with ipsilateral (same side) ICA occlusion depends on the resistance in the ECA; high resistance will result in low diastolic flow in the CCA. Conversely, low resistance in the ECA will elevate CCA diastole. The CCA waveform appearance is variable between patients with ICA occlusions, so compare to the contralateral CCA.

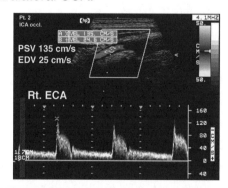

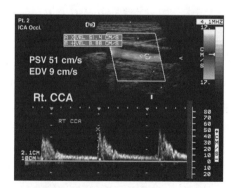

In the figure above, the ICA is occluded. The waveform morphology of the CCA (above) will resemble that of the ECA in the presence of an ICA occlusion, as the ECA and CCA are now essentially the same vessel.

◆ In the presence of an ICA occlusion, the ECA may function as a collateral pathway to the distal ICA. On some patients this pathway (see below) is well-developed via the facial and superficial temporal arteries that anastomose with the supraorbital and supratrochlear arteries, branches of the ophthalmic artery. Blood flows in a retrograde fashion in these arteries to reconstitute the distal ICA. If this occurs, the ECA waveform changes and may demonstrates low resistance instead of the expected high resistance. It may look like the ICA waveform, so BEWARE.

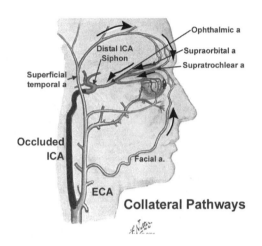

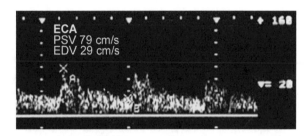

Collateral pathway via the ECA is well developed in this patient with ICA occlusion

UNCOMMON AND ATYPICAL DISEASE CONDITIONS

> 95% diameter stenosis

In some very high-grade stenoses, velocity parameters and ratios may not be useful in grading the severity of disease. The diagram on the right depicts a decrease in velocity at stenosis greater than 95%. Velocities may be elevated, but may be less than the range useful for quantifying disease.   Often, a very low-flow situation can occur due to the high resistance of the residual lumen diameter and length.

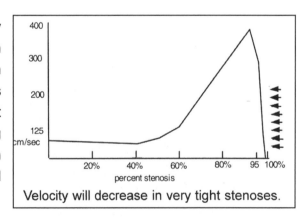

Velocity will decrease in very tight stenoses.

Subjective findings that can assist in identifying this situation include:

• Difficulty in obtaining a complete spectral waveform from the region of maximum stenosis. Reduced blood volume passing through the tight stenosis reduces the number of "reflectors" and the Doppler signal becomes weak.

- Low velocity proximal to the stenosis.

- The observation of low flow velocity distal to the stenotic region.

Very low velocity may occur in a near total occlusion. In this "trickle flow" condition, a low pulse repetition frequency (PRF) or color scale must be employed to detect flow. The residual lumen in this situation may be less than 0.5 mm.

The case below demonstrates a >95 % stenosis.

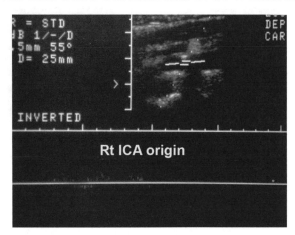

Unable to detect flow on the initial spectral assessment. Calcified plaque could be blocking the Doppler signal.

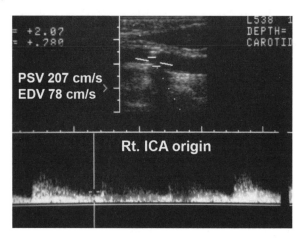

Reverse Doppler steering angle was used in an attempt to get underneath the calcified plaque. It was difficult to obtain a good waveform (high frequency "wisp", then nothing), but the spectra above were the best acquired: PSV 207 cm/sec, EDV 78 cm/sec.

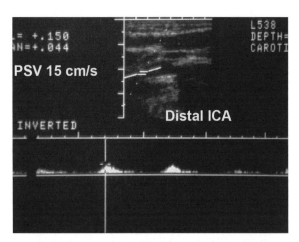

Tardus-parvus flow was detected distal to the stenosis with PSV only 15 cm/sec.

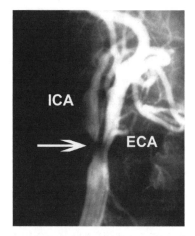

Angiogram demonstrating the severe (>90%) ICA stenosis.

Subjective findings suggested a very severe stenosis, confirmed by contrast digital angiography. If only velocity criteria were used, this >95 % stenosis would have been grossly underestimated.

Occluded Common Carotid Artery

Total occlusion of the internal carotid artery (ICA) is a common finding and is usually not amenable to surgical correction. Occasionally, it is found that the common carotid artery (CCA) is occluded and the ICA distal to the bifurcation remains patent. This scenario is usually enabled by retrograde flow in the external carotid artery (ECA) feeding the patent ICA. If CCA occlusion is found, it is essential to scan the ICA and ECA. In the angiogram on the right, the ECA flow is via an ECA branch connection with a vertebral artery.

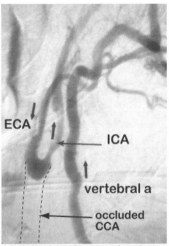

Vertebral angiogram showing retrograde ECA flow and patent ICA in the presence of CCA occlusion.

There have been a few reported cases of retrograde ICA flow supplying the ECA, so a careful assessment of patency and flow direction is warranted in the case of CCA occlusion. When the CCA is occluded branches of the vertebral system that anastomose with ECA branches often supply the ECA.

External Carotid Artery Occlusion

This rarely occurs due to the numerous branches of the ECA. ECA patency is maintained by retrograde flow in the proximal branches. If you are suspicious of ECA occlusion, palpate the superficial temporal artery or facial artery; if a pulse is present, it's unlikely that the ECA is occluded.

Fibromuscular Dysplasia

Fibromuscular Dysplasia (FMD) is a non-atherosclerotic disease that affects the media of the arterial wall. It is found in the renal arteries and in the internal carotid arteries and occurs predominately in women.

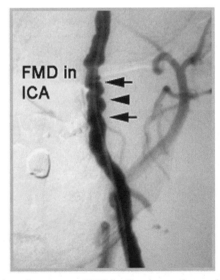

Angiogram of ICA: "string of pearls" appearance is consistent with FMD.

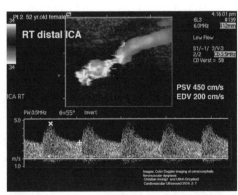

High velocity in distal ICA with FMD

Image courtesy of Christian Arning & Ulrich Gryyska, Cardiovascular Ultrasound 2004,2:7

There are four types of FMD:

      1) intimal fibroplasia

      2) medial fibroplasia - most common form

      3) medial hyperplasia

      4) perimedial dysplasia

The natural history of FMD is unknown. It occurs in the distal segment of the cervical portion of the ICA. The proximal ICA and distal cavernous portion are usually spared. It may not be detected with duplex scanning unless one evaluates the extracranial ICA as distal as possible. The appearance of turbulent flow by color Doppler along the arterial wall and focal velocity increases in the absence of atherosclerotic lesions in the more proximal ICA should raise the question of the presence of FMD, especially in women patients. The wall irregularity is difficult to image with ultrasound due to the depth and angle of the ICA. The most common referral for those with FMD is asymptomatic cervical bruit.

> NOTE: It is imperative that the distal extracranial ICA be carefully evaluated with spectral and color Doppler, particularly in women, to detect FMD.

Carotid Dissection

Carotid dissection is an uncommon condition in which a "delamination" occurs between the intimal and medial layers of the arterial wall presumably by blood flowing through a tear in the intimal wall.

There are basically two types of dissections found in the carotid arteries:

Proximal dissection

⇒   This may occur in conjunction with a thoracic aortic dissection in which the dissection extends into the common carotid artery. Often a separate flow channel occurs within the dissected wall and this can be discerned with spectral and color Doppler. This type of proximal carotid dissection usually does not extend into the ICA.

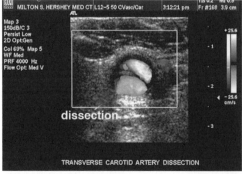
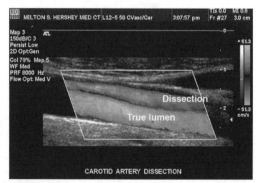

CCA Dissection

Figure pg. 48:1-2. *See Color Plate #5: C-D.*

Distal ICA dissection

⇒   This is also uncommon but can cause cerebral hypo perfusion and significant neurologic sequelae. The mechanism is not well understood, but a intimal tear may cause a "hematoma" in the wall of the artery causing the intima to press inward and encroach on the ICA lumen. There is no false lumen with this type of dissection.

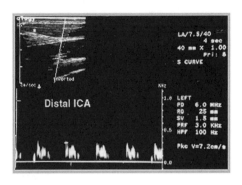

Several conditions have been suggested for its etiology:
- Fibromuscular Dysplasia.
- Blunt trauma to head and neck.
- Congenital defects in the media or internal elastic membrane.
- Chiropractic manipulation.
- Idiopathic.

Symptoms include:
- Hemispheric ischemia and stroke.
- Headache.
- Ipsilateral neck pain.

⇒   This condition seems to be gender specific, occurring more frequently in women than men. The typical Doppler finding in the ICA is a high resistant waveform pattern with low systolic velocity and absent or reduced diastolic flow.

⇒   Flow comparison to the contralateral ICA is important. On angiography, this condition appears as a "string sign" with tapering lumen in the distal ICA to a very small diameter. The dissection has encroached on the lumen to a point where the artery is functionally occluded. These distal ICA dissections often resolve and vessel patency is restored.

⇒   A high resistance ICA waveform may also occur with severe atherosclerotic disease in the distal ICA (siphon region). However, this condition usually coexists with extensive disease in the proximal ICA; this is not typical with dissections.

⇒   Dissections can also occur in the vertebral arteries.

Proximal Disease: CCA or Innominate

Although atherosclerosis predominantly affects the bifurcation region in the neck, occasionally it affects the innominate, subclavian, or common carotid artery origins. Innominate and subclavian disease is addressed in Chapter 4. In the CCAs, the appearance of a rounded waveform with prolonged rise time and low amplitude is often indicative of significant proximal CCA disease, or more likely, innominate artery obstruction, particularly if the phenomenon is observed unilaterally.

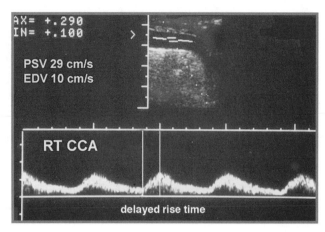

Rt. CCA waveform with innominate artery stenosis.

CAROTID STENTS

Carotid angioplasty with stent placement is alternative to carotid endarterectomy in certain high-risk patients. Intravascular stents can be either self-expanding devices, or balloon deployed; they may be "covered" or open mesh design made of stainless steel or Nitrinol. As with carotid endarterectomy, re-stenosis can occur following the procedure, and serial follow-up exams are recommended for detecting stent complications.

Complications that can be detected with ultrasound include:

⇒   Poor initial stent deployment.

⇒   Re-stenosis by intima hyperplasia.

⇒   Progressive stenosis distal to the stent due to athero disease.

⇒   Stent positional shift.

⇒   Stent kinking.

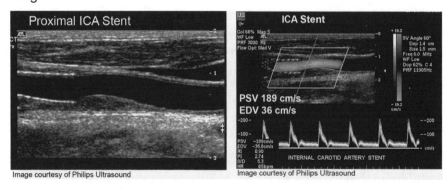

Flow into the ECA depends on the type of stent: a covered stent will block the ECA origin, while a non-covered stent will allow flow through the mesh into the ECA.

Stent Imaging Protocol

⇒   Perform a complete bilateral carotid ultrasound exam.

⇒   On B-mode ultrasound, note the stent position and record images.

⇒   Note whether the stent was fully deployed, and the relationship of the stent to the wall; is there a gap?

⇒   Obtain Doppler samples in the CCA, just proximal to the stent, throughout the stent and distal to the stent. Measure PSV and note where the samples were obtained for comparison to future exams.

⇒   Pay specific attention to the ICA distally, at least 1 cm distal to the stent.

Image courtesy of Dr.Ann Marie Kupinski

⇒   Demonstrate smooth velocity increase into the stent (expected).

⇒   Document any regions of abrupt increased velocity and post-stenotic turbulence.

⇒   Assess the ECA origin for flow irregularities or occlusion.

⇒   Because peak systolic velocity within a stent is somewhat unpredictable, obtain spectral waveforms from easily-reproduced sites within the stent. Measure peak systolic velocity and record Doppler angle and steering position (steered left, center or right). These measurements should be used as a baseline or "benchmark" for comparison during subsequent follow-up exams. During follow-up exams, use the same Doppler and steering angles and measure PSV from the same locations as before.

> NOTE: Velocity parameters used to grade "garden variety" carotid stenosis are not valid for post-stent evaluation. Because wall elasticity is reduced or eliminated by the stent, and the fact that the stent does not restore the original arterial lumen, velocities tend to be higher than thresholds for disease. See carotid interpretation chapter for more detail.

Carotid Rules of the Road Summary:

♦   Always optimize B-mode image: the better the image, the better the color and spectral Doppler.

♦   Use color Doppler to assist in determining anatomy and finding vessels if necessary.

♦   Use color Doppler to identify regions of stenosis and flow disturbance.

♦   Use spectral Doppler angles of 60 degrees or less for accurate velocity estimation and subsequent disease classification.

♦ To avoid adding Doppler variables that may affect velocity measurements, in follow-up exams reproduce the previous Doppler angle and the steering direction (e.g., Doppler steered left to right, right to left, etc.) within the stenotic region.

♦ Obtain 3 or more Doppler samples in a hemodynamically significant stenosis; values should be consistent for the same category for disease. (Know your carotid criteria!)

♦ Doppler information is more reliable than image information in stenoses exceeding 50% diameter. Image is more reliable in stenoses less than 50%.

♦ Do not rely on a single velocity measurement for the presence of disease; use focal velocity acceleration, post-stenotic turbulence, and plaque image as well as objective parameters.

♦ Compare duplex results with angiographic findings, MRA or CTA results and learn from your successes and your mistakes. Be certain that the person "reading" the comparative tests is using the same stenosis measurement method as you're using.

REFERENCES

1. Daigle RJ, Stavros AT, Lee RM. Overestimation of Velocity and Frequency Values by Multi-element Linear Array Dopplers. J Vasc Technol, 14(5):206-213,1990

CHAPTER 3: CAROTID INTERPRETATION

INTRODUCTION

Traditional Duplex Ultrasound Criteria

One of the first documents on duplex ultrasound criteria for stenosis categorization was published in the early 1980s by D.E.S. Strandness Jr. MD at the University of Washington, Seattle WA.[1] The criteria were based on Doppler-derived maximum frequency shift, and on spectral broadening of the Doppler waveform. Frequency parameters were limited, however, by the necessity of a constant, or fixed Doppler angle, and a standard (5.0 MHz) Doppler frequency to avoid variability. (Remember, Doppler frequency shift is related to speed of blood, Doppler angle, and the transmitted frequency). In later years these criteria were converted to velocity parameters.

The stenosis categories included: Normal, 1-15%, 15-49%, 50-99%, and total occlusion. Later, an additional category, >80 %, was established.[2] These categories were based exclusively on spectral Doppler information, including the dubious ability to differentiate normal from 1-15% stenosis based on spectral broadening. When asked by this author why B-mode image information was not included when criteria was established, Dr. Strandness stated that the early duplex systems in their possession had resolution sufficient to see the artery and place a sample volume, but insufficient to accurately image plaque. Hence, the reliance on spectral broadening for lesser degrees of stenosis. These parameters became known as the University of Washington Criteria, or the "Strandness Criteria".

In 1983 Dreisbach et al., from Swedish Medical Center in Englewood, CO., published duplex ultrasound criteria based on velocity parameters and high-resolution B-mode image.[3] Using high frequency (10 MHz) transducers, the study demonstrated the ability to categorize "hemodynamically significant stenosis" (as well as occlusion); it also accurately defined categories of 20% stenosis, e.g., 0-19% (normal), 20-39%, 40-59%, based on cross-sectional diameter measurements of residual and true lumen. Categories of 60-99% were based on elevated peak systolic velocity and velocity ratios (ICA/CCA ratio). R. Daigle, & T. Stavros, from the same institution, established velocity criteria for the differentiation of 60-79% from ≥80% diameter stenosis in 1988.[4] These criteria were included in a consensus paper published in Radiographics in 1988 and became known as the "Bluth Criteria", named after the first (alphabetical) author.[5]

Although other criteria appeared over the years, the majority of those performing and interpreting carotid ultrasound used one of these sets of criteria, until the results of the North American Symptomatic Carotid Endarterectomy Trials (NASCET) were published in 1991.

The University of Washington studies and those of the Bluth consensus, were performed by correlating various Duplex ultrasound parameters to biplane, contrast angiography. The percent diameter reduction on the angiogram was obtained by measuring the smallest residual lumen and the estimated true diameter of the vessel at the same location, aka, <u>bulb diameter stenosis</u>.

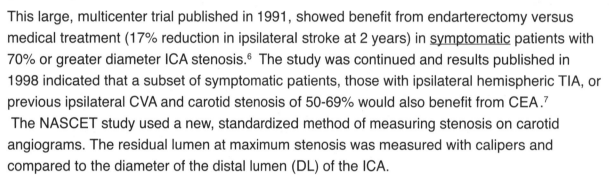

$$\% \text{ stenosis} = 100 \times \left(1 - \frac{\text{residual lumen}}{\text{true lumen}} \right)$$

CAROTID CRITERIA BASED ON CLINICAL STOKE TRIALS

The North American Symptomatic Carotid Endarterectomy Trial (NASCET)

This large, multicenter trial published in 1991, showed benefit from endarterectomy versus medical treatment (17% reduction in ipsilateral stroke at 2 years) in <u>symptomatic</u> patients with 70% or greater diameter ICA stenosis.[6] The study was continued and results published in 1998 indicated that a subset of symptomatic patients, those with ipsilateral hemispheric TIA, or previous ipsilateral CVA and carotid stenosis of 50-69% would also benefit from CEA.[7] The NASCET study used a new, standardized method of measuring stenosis on carotid angiograms. The residual lumen at maximum stenosis was measured with calipers and compared to the diameter of the distal lumen (DL) of the ICA.

Asymptomatic Carotid Atherosclerosis Study (ACAS)

The ACAS trial, published in 1994, demonstrated that carotid endarterectomy reduced stroke risk by 5.8% over <u>5 years</u> in <u>asymptomatic</u> male patients with 60% or greater diameter ICA stenosis.[8] There was no benefit shown for women in this study. Percent stenosis was measured in the NASCET fashion with residual lumen compared to ICA diameter distal to stenosis (DL).

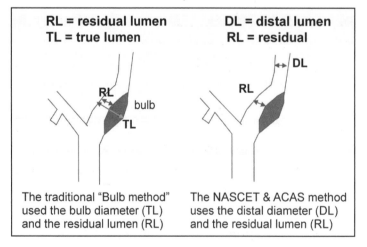

Comparison of the traditional angiographic measurement method and the "new" NASCET method.

Although the NASCET angiographic measurement method eliminates the difficulty in estimating the true vessel diameter in the bulb region, it does not account for stenosis in which the residual lumen is the same as the distal lumen. For example, if the bulb is 8 mm in diameter, the residual lumen is 4 mm and distal ICA diameter is 4 mm, NASCET standard will be <u>0% stenosis</u>. In fact with the NASCET method it is possible to have a negative percent stenosis! <u>It is important to note that the NASCET angiographic measuring method has now been adopted by most radiologists</u>. ***Consequently, most traditional duplex ultrasound criteria do not agree with the NASCET angiogram percent diameter stenosis.***

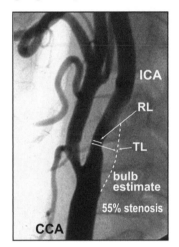   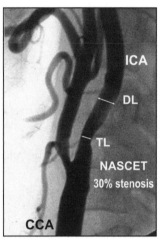

This hemodynamically significant ICA stenosis, (based on Doppler criteria), measures **55%** on the angiogram if calculated via the traditional method, and **30%** if measured with the NASCET method.

Following the publication of the NASCET, ACAS and a large European carotid surgery trial (ECST),[9] several investigators established criteria to define the new NASCET/ACAS percent stenosis.

NASCET CRITERIA FOR > 70% STENOSIS				
Author	**PSV cm/s**	**EDV cm/s**	**ICA/CCA**	**PSV ICA/EDV CCA**
Moneta[10] 70-99%	> 325		> 4.0 (best)	
Fraught[11] 70-99%	>130 Plus EDV	> 100		
Neale[12] 70-99%	>270 Plus EDV	> 110		
Hood[13] 70-99%	>130 Plus EDV	>100		
Dhanjil[14]				>15 = > 70%, < 10 = < 70%, 10 -15= use other criteria
Winkelaar[15]			> 3.6	

The studies above used the NASCET measurement method. Other studies were published for 60% stenosis, and combined with the above parameters and old traditional criteria, ***things got pretty confusing.***

THE SRU CONSENSUS CONFERENCE RECOMMENDATIONS FOR CAROTID ARTERY CRITERIA- 2003.[16]

In September of 2003, the Society of Radiologists in Ultrasound (SRU) convened a multidisciplinary panel of experts to establish a consensus and a recommendation for carotid duplex ultrasound criteria. The goal was to simplify the confusing array of various criteria and to standardize categories and thresholds.

The points of the consensus are as follows:

1) Carotid artery ultrasound examinations should include B-mode (gray-scale) image, color Doppler and spectral Doppler.

2) The degree of stenosis should be stratified into the following categories:
   * Normal (no stenosis)
   * < 50% stenosis
   * 50-69% stenosis
   * ≥ 70% stenosis to near total occlusion
   * Total occlusion

The panel recommended standardization of a number of specific areas of testing and interpretation.

* Exams should be performed with gray scale imaging, color and spectral Doppler in a protocol recommended by an accrediting organization.

* Doppler waveforms should be obtained at angles of 60 degrees or less.

* The ICA should be interrogated with the Doppler sample volume from the bulb region to the distal segment so that the maximum stenotic region can be located.

* The final report should discuss the velocity measurements, B-mode image and color Doppler findings and comments on any technical limitations that may have occurred or be present.

* Comparisons to previous studies, if available, should be contained in the body of the report.

* The conclusion or final impression should contain an estimate of the degree of ICA stenosis according to the stratification parameters illustrated below.

* On angiograms, the carotid stenosis should be measured according to the NASCET method.

* Every test center should have systems in place for both quality assurance and internal validation.

* **Velocity measurements for ICA stenosis should be obtained from the point of maximum stenosis (added by rjd).**

Also, the ICA/CCA ratio is intended to mean "maximum peak systolic velocity (PSV) from the maximum stenotic region divided by a PSV obtained in a disease-free portion of the mid CCA.

SRU CRITERIA TABLE.[16]

Primary Parameters			Additional Parameters	
Degree of stenosis (%)	ICA PSV (cm/s)	Plaque Estimate (%) *	ICA/CCA PSV Ratio	ICA EDV (cm/s)
Normal	< 125	None	< 2.0	< 40
< 50	< 125	< 50	< 2.0	< 40
50 - 69 ##	125-230	> 50	2.0 - 4.0	40-100
≥ 70, but < near total occlusion	> 230	> 50	> 4.0	> 100
Near occlusion	High, low, or undetectable	Visible	Variable	Variable
Total occlusion	Undetectable	Visible, no detectable lumen	N/A	N/A
* Plaque estimates (diameter reduction) with gray scale and color Doppler US				

The velocity and ratio values adopted by the consensus panel for the 50 - 69 % category are controversial. The criteria values appear to be those previously used in traditional criteria (established against the "Bulb Method" of angiographic correlation). The widely-used University of Washington criteria lists ≥125 cm/s for a ≥50% ICA stenosis[1,2], and the "Bluth" criteria uses ≥125 cm/s and a 2.0 ratio for a ≥60% stenosis.[3,4,5] It is likely that the use of 125 cm/ s and a ratio of 2.0 will result in overcalling a stenosis category compared to NASCET angiograms. (An analogy to this situation is mixing Celsius and Fahrenheit values for temperature reporting!)

A number of studies have been published, some since the issuance of the SRU recommendations, that provide more realistic criteria for the 50-69% category. All have correlated velocity and velocity ratios to NASCET angiographic methods.

Criteria for 50-69% "NASCET" carotid stenosis			
Author	PSV cm/s	EDV cm/s	ICA/CCA Ratio
AbuRahma[17]	≥ 140 *	≥ 60	≥ 2.12
Filis[18] (50-59%)	150-200	50-70	≥ 2.2
Winkelaar[19]	≥ 150		≥ 2.0 *
Sabeti[20]	150-249		2.0-3.9
* = Best criteria (most accurate within the respective study)			

Of interest is the similarity of values from the different studies for 50-69% category: >140 or 150 cm/s and ratios of 2.0 or 2.2.

REVISED (BY AUTHOR) SRU CRITERIA TABLE

This table includes a 50-69% criteria based on NASCET measured angiograms from studies listed on the previous page.

Degree of stenosis (%)	ICA PSV (cm/s)	Plaque Estimate (%) *	ICA/CCA PSV Ratio	ICA EDV (cm/s)
Normal	< 125	None	< 2.0	< 40
< 50	< 150	< 50	< 2.0	
50 - 69	> 150	> 50	2.0 - 4.0	60-100
≥ 70, but < near total occlusion	>230	> 50	> 4.0	> 100
Near occlusion	High, low, or undetectable	Visible	Variable	Variable
Total occlusion	Undetectable	Visible, no detectable lumen	N/A	N/A

* Plaque estimates (diameter reduction) with gray scale and color Doppler US

KEY INTERPRETATION POINTS

Several important principles must be understood for interpretation of color duplex findings:

1. According to the Bernoulli principle, significant velocity increase will occur over a lesion that is greater than 50% diameter stenosis, with residual lumen and true diameter measured at the same location.

2. Turbulent, chaotic blood flow is almost always present immediately distal to a 50% or greater stenosis; this appears as spectral broadening in the Doppler waveform.

3. Caliper-determined estimate of percent stenosis from the B-mode image works best if the stenosis is less than 50%. Velocity criteria work best and are essential when the stenosis exceeds 50%.

    Therefore:

    a. If a stenosis measures 50% or greater from the B-mode image (using measurement calipers), but there is no focal velocity acceleration over the plaque, that stenosis is less than 50% in diameter.

    b. If a stenosis measures or appears less than 50% by image/caliper method but velocity acceleration with post stenotic turbulence occurs, that lesion is greater than 50%.

> *Carotid criteria should be used to categorize disease, not to determine normalcy.*

Carotid criteria is meaningless, unless the following 3 conditions exist:
- 1) You can visualize plaque within the artery.
- 2) There is focal velocity acceleration over the plaque.
- 3) Post-stenotic turbulence exists distal to the plaque.

Once these conditions have been recognized, then criteria can be applied.

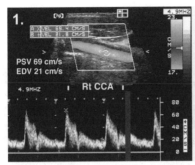 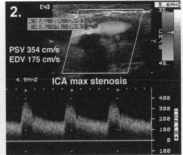 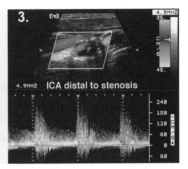

Figure pg. 59: 1-3

Key information in "mapping" a stenosis: 1) mid CCA velocity, 2) spectrum from maximum stenosis, and 3) post-stenotic turbulence. Measurements indicate a >70% stenosis. ***See Color Plate #4: A-F, Plate #5, G-H.***

Difficult diagnoses: >95% stenosis

In some very high-grade stenoses, velocity values and ratios may not be useful in grading the severity of disease. Velocities may be elevated, but may be less than the range used for quantifying disease. Often a trickle flow situation can occur due to the high resistance of the small residual lumen diameter and length of stenosis.

Subjective findings that can assist in identifying this situation include:

- Difficulty in obtaining a complete spectral waveform from the region of maximum stenosis. (Reduced blood volume passing through the tight stenosis yields a weaker returning Doppler signal).

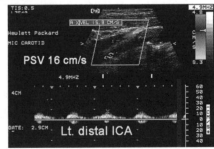

- Low velocity distal to the stenotic region.

Low flow velocity (PSV 16 cm/s) distal to a >90% ICA stenosis.

Very low velocity may occur in a near total occlusion. In this "trickle flow" condition a low pulse repetition frequency (PRF) or color scale must be employed to detect flow. Power Doppler may be useful in this situation. <u>The residual lumen in this situation may be less than 0.5 mm.</u>

Internal Carotid Occlusion

The ability of duplex imaging to accurately diagnose total ICA occlusion is improved by using color Doppler and color power Doppler. However, the overall accuracy of this category of disease remains sub-optimal, as there are a number of pitfalls. There is no substitute for experience in this often-difficult determination. Technologists and interpreting physicians should err on the side of caution if not absolutely sure of total occlusion, and recommend angiography, MRA or CTA in symptomatic patients.

ICA total occlusion

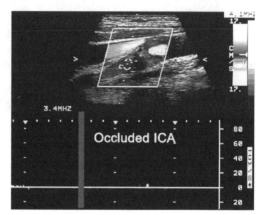

Occluded ICA

- Determine that there is no flow in the ICA, sample at multiples ICA sites.

- Use color Doppler (and power Doppler if available) at normal and low PRF.

- Observe extensive thrombus within the ICA.

- The ICA may be contracted in appearance if chronically occluded; look carefully.

- Technical problems such as inappropriate color Doppler gain, PRF, and steering angle must be avoided.

- Observe carefully in transverse plane to determine the course of a tortuous ICA.

As mentioned in Chapter 2, the presence or absence of diastolic flow in the CCA, when the ICA is occluded, depends on resistance in the ECA; if collateral pathways are well developed, low resistance in the ECA will result in near normal CCA flow. Therefore, CCA waveform appearance may be variable between patients with ICA occlusions. Compare to the contralateral CCA.

CCA stenosis/occlusion

To date there are no specific criteria for stenosis in the CCA. However, a rule of thumb in most arterial systems applies; if the PSV doubles over the stenosis, and there is post stenotic turbulence, this is consistent with a 50% or greater stenosis.

Occasionally, an occluded CCA is found during a carotid ultrasound exam. It's important that the sonographer establish whether there is flow in the ICA. Often the ECA flow will be reversed and fed by an anastomosis between an ECA and a vertebral artery branch. The resulting retrograde ECA flow supplies the patent ICA. See panel below. Although this flow pattern is the most common, the opposite can occur. Retrograde ICA flow can supply the ECA.[21]

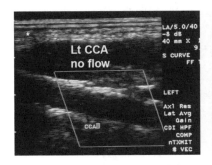 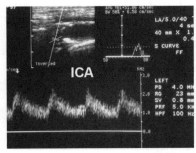 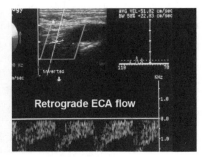

Occluded CCA with patent ICA. ICA flow is supplied by retrograde ECA flow.

ECA stenosis/occlusion

There are no published criteria for ECA stenosis, but a focal increase in velocity followed by turbulence indicates a ≥ 50% stenosis. ECA occlusion is rare, and when it does occur, it's reconstituted soon after its origin by retrograde flow in the proximal ECA branches.

Criteria for Carotid Artery Stents (CAS)

Carotid artery stenting has gained acceptance as an effective alternative for carotid endarterectomy (CEA) in certain high risk patients. These include patients with significant medical comorbid conditions, anatomically inaccessible stenoses, radiation-induced stenoses, and recurrent stenosis following endarterectomy.[22,23,24] The number of patients undergoing CAS is increasing rapidly, and many investigators are recommending periodic follow-up to monitor for stent complications and in-stent stenosis.[25,26,27]

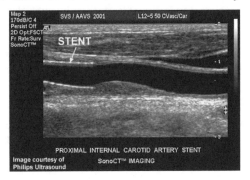

Post-op Carotid Stent Ultrasound Exam

- Expect higher velocities in an ICA stent. Stents usually do not restore arterial lumen diameter to normal size so velocities tend to be higher than in a normal carotid.

- The increased "stiffness" and loss of compliance may also contribute to higher velocities in normal stents.

- Flow may or may not be present in the ECA; it depends on the type of stent.

- Check for stent "shift", re-stenosis and increased distal disease

Soon after stent surveillance became common, investigators found that if standard velocity criteria were used for stent evaluation, stents would be falsely classified as having stenoses when in fact the stents were normal. [28,29]

Ringer et al.,[26] recommends the following: "Blood flow velocity (BFV) criteria for re-stenosis after carotid artery stenting are less reliable than is the change in BFV over time. An immediate post-stenting Doppler study must be obtained to serve as a reference value for future follow-up evaluation."

The following is a table of some of the recently published velocity criteria for CAS. The "ratio" refers to the maximum stent PSV divided by the PSV of the CCA.

Criteria for Carotid Stent Re-stenosis				
	50-69%		≥ 70 %	
Author	PSV cm/s	Ratio	PSV cm/s	Ratio
AbuRahma[29] (>30%)	>155			
Chi [30]	> 240	> 2.45	> 450	> 4.3
Stanziale [31]	> 225	> 2.5	> 350	> 4.75
Armstrong [27]	> 150	> 2	(75%) > 300	> 4

Criteria for Contralateral Carotid Stenosis

In patients with significant bilateral carotid stenosis or occlusion, increased (compensatory) flow in the side with the lesser stenosis can occur. The increased flow volume can result in higher stenotic velocity than expected; this may result in an overestimation of the stenosis.[32,33] Unfortunately for consistency within our diagnostic criteria, the effect does not always occur, and the compensatory effect is variable.

Everdingen et al., demonstrated that increased flow volume on the side opposite the high grade ICA stenosis or occlusion caused PSV to be higher than expected for a particular diameter reduction. This is perhaps a result of a tenet of Poiseuille's Law: a pressure gradient across a stenosis becomes more pronounced with increased flow volume.[34]

Some authors have shown that the use of the velocity ratio is advantageous in this situation. Ray et al., found the use of the ICA/CCA velocity ratio prevented overestimation in eight of the 14 patients with bilateral ICA stenosis.[35]

Other investigators, demonstrating overestimation of stenosis severity in the contralateral carotid due to elevated Doppler flow velocities, have recommended that these patients receive a repeat carotid ultrasound following the intervention, whether endarterectomy or stenting, to assess the true grade of stenosis.[36]

However, it appears that contralateral compensatory flow may or may not be reduced following intervention on the ipsilateral side. In a study published by Roddy et al., in 1999 [37], the contralateral systolic velocity and diastolic velocities did not change following ipsilateral carotid endarterectomy (CEA). They identified no statistical difference in measured contralateral velocities after surgical intervention.

In a large multicenter study including 350 consecutive symptomatic patients who underwent bilateral duplex ultrasonography and digital subtraction angiography, Heijenbrok-Kal et al., evaluated duplex ultrasound thresholds for 70%-99% stenosis of the ipsilateral and contralateral internal carotid arteries. Their assessment of criteria included "optimum" velocity parameters (the SRU criteria for 70-99%), values that were found to be the most accurate, and those that were the most cost-effective (cost of clinical consequences of missed diagnoses and unnecessary endarterectomies). In their report, maximum accuracy for ipsilateral (the symptomatic side) 70-99% carotid stenosis was obtained with PSV ≥ 280 cm/s and for contralateral stenosis, ≥ 370 cm/s. It appears that the contralateral side exhibited velocities that were 24% higher.[38]

Heijenbrok-Kal Criteria Set for 70-99% Carotid Ipsilateral & Contralateral Stenosis.[38]				
"Optimum" (SRU) Threshold	PSV cm/s	Sens. %	Spec. %	Acc. %
Ipsilateral	230	95.4	51.4	75.8
Contralateral	230	92.1	86.5	87.3
Cost effective				
Ipsilateral	220	96.2	55.5	75.8
Contralateral	290	84.2	91.4	90.3
Maximum Accuracy				
Ipsilateral	280	84.7	69.5	78
Contralateral	370	71.1	97.8	94
Sens. = Sensitivity. Spec. = Specificity, Acc = Accuracy				

Plaque Morphology Discussion

In addition to the degree of stenosis, ultrasound characteristics of plaque composition and surface contour have been investigated as a possible risk factor for cerebrovascular events. Gray-Weale and Lusby in 1988 classified plaques into heterogeneous and homogeneous based on B-mode ultrasound image, and compared the classification to surgical specimen pathology following carotid endarterectomy.[39] They found a strong correlation between heterogeneous lesions and the presence of intraplaque hemorrhage or ulceration in the endarterectomy specimen of symptomatic patients. They also established a rating scale of B-mode-derived plaque composition, referred to as the Gray-Weale scale.

Categories:

1. Dominantly echolucent.

2. Substantially echolucent with small areas of echogenicity.

3. Dominantly echogenic with small areas (<25%) of echolucency.

4. Uniformly echogenic
5. Invisible because of heavy calcification

Terminology-definitions

ANECHOIC - Describes the property of being echo-free or without echoes (e.g., a fluid-filled cyst).

SONOLUCENT - Same as anechoic.

ECHOLUCENT - Same as anechoic.

ECHOGENIC - The ability to create an ultrasound echo.

HYPERECHOIC - Producing echoes of higher amplitude than normal for the surrounding medium.

HYPOECHOIC - Producing echoes of lower amplitude than normal for the surrounding medium.

ISOECHOIC - Areas which have similar echogenicity to each other. An isoechoic "property" makes it more difficult to see the desired tissue structure.

HETEROGENEOUS - mixed echoic pattern within plaque- areas of sonolucence and echogenicity.

HOMOGENEOUS - uniform plaque texture.

While some investigators have shown that heterogeneity (mixed hyperechoic, hypoechoic) or echolucency of the plaque was more positively correlated with symptoms than was any degree of stenosis,[40,41] others have indicated that a combination of 50-100% stenosis and hypoechoic plaque are risk factors for CVA in asymptomatic patients.[42]

Computer-Assisted Characterization

Lal et al., found that initial attempts at characterizing echogenicity of carotid plaque were not successful due to variability in ultrasound image settings. They resorted to computer assisted, offline image analysis of ultrasound images using graphic imaging software. Using Gray Scale Median (GSM) "pixel distribution analysis" to standardize the GSM of blood, lipids, muscle, fibrous tissue and calcium, they applied the standard GSM to plaque composition. They reported that large amounts of lipids and intraplaque hemorrhage were found in symptomatic plaques, while a larger amount of calcification and fibromuscular tissue where found within asymptomatic plaques.[43]

Nicolaides' group at St. Mary's Hospital in London has published a series of papers supporting the offline GSM plaque analysis. They report that GSM is an accurate method for assessing plaque composition and that hypoechoic plaques are more likely to be symptomatic for cerebrovascular events.[44,45]

So there appears to be general, but not unanimous, agreement that echolucent, heterogeneous plaques on ultrasound images, indicate a "high-risk" lesion. This determination is more accurately performed with computer-assisted, offline analysis.[46]

The Non-Believers

Not all are in agreement that plaque morphology can be identified by ultrasound, nor can plaque morphology be used to predict risk for cerebrovascular events. Hatsukami et al., analyzed atherosclerotic plaques sonographically and histologically in 43 patients undergoing CEA. There was no difference between plaques removed from asymptomatic and symptomatic patients with regard to the presence and volume of fibrous intimal tissue, intraplaque hemorrhage, the lipid core, the necrotic core, or calcification. They concluded that in patients with highly stenotic carotid lesions, gross plaque composition is similar between symptomatic and asymptomatic patients.[47]

Lovett et al., reported that pathological correlation in studies of carotid plaque imaging cannot be reliably interpreted or compared because of incomparable and poorly reported histology methods.[48]

In a recently published report in Stroke, Reiter et al., found that neither objective echolucency grading of carotid plaque with offline GSM pixel analysis, nor subjective assessment from the ultrasound image could identify patients with an increased risk of peri-interventional neurological events. "Evaluation of plaque echolucency therefore cannot be recommended for risk stratification in CAS patients." [49]

Surface Contour

There are also conflicting reports about the significance of plaque surface characteristics. AbuRahma et al.,[50] found that heterogeneous and/or irregular plaques were more often associated with both neurological symptoms and infarctions than smooth or homogeneous plaques. However, a report by Tegos et al.,[51] suggested that echogenic characteristics and degree stenosis, NOT surface contour, predicted plaque behavior.

Plaque Characterization and Morphology

- **Smooth**: the surface of the plaque appears continuous and shows no irregularities. This plaque is uniformly echogenic and homogeneous: on the Gray-Weale scale, category 4.

- **Irregular**: plaque surface is discontinuous and irregular. It that may contain ulceration.

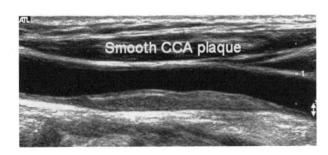

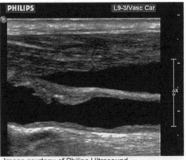

Image courtesy of Philips Ultrasound

- Heterogeneous, echolucent plaque: substantially echolucent with small areas of echogenicity. Echolucent plaques, like the one below, are often difficult to visualize on B-mode ultrasound. Gray-Weale scale-Category 1 or 2.

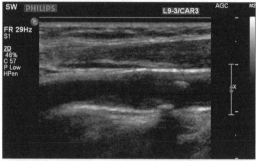

Predominately echolucent ICA 50% plaque

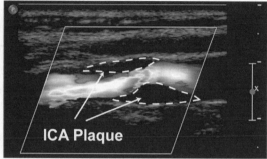

Color Doppler with filling defect in areas of plaque

Figure pg. 66:1-2   This plaque has mixed echogenicity with hypoechoic areas. The plaque appears minor, but color Doppler defines the contour of a more significant plaque. ***See Color Plate #5: E-F.***

- Heterogeneous: predominantly echogenic plaque with small areas of echolucency and calcium. Note the acoustic shadowing caused by plaque calcification. Gray-Weale scale-Category 3.

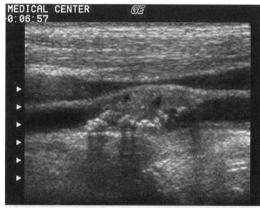

Heterogeneous plaque w/ mixed echogenicity

- *Intraplaque hemorrhage (IPH)*: results from a rupture of a small artery within either the artery wall or plaque (vasa vasorum), with subsequent bleeding into the plaque itself. This phenomenon may cause the plaque to increase in size faster than it would with the non-hemorrhagic atherosclerotic process. The ultrasonic appearance of a large sonolucent region with a thin echogenic cap separating it from the arterial lumen (egg-shell appearance), with no flow detected within the plaque, is suggestive of IPH.   However, lipid deposits, micro-calcification and other effects also cause anechoic regions within plaque image, so the determination of IPH based on standard ultrasound is not always reliable.

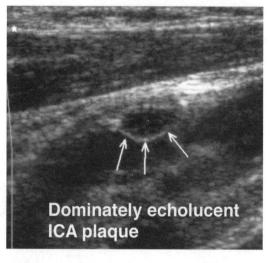

Dominately echolucent ICA plaque

- Calcified plaque: Calcium deposits within plaque may either prevent ultrasound from passing through the plaque, or prevent the weaker echo from returning. The result is an acoustic shadow deep to the plaque. If the calcified plaque is located in the near wall, the shadow obliterates the image below (see image on left below). If the calcified plaque is in the far wall, it may not interfere with the B-Mode or Doppler signals (see below on right).

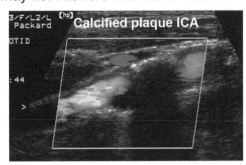 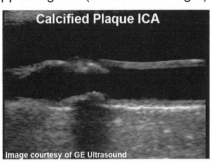

- Plaque Ulceration: an erosion, cavity or excavation within the plaque that may contain atheromatous debris, platelet aggregates or thrombus. The etiology is not clearly understood, but plaque necrosis and/or ruptured IPH are likely causes. When an ulcer is clearly seen on ultrasound, and if the depth of the depression exceeds 2 mm, it should be reported. The ability to characterize plaque is somewhat controversial.

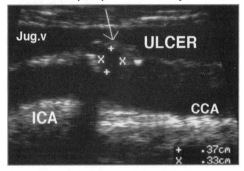

- The sonographic image of a severely diseased artery is often of insufficient clarity to enable morphology assessment. It is also a very subjective "science"; what may be smooth surface to one interpreter, may be irregular to another. Although there is controversy in the literature regarding the importance of plaque characterization, the predominant opinion is that hypoechoic plaques are more likely to be associated with symptoms.

REFERENCES

1. Roederer GO, Langlois YE, Jager KA, Lawrence RJ, Primozich JF, Phillips DJ, Strandness DES. A simple parameter for accurate classification of severe carotid disease: Bruit 8: 174-178, 1984

2. Roederer GO, Langlois YE, Primozich JF, Beach KW, et al. The natural history of carotid disease in asymptomatic patients with cervical bruits. Stroke 15: 605-613, 1984

3. Dreisbach JD, Seibert SE, Stavros AT, Daigle RJ. Duplex sonography in the evaluation of carotid artery disease. AJNR 4 :678-680 1983

4. Daigle RJ, Stavros AT, et al. Velocity criteria for differentiation of 60-79% carotid stenosis from 80% or greater...J Vasc Technol 12:177-183, July 1988

5. Bluth EI, Stavros AT, Marich KW, Wetzner SM, Baker JD. Carotid Duplex Sonography: A multicenter recommendation for standardized imaging and Doppler criteria. Radiographics 8 487-506. 1988

6. North American Symptomatic Carotid Endarterectomy Trial Collaborators. Beneficial effect of carotid endarterectomy in symptomatic patients with high grade stenosis. N.ENGL J Med 1991;325:445-53

7. North American Symptomatic Carotid Endarterectomy Trial Collaborators. Beneficial effect of carotid endarterectomy in patients with symptomatic moderate or severe stenosis. N.ENGL J Med 1998;339:1415 –25

8. National Institute of Neurological Disorders and Stroke. Clinical Advisory: carotid endarterectomy for patients with asymptomatic internal carotid artery stenosis. Stroke 1994;25:2523-4

9. ECSTs Collaborative Group: Randomized trial of endarterectomy for recently symptomatic carotid stenosis: Final results of the MRC European Carotid Surgery Trial (ECST) Lancet 351:1379-1387, 1998

10. Moneta GL, Edwards JM, et al. Correlation of the north american symptomatic carotid endarterectomy trial (nascet) angiographic definition of 70% to 99% ica stenosis with duplex scanning. J Vasc Surg 1993; 17:152-9

11. Fraught WE, Mattos MA, Sumner DS, et al. Color flow duplex scanning of carotid arteries: New velocity criteria... J Vasc Surg 1994:19; 818-28

12. Neale ML, Chambers JL, Kelly A, et al. Reappraisal of duplex criteria to assess significant carotid stenosis. J Vasc Surg 1994;20, 642-49

13. Hood DB, Mattos MA, Mansour A, Sumner DS. Prospective evaluation of new duplex criteria to identify 70% internal carotid artery stenosis. J Vasc Surg 1996:23: 254-262

14. Dhanjil S, Jameel M, Nicoladides A, Belcaro G, Williams M, Griffin M, Ramaswami G. Ratio of peak systolic velocity of the ICA to end diastolic velocity of the common carotid: new duplex criteria for grading internal carotid stenosis. J Vasc Technol 21(4):237-240,1997

15. Winkelaar GB, Chen JC, Salvian AJ, et al. New duplex ultrasound scan criteria for managing symptomatic 50% or greater carotid stenosis. J Vasc Surg 1999;29:986-94

16. Grant EG, et al. Carotid Artery Stenosis: Gray-scale and Doppler US diagnosis-Society of Radiologists in Ultrasound Consensus Conference. Radiology 2003;229:340-346

17. AbuRahma AF, Robinson PA, Strickler DL, Alberts S, Young L. Proposed new duplex classification for threshold stenoses used in various symptomatic and asymptomatic endarterectomy trials. Ann Vasc Surg 1998; 12:349–358

18. Filis KA, Arko FR, Johnson BL, et al. Duplex ultrasound criteria for defining the severity of carotid stenosis. Ann Vasc Surg 2002; 16:413–421

19. Winkelaar GB, Chen JC, MD, Salvian AJ, Taylor DC, Teal PA, York N. Hsiang YH. New duplex ultrasound scan criteria for managing symptomatic 50% or greater carotid stenosis. J Vasc Surg 1999;29:986-94

20. Sabeti S, Schillinger M, Mlekusch W, et al. Duplex us of carotid artery stenosis quantification of internal carotid artery stenosis with duplex us: comparative analysis of different flow velocity criteria. Radiology 2004; 232:431-439

21. Daigle RJ, Stavros AT, Seibert CE .External carotid artery "steal" from the internal carotid artery following iatrogenic common carotid dissection.. Video Journal of Color Flow Imaging;Vol 2., No.1, pp. 21-28;January 1992

22. Hobson RW, Goldstein JE, Jamil Z, Lee BC, Padberg FT Jr, Hanna AK, et al. Carotid restenosis: operative and endovascular management. J Vasc Surg 1999;29:228-35.

23. New G, Roubin GS, Iyer SS, Vitek JJ, Wholey MH, Diethrich EB, et al. Safety, efficacy, and durability of carotid artery stenting for restenosis following carotid endarterectomy: a multicenter study. J Endovasc Ther 2000;7:345-52.

24. Veith FJ, Amor M, Ohki T, Beebe HG, Bell PR, Bolia A, et al. Current status of carotid bifurcation angioplasty and stenting based on a consensus of opinion leaders. J Vasc Surg 2001;33 (suppl 2):S111-6.

25. Hobson RW, Lal BK, Chaktoura E, Goldstein J, Haser PB, Kubicka R,et al. Carotid artery stenting: analysis of data for 105 patients at high risk. J Vasc Surg 2003;37:1234-9.

26. Ringer AJ, German JW, Guterman LR, Hopkins LN. Follow-up of stented carotid arteries by Doppler ultrasound. Neurosurgery 2002;51:639-43.

27. Armstrong PA, Bandyk DF, Johnson BL. Shames ML. Zwiebel BR. Back MR . Duplex scan surveillance after carotid angioplasty and stenting: a rational definition of stent stenosis. J Vasc Surg 2007;46 (3):460-5

28. Lal BK, Hobson RW, Goldstein J, Chakhtoura EY, Duran WN. Carotid artery stenting: Is there a need to revise ultrasound velocity criteria? J Vasc Surg 2004;39:58-66.

29. AbuRahma AF, Maxwell D, Eads K, Flaherty SK, Stutler T. Carotid duplex velocity criteria revisited for the diagnosis of carotid in-stent restenosis vascular. Vascular. 2007;15(3):119-125

30. Chi YW, White CJ, Woods TC, Goldman CK. Ultrasound velocity criteria for carotid in-stent restenosis. Catheter Cardiovasc Interv. 2007 Feb 15;69(3):349-54

31. Stanziale SF, Wholey MH, Boules TN, Selzer F, Mararoun MS. Determining in-stent stenosis of carotid arteries by duplex ultrasound criteria. J Endovasc Ther. 2005 Jun;12(3):346-53.

32. Cato RF, Bandyk DF, et al. Carotid Collateral Circulation Decreases the Diagnostic Accuracy of Duplex scanning Bruit Vol X, 1986 p 68-73

33. Fujitani RM, Mills JL, et al. The effect of unilateral carotid occlusion upon contralateral duplex study: Criteria for accurate interpretation. J Vasc Surg 1992;16:459-68

34. Everdingen KJ, van der Grond, J, Kappelle LJ. Overestimation of a stenosis in the ICA by duplex sonography caused by an increase in volume flow. J Vasc Surg 1998;27:479-85

35. Ray SA, Lockhart SJM, Dourado R, Irvine AT, Burnand KG. Effect of contralateral disease on duplex measurements of internal carotid artery stenosis as Br J Surg 1999; 86: 705

36. Sachar R, Yadav JS, Roffi M, Cho L, Reginelli JP, Abo¨u-Cheb A, Bhatt DL, Bajzer CT. Severe bilateral carotid stenosis: The impact of ipsilateral stenting on Doppler-defined contralateral stenosis J Am Coll Cardiol, 2004;43: 1358 – 1362

37. Roddy SP, Estes JM, Harrington AP, Heggerick PA, O'donnell TF, Mackey WC. Comparison of preoperative and postoperative duplex ultrasound evaluation of the contralateral carotid artery. Vasc Endovascular Surg 1999 33: 663-669

38. Heijenbrok-Kal MH, Nederkoorn PJ, Buskens E, van der Graaf Y, Myriam –Hunink MG. Diagnostic performance of duplex ultrasound in patients suspected of carotid artery disease: the ipsilateral versus contralateral artery. Stroke 2005;36;2105-2109;

39. Gray-Weale AC, Graham JC, Burnett JR, Byrne K, Lusby RJ. Carotid artery atheroma: comparison of preoperative B-mode ultrasound appearance with carotid endarterectomy specimen pathology. J Cardiovasc Surg (Torino). 1988 Nov-Dec;29(6):676-81

40. AbuRahma AF, Wulu JT Jr, Crotty B. Carotid plaque ultrasonic heterogeneity and severity of stenosis. Stroke. 2002 Jul;33(7):1772-5

41. Mathiesen EB, Bønaa KH, Joakimsen O. Echolucent Plaques Are Associated With High Risk of Ischemic Cerebrovascular Events in Carotid Stenosis. Circulation. 2001;103:2171-2175

42. Polak JF, Shemanski L, O'Leary DH, Jerkewitz D, Price TR, Savage PJ, Brant WE, Reid C. Hypoechoic plaque at US of the carotid artery: an independent risk factor for incident stroke in adults aged 65 years or older. Radiology. 1998 Sept ;208(3):649-54

43. Lal BK, Hobson RW, Pappas PJ, et al. Pixel distribution analysis of B-mode ultrasound scan images predicts histologic features of atherosclerotic carotid plaques. J Vasc Surg. 2002;35:1210-1217.

44. Tegos TJ, Sabetai MM, Nicolaides AN, Pare G, Elatrozy TS, Dhanjil S. Griffin M. Comparability of the ultrasonic tissue characteristics of carotid plaques. Journal of Ultrasound in Medicine, Vol 19, Issue 6 399-407, 2000 AIUM

45. Sabetai MM, Tegos TJ, Nicolaides AN, El-Atrozy TS, Dhanjil S, Griffin M, Belcaro G, Geroulakos G. Hemispheric symptoms and carotid plaque echomorphology. J Vasc Surg. 2000 Jan;31(1 Pt 1):39-49

46. Hayward JK, Davies AH, Lamont PM. Carotid plaque morphology: A review. Eur J Vasc Endovasc Surg. 1995;9:368–374

47. Hatsukami TS, Ferguson MS, Beach KW, Gordon D, Detmer P, Burns D, Alpers C, Strandness DE Jr. Carotid plaque morphology and clinical events. Stroke. 1997 Jan;28(1):95-100

48. Lovett JK, Redgrave JNE, Rothwell PM. A Critical Appraisal of the Performance, Reporting, and Interpretation of Studies Comparing Carotid Plaque Imaging With Histology. Stroke. 36(5):1091-1097, May 2005.

49. Reiter M, Bucek RA, Effenberger I, Boltuch J, Lang W, Ahmadi R, Minar E, Schillinger M. Plaque Echolucency Is Not Associated With the Risk of Stroke in Carotid Stenting (Stroke. 2006;37:2378.

50. AbuRahma AF, Covelli MA, Robinson PA, Holt SM. The Role of Carotid Duplex Ultrasound in Evaluating Plaque Morphology: Potential Use in Selecting Patients for Carotid Stenting. Journal of Endovascular Surgery: Vol. 6, No. 1, pp. 59–65 1999

51. Tegos TJ, Kalomiris KJ, Sabetai MM, Kalodiki E, Nicolaides AJ .Tissue and Surface Characteristics of Carotid Significance of Sonographic Plaques. AJNR Am J Neuroradiol 22:1605–1612, September 2001

CHAPTER 4: VERTEBRAL & SUBCLAVIAN ARTERY IMAGING

INDICATIONS

Vertebral exam:

- Flow direction analysis during routine carotid duplex exam.
- Vertigo.
- Syncope.
- Drop attacks.
- Diplopia (double vision).
- Other vertebro-basilar symptoms.

Subclavian exam:

- Supraclavicular bruit.
- Reduced arm blood pressures.
- Abnormal vertebral spectra or abnormal vertebral artery flow direction.
- Arm weakness.
- ICAVL accreditation requirement.

VERTEBRAL IMAGING PROCEDURE

The vertebral arteries are assessed with the patient in a position similar to the carotid exam, but with the head turned <u>slightly</u> away from the side to be evaluated. The arteries are accessed between the transverse process of the vertebrae. Because it is often difficult to image the origin of the vertebral vessels, especially on the left side, careful attention to the morphology of the waveform is necessary to detect proximal disease.

- Identify the CCA in longitudinal view from an anterolateral position.
- Scan in a posterior direction to identify the "shadowed" vertebrae (see below).
- Color may be helpful in identifying the vertebral artery and vein between the transverse processes of the vertebrae, but caution is recommended for determining flow direction.

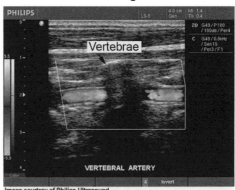

Vertebral artery with flow demonstrated on the proximal and distal sides of the vertebrae. *See* ***Color Plate #6: A-B.***

Figure pg. 71:1

- Place the Doppler sample volume between a vertebral segment lying between two vertebrae; be careful that the Doppler beam (which is wider than the cursor line) does not come through the bone of the vertebrae as this will weaken the strength of the Doppler signal.

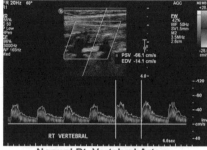

- The Doppler gain usually needs to be increased due to the increased depth of the vessel.

- Record spectral waveforms, and pay close attention to the flow direction.

Normal Rt. Vertebral Artery

- The vertebral artery analysis on many elderly patients is difficult due to the close spacing of the vertebra. An attempt should be made to image the proximal vertebral artery on <u>symptomatic</u> patients, although this is a difficult undertaking on many.

> The origin of right vertebral artery off the subclavian artery.

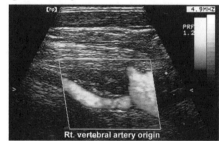

Figure pg. 72:1-2

See Color Plate #6: C-D.

⇒ The most common vertebral pathophysiology is subclavian steal. This occurs more commonly on the left side, but can occur on the right.

⇒ Proximal subclavian stenosis or occlusion can cause ipsilateral vertebral flow to reverse (retrograde), completely or partially, to supply blood flow to the arm. Generally the contralateral vertebral flow increases to provide the flow volume to the arm.

⇒ Usually subclavian steal does not cause neurological deficit or symptoms.

⇒ However, in the presence of severe carotid disease, flow in the basilar artery may reverse direction, causing neurologic symptoms related to the posterior hemisphere. This is known as Subclavian Steal <u>Syndrome.</u>

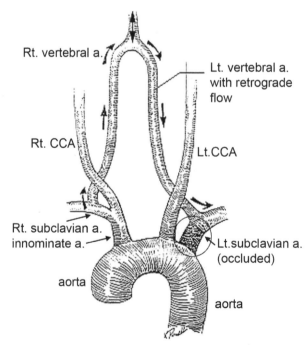

Lt. subclavian "steal": blood flow from the right vertebral artery supplies the left subclavian artery.

⇒   Although subclavian steal is frequently detected with duplex ultrasound, the steal "syndrome" is less common.

⇒   In the presence of innominate or subclavian artery obstruction on the right side, the right vertebral flow can reverse direction to perfuse the right arm. If retrograde flow is detected in the right vertebral artery, the subclavian and innominate arteries should be carefully evaluated.

⇒   Retrograde flow in the right vertebral artery and proximal subclavian artery usually indicates innominate obstruction. The right CCA is often supplied by retrograde flow in the subclavian artery. In this scenario, the proximal CCA should be evaluated as well. The CCA flow is often abnormal and may display a waveform of low amplitude and rounded contour.

⇒   If CCA flow is normal, the stenosis/occlusion is probably restricted to the proximal right subclavian artery.

⇒   The diagram below demonstrates retrograde flow in the right vertebral artery, and subclavian artery in the presence of an innominate artery obstruction. Note that the CCA is being supplies by the right vertebral artery.

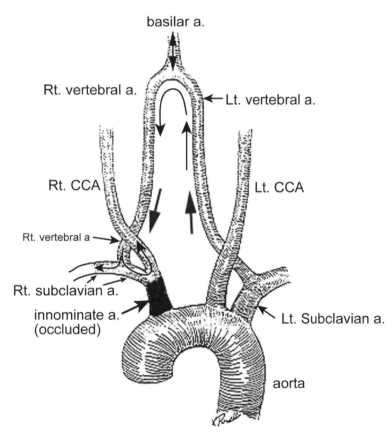

Rt. subclavian "steal"

⇒ Right CCA waveforms are usually abnormal in the presence of right vertebral steal.

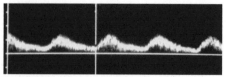

Rt. CCA with innominate stenosis.

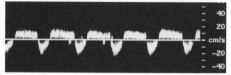

Rt. CCA with innominate occlusion.

⇒ Vertebral arteries are often of different size, bilaterally, and consequently flow velocities may be asymmetrical. One vertebral artery is often dominant in terms of flow and velocity.

⇒ The vertebral origin should be scanned if mid -vertebral waveforms are abnormal. Although the origins are difficult to image on many patients, the right side is often easier than the left.

VERTEBRAL INTERPRETATION

1. Normal mid vertebral artery waveform

Waveform reflects low resistance flow and is similar to the CCA. Normal flow is in an antegrade direction.

See Color Plate #6: D.

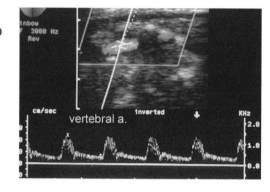

2. Resistive Spectra

This pattern is often seen with distal obstruction in the vertebral or basilar arteries. Vertebral dissection can also cause this high resistance waveform pattern.

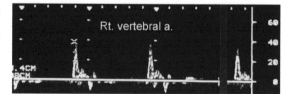

3. Tardus Parvus waveform

The waveform is of low amplitude and has a pronounced delay in the rise time from the onset to completion of systole. The waveform looks somewhat rounded. This pattern is consistent with proximal vertebral artery obstruction.

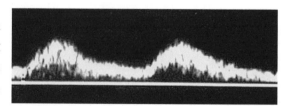

4. Early systolic deceleration

Also known as the "Bunny Rabbit" waveform. This waveform is consistent with subclavian stenosis. It is a more sensitive indicator of subclavian stenosis than arm pressure differentials.

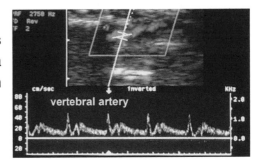

5. Progressive early systolic deceleration

Late systolic flow reverses for a brief period: a 'dip" below baseline. Diastolic flow is antegrade. Brachial systolic pressures in this case are most likely still symmetrical.

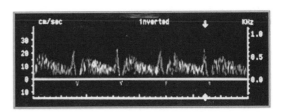

6. "To & Fro" pattern

This results from increasing degree of subclavian stenosis. Flow is retrograde in systole but returns to an antegrade direction in diastole. Brachial pressure gradient will probably exist.

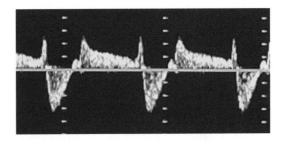

7. Retrograde flow

Complete reversal of vertebral artery flow in a full subclavian steal. The contralateral vertebral artery flow volume and velocity has increased, as this artery is now supplying flow to the ipsilateral arm, i.e., if the subclavian steal is on the left side, the right vertebral artery will be supplying flow volume to the left arm. A substantial brachial pressure differential usually will exist.

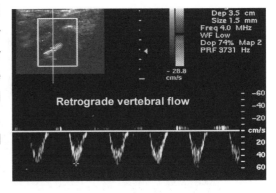

8. Post-stenotic vertebral flow

A turbulent flow pattern in spectral Doppler, or in color Doppler, usually indicates that there is a stenosis proximal to that location. Assess the vertebral artery proximally with spectral Doppler to detect the source of the turbulence.

Reactive Hyperemia: optional stress test of arm perfusion.

This test is sometimes used to detect complete reversal of flow with left arm exercise in patients with early systolic deceleration or "to and fro" flow. It's a useless and obsolete exercise. Better to spend the time evaluating the subclavian artery directly with ultrasound.

SUBCLAVIAN ARTERY ASSESSMENT

Subclavian arteries are assessed by either duplex imaging or by obtaining bilateral arm blood pressures. A pressure differential of 20 mmHg or more suggests the presence of subclavian obstruction on the side with the lower pressure. If this gradient is present, repeat the pressure tests to confirm.

SUBCLAVIAN SCAN PROCEDURE

Color duplex imaging of the right subclavian.

⇒   In transverse view identify the CCA and follow it proximally to or near its origin at the Innominate artery. The subclavian artery will be seen in long view coursing away from the innominate artery.

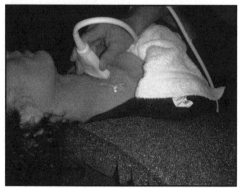

Transverse transducer position on CCA: follow proximally to the innominate artery.

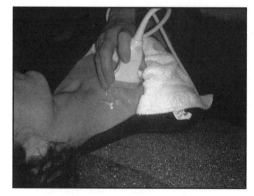

Transducer longitudinal over distal subclavian-axillary artery.

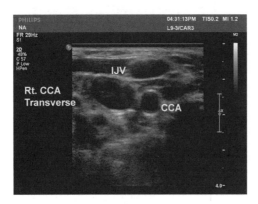
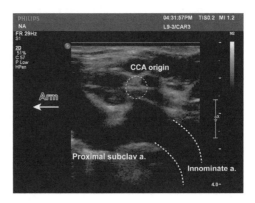

Transverse Rt. CCA with appropriate orientation. Scan proximally along the course of the CCA to identify its origin, the innominate artery and the proximal subclavian artery.

⇒ Obtain spectral waveforms and assess for normal or abnormal patterns. If abnormal, try to identify the stenotic region. If flow is retrograde, evaluate the vertebral, the innominate and the CCA. Retrograde flow in the right proximal subclavian artery usually indicates innominate stenosis or occlusion. Common carotid artery flow is supplied by retrograde right vertebral and retrograde subclavian artery flow.

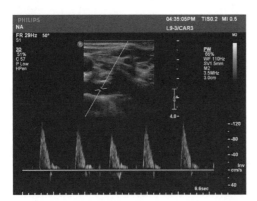
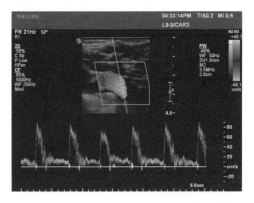

Rt. proximal subclavian artery waveform; note the typical high resistance waveform.

By contrast, a lower resistance normal innominate artery that feeds the CCA and the subclavian.

Color Duplex imaging of the left subclavian.

⇒ Place the transducer along the superior border of the clavicle and aim the transducer down in a caudal direction.

⇒ Obtain Doppler waveforms.

⇒ If abnormal (disturbed, turbulent flow pattern) proceed proximally and identify the actual stenosis. Color Doppler is useful in identifying the proximal subclavian artery on the left side.

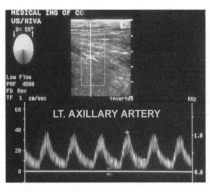

Abnormal axillary artery waveform caused by proximal subclavian artery stenosis (see below).

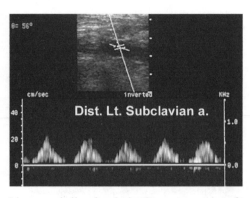

Abnormal distal subclavian artery waveform resulting from a proximal stenosis (see below). Note the delayed rise time to peak systole.

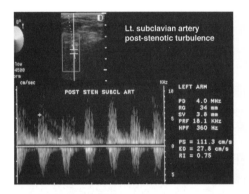

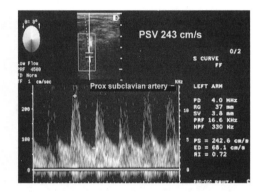

Severe post-stenotic turbulence in the proximal left subclavian artery. Deeper placement of the Doppler sample volume identified the stenotic region. Patient had abnormal left vertebral artery flow as well.

⇒ Be careful not to mistake the very pulsatile subclavian vein for the artery. The venous signal will have a respiratory pattern and be flowing centrally, or towards the heart.

⇒ Subclavian arteries should be carefully evaluated for the presence of aneurysms if emboli to the digits is suspected.

⇒ Subclavian artery aneurysms can result from chronic thoracic outlet compression.

CHAPTER 5: VENOUS ANATOMY AND HEMODYNAMICS

ANATOMY

The veins of the lower extremity consist of the deep venous system, the superficial system, the dermal veins, the perforating veins and the muscle tributaries. In the interest of clarity, *distal* refers to "away from the heart", and *proximal* means closer to the heart.

Deep venous system

- Veins course adjacent to major arteries and have the same names (exception- inferior vena cava).

- Deep veins carry 85% of blood volume in the legs.

The deep system consists of:

- Inferior vena cava (IVC)
  - from the confluence of both CIVs to the right atrium of the heart.

- Common iliac vein (CIV)
  - from the confluence of the internal and external iliac veins to the IVC.

- Internal iliac vein (IIV) (aka, hypogastric vein)
  - drains the pelvic and buttock regions.

- External iliac vein (EIV)
  - from the inguinal ligament to the CIV, drains the leg.

- Common femoral vein (CFV)
  - from the confluence of the deep femoral and femoral vein, it extends 2-3 cm to the groin crease.
  - confluence of the great saphenous vein (saphenofemoral junction).

- Femoral vein (previously known as the superficial femoral vein)
  - from the adductor canal in the distal thigh, to the CFV; main conduit of blood out of the lower leg.

- Deep femoral vein (DFA) (aka, profunda femoris vein, PFA)
  - drains the thigh and lower pelvic regions.

- Popliteal vein (POP V)
  - from the anterior tibial vein confluence to the femoral vein at the adductor canal.
  - receives the gastrocnemius veins, the small saphenous vein (exceptions), and drains the calf muscle veins.

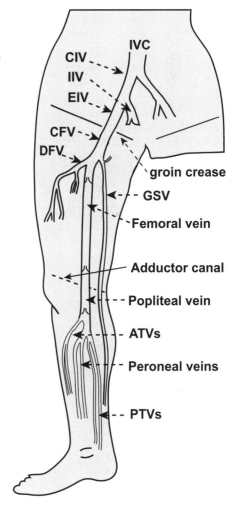

Deep venous anatomy

- Anterior tibial veins (paired) (ATV) - Drains anterior calf muscles and the foot.
- Posterior tibial veins (paired) PTV) - Drains medial and posterior calf muscles and the foot.
- Peroneal veins (paired) (PER) - Drains medial and posterior calf muscles.

Common popliteal vein anatomy variants

1. Typical anatomy with tibioperoneal trunk.

2. Proximal confluence of a common posterior tibial vein trunk and a common peroneal trunk.

3. High confluence of anterior tibial vein with popliteal vein. A common variant that is often mistaken for a "bifed" popliteal vein.

> *Small saphenous vein (SSV) is the new nomenclature for the lesser saphenous vein (LSV).*[1]

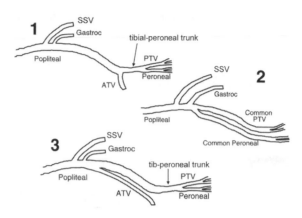

Common popliteal variants

Cross sectional mid-calf anatomy, right leg.

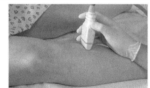

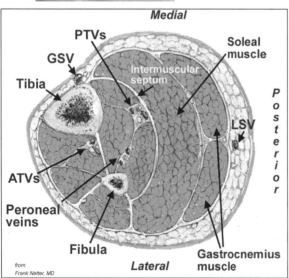

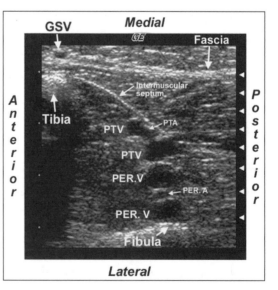

- The posterior tibial complex (paired veins, artery and nerve) lies along the intermuscular septum, and posterior to the tibia.

- The peroneal complex (paired veins, artery and nerve) lies close to the medial aspect of the fibula. Peroneal veins lie deep to the PTVs when imaged from the medial calf. They are difficult to image distally. It's best to start in mid-calf, medial side and work proximally.

- The anterior tibial complex lies just above the interosseous membrane and between the tibia and fibula. These can be imaged from an anterior approach and lateral to the tibia. Don't bother to image these veins (unless compartment syndrome is suspected).

Calf muscle veins

- Gastrocnemius veins (AKA, gastrocs) lie in the gastrocnemius muscles and drain into the popliteal vein (some consider these deep veins).

- Soleal veins or soleal sinuses lie in the deeper soleal muscle and drain into the posterior tibial or peroneals veins.

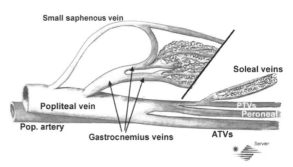

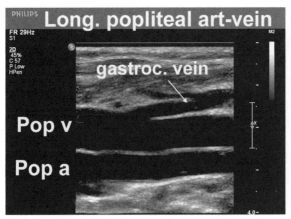

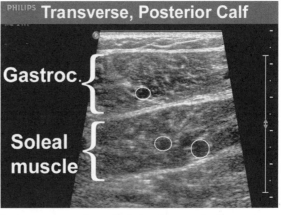

· The gastrocnemius vein confluence with the popliteal vein. To confirm that the vein is the gastroc, follow its course into the gastrocnemius muscles.

In transverse plane, in lateral or posterior scan positions, the gastroc muscles are superficial to the soleal muscle groups.

- Soleal veins drain into the posterior tibial and peroneals veins. It's not necessary to scan these veins routinely. However, if the patient complains of pain/tenderness in the calf region, scan and look for thrombosed soleal or gastrocnemius veins. Because they lie within muscle tissue, if thrombosed, they can be the source of considerable pain when the patient walks.

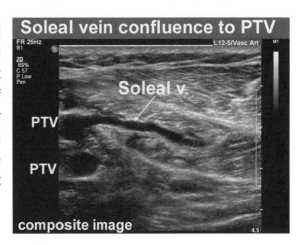

- If thrombus is found in the gastrocnemius veins, follow to the popliteal confluence and determine if the thrombus extended into the popliteal vein (a more serious condition).

Superficial system

Veins do not have an accompanying artery.

- Saphenous veins carries only about 15% of leg blood volume.

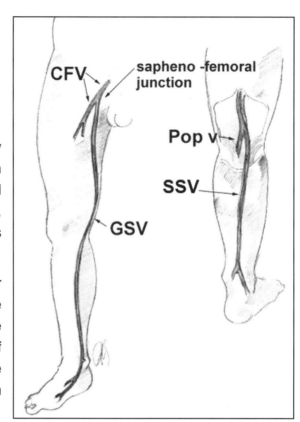

Superficial system consists of:

- Great saphenous vein (GSV) courses medially and enters deep system at the common femoral vein. The GSV lies within a fascial envelope. When imaged in transverse plane, the appearance is sometimes referred to as the "Egyptian eye" or "Cleopatra's eye".

- Small saphenous vein (SSV) (aka, lesser saphenous vein) courses posteriorly in the calf and usually enters the deep system at the popliteal vein. In approximately 20-30% of patients, SSV will enter the deep system above the popliteal vein via the intersaphenous vein (Giacomini vein).

- Lateral subdermic system is an extensive network of small superficial veins lying superficial to fascial plane. This is the source of "spider veins" or telangiectasia.

- An accessory saphenous vein courses along the anterior aspect of the thigh and drains into the GSV or the CFV. This is usually small and not well-seen, unless it dilates in venous insufficiency. It can be the source of prominent, anterior thigh varicosities.

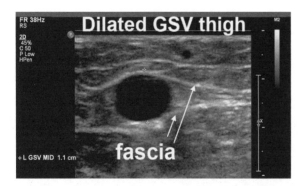

Dilated (11 mm) GSV seen in transverse in mid-thigh. Note the encompassing deep and superficial fascial layers.

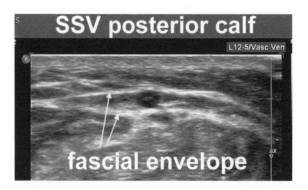

Superficial SSV in mid calf. As with the GSV, it is enclosed by a deep and superficial fascial layer.

Perforating veins (PV)

- PVs course between the superficial and deep systems through the deep fascia.

- Normal flow is from the superficial to the deep veins.

- Perforating veins have valves to prevent flow from moving from deep to superficial.

- Most commonly found in medial aspect of lower calf (Cockett's perforators). Perforators occur in the thigh as well (Dodd's and Hunterian perforators), and in the lateral aspect of the calf. (The location of Dodd and Hunterian perforators varies in the medical literature).

- Normal, competent perforating veins are small and difficult to see with ultrasound.

- Perforating veins often originate in the posterior arch vein, a tributary of the GSV in the calf.

- Perforators can also exist between the gastroc veins and the GSV or SSV, and between the soleal veins and the superficial system.

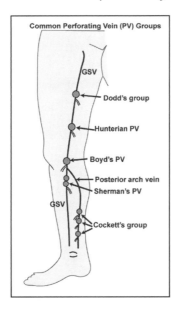

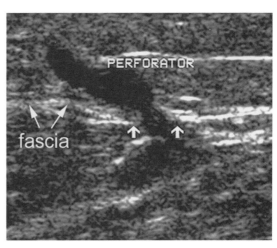

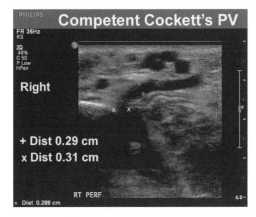

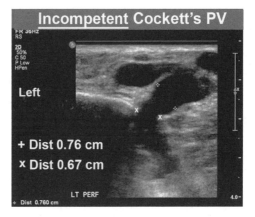

Image on left is a large (3.1 mm), competent Cockett's PV. PV in right image is large (7.6 mm) and incompetent. Images courtesy of James Moore, RVT, RDMS, Vascular lab, Kaiser Permanente, Irvine, CA

VENOUS HEMODYNAMICS

Venous Resistance

⇒ Blood flow to tissue in the upper and lower extremities is governed by:

  • contractility of the heart.

  • intraluminal blood pressure.

  • peripheral resistance in the distal end of the arterial "tree", the capillary bed.

⇒ Small arterioles leading into capillary beds in tissue are constricted in the basal state.

⇒ During exercise, peripheral resistance in these capillary beds <u>decreases</u> dramatically as vasodilatation occurs in the arterioles.

⇒ This allows more blood volume to enter muscle tissue to support increases in metabolic activity related to the exercise. More red blood cells with hemoglobin and oxygen <u>in</u>, more metabolic waste, including lactic acid, <u>out</u>.

⇒ This increase in flow volume during exercise can be as much as 10 times the resting inflow volume.

⇒ Peripheral resistance in capillary beds may <u>decrease</u> in response to heat, inflammation and infection. This causes a marked increase in blood flow volume to the limb.

⇒ More blood entering the limb means more blood volume for the venous system to transport back to the "old ticker".

⇒ Exposure to cold, emotional stress, and ingestion or inhalation of certain chemicals (nicotine for one) may cause an increase in vasoconstriction, an increase in resistance, thus reducing blood volume passing to the capillary beds.

⇒ A pressure gradient exists across all capillary beds with high pressure occurring in the arterial side (arterioles) and low pressure in the venous side (venules). This phenomenon allows blood to perfuse through tissue.

⇒ If venous pressure in the venules is equal to or higher than pressure in the arterioles, we're in trouble, as little or no perfusion will occur in the capillary bed.

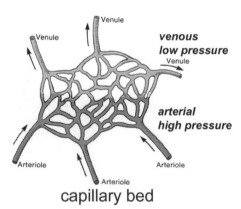

capillary bed

Hydrostatic pressure

In the lower extremities once blood passes across to the venous side of the capillaries, it has got a real uphill battle. A significant impediment for blood getting back to the heart is hydrostatic pressure (HP). This is old gravity at work pulling this column of blood volume back down to the feet (or down to the hands).

The amount of hydrostatic pressure (HP) is related to a person's height and to body position. When standing, a taller individual will have higher HP in the lower leg than a shorter person. <u>For every 12 inches of vertical distance below the heart, there are 22 mmHg of hydrostatic pressure.</u>

Hydrostatic pressure

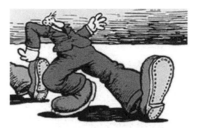

Venous intraluminal pressure in the legs is affected by body position and activity. Individuals who stand for a significant amount of the day are more susceptible to the effects of HP.

Venous intraluminal pressure is approximately 10 mmHg when one is lying supine, and about 80 mmHg when standing. This increase in transmural pressure in the veins leads to vessel distention and a pooling of blood in the lower leg and foot. Walking reduces the distal venous pressure.

Distal venous pressure:

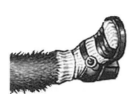
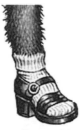
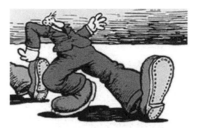

Lying - 10 mmHg   Standing - 80 mmHg   Walking - 25 mmHg

Venous pooling reduces venous return to the heart and results in a decrease in cardiac output. If you don't have a sizable volume of blood getting to the heart, you won't have a sizable volume pumped out. Additionally, this decrease in cardiac output may lead to hypotension. This is why soldiers standing at attention for too long occasionally faint and "face plant" into the concrete. Once they're lying prone on the concrete, hydrostatic pressure is significantly reduced, venous return increases, the soldier becomes normotensive and wakes up.

> **Hydrostatic Pressure**
> ⇧ transmural pressure
> ⇩ capillary perfusion
> ⇧ vein distention & blood pooling
> ⇧ filtration of fluids into tissue
> ⇩ venous return
> ⇩ cardiac output
> **Hypotension**

Because arterial pressure is transmitted through the capillary beds, blood does flow upward to the heart when one is standing, but it flows very slowly. If only there was some way to pump all this blood back to the heart!

Phasic changes in venous flow

Cardiac influence

*   Changes in venous pressure and flow occur in response to cardiac activity and changes in intra-thoracic and intra-abdominal pressure.

*   Atrial contraction and relaxation increase and decrease venous flow in the thoracic vessels.

*   Pulsatility is more readily seen in the upper extremities since the effects of right sided heart contractions are often transmitted to the large veins of the neck and arms. Respiratory phasicity is opposite from the legs.

*   These changes in venous pressure are usually not evident in the peripheral veins of the lower extremities because the high distensibility, or compliance, of the large veins dampen the appearance of pulsatility.

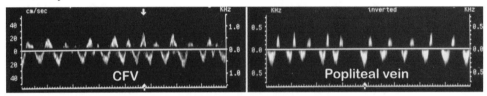

Pulsatile upper extremity venous flow due to cardiac influence.

*   High pressure in the right side of the heart can cause pulsatility at the level of the CFV and below. This phenomenon is most evident in congestive heart failure (CHF); if present, it will occur bilaterally.

Pulsatile flow in the common femoral vein and ipsilateral popliteal vein in a patient with congestive heart failure (CHF).

Respiratory variation

*   Venous blood flow in the extremities is affected by respiration. When one inspires the diaphragm mores down and increases intra-abdominal pressure.

*   This increase in intra-abdominal pressure compresses and collapses the inferior vena cava in the abdomen, and venous outflow in the lower extremities is temporarily reduced.

*   In addition, the venous intramural pressure is increased distally, and the pressure gradient across the capillary bed is decreased. This results in a slight reduction in capillary perfusion.

*   When one exhales, the intra-abdominal pressure is reduced, the inferior vena cava (IVC) distends and venous outflow increases.

*   The effects of respiration provide a clear, phasic Doppler signal in a normal venous system. See image on right.

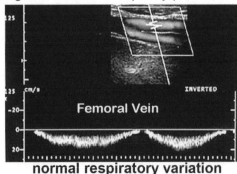

normal respiratory variation

- Respiratory changes in flow (phasicity) may be reduced or absent when in a supine position, or in patients who are shallow breathers. It also may be damped out in the calf veins,

> The presence of respiratory variation and/or cardiac pulsatility demonstrated in the Doppler waveform is a reliable sign (although not 100%) of vein patency proximal to the Doppler site. However, this does not infer distal patency.

- High venous outflows due to arterial hyperemia or arteriovenous fistula in the legs may override the effects of respiration on venous return.

- So, in a nutshell, when you breathe in, flow out of the legs slows or stops; when you breathe out, flow resumes.

Venous Return - The Pump System

There are 3 "pump systems" in lower extremity venous return.

1. The foot pump: during plantarflexion venous blood in the foot is moved into the calf veins. The foot pump "primes" the calf veno-motor pump. It's a low volume system compared to the calf pump.

2. The thigh pump: venous volume in the thigh, primarily in the deep femoral vein network, is ejected upwards with thigh muscle contraction.

3. The calf veno-motor pump: the primary venous return mechanism, described in detail below.

<u>The Calf Pump</u>

- Venous blood is propelled towards the heart by the calf "veno-motor" pump.

- There are numerous veins in the calf (paired posterior tibial, anterior tibial, peroneal, gastrocnemius, and soleal veins) and each has numerous valves. When the skeletal muscles are contracted in walking or running, the following events occur:

1. During muscle contraction, the large blood volume residing in the deep calf veins and soleal sinuses is literally squeezed up and out of the calf.

2. The proximal valves of the deep veins are forced open.

3. The distal valves close to prevent caudal flow.

4. The perforator valves close to prevent flow into the superficial venous system.

5. During muscle relaxation, the proximal valves close due to the hydrostatic pressure forcing blood back down the veins to the level of the valve.

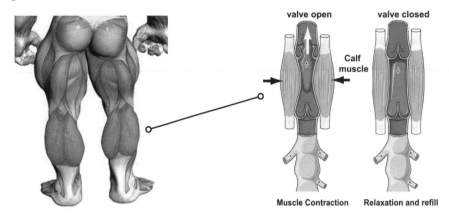

valve open   valve closed

Calf muscle

Muscle Contraction   Relaxation and refill

6. During relaxation, the distal and perforator valves open, and blood flows into the calf deep veins.

•   Due to this pump action, the hydrostatic pressure column is interrupted and distal intraluminal pressure is reduced.

•   The muscles in the thigh and buttock also contribute to the venous return "pump".

VENOUS INSUFFICIENCY

The efficiency of the calf veno-motor pump is dependent upon:

1. The ability of the calf skeletal muscles to contract.

2. The competency of the venous valves.

3. The patency of outflow veins.

If there is no muscle contraction, there is no pump action. The resulting stagnation of blood increases the risk for deep venous thrombosis.

Symptomatic venous insufficiency is a chronic condition and usually takes years to develop. It can be a very disabling condition.

Deficiency in valve function may be due to:

1. <u>Primary venous insufficiency</u>: A congenital absence of valves, or defects in valve structure.

2. <u>Secondary venous insufficiency:</u> Dysfunctional, damaged valves as a result of previous thrombophlebitis. This "post-phlebitic" condition is devastating to the venous return system.

⇒   When valves are not working, blood volume that is squeezed upward by muscle contraction simply flows back down during muscle relaxation.

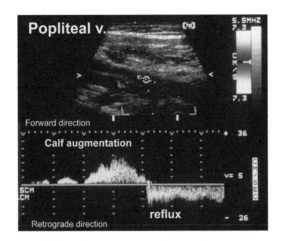

Antegrade popliteal venous flow during calf compression, then retrograde flow (reflux) with cessation of compression.

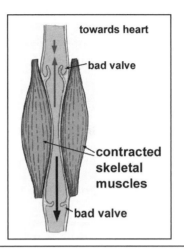

During muscle contraction, blood may be forced downward if distal valves are incompetent.

⇒   Calf muscle contraction can also force blood volume back down the veins toward the foot. This increases intraluminal venous pressure distally, and a myriad of symptoms may occur.

⇒   Perforating veins may dilate (due to high intramural pressure in the deep system) to a point where the valves become incompetent. The valve leaflets, although present, may not touch due to vein distention.

⇒   When perforating veins are incompetent, intramural pressure may increase in the superficial venous system. This may to contribute varicose vein formation.

Venous insufficiency can result from either single system incompetence, i.e., deep, superficial or perforating system, or from a combination of dysfunctional systems, e.g., incompetent great saphenous vein AND perforating veins.

Chronic outflow obstruction

Venous insufficiency may also result from chronic outflow obstruction in the iliofemoral veins following an episode of deep venous thrombosis. Venous outflow is restricted by partially recannalized iliac veins or by flow through small collateral pathways. The resulting increase in venous intraluminal pressure is exacerbated during exercise; inflow blood volume increases dramatically, but the veins cannot accommodate the required outflow. Limb swelling, discomfort and venous "claudication" are often the result.

Symptoms of venous insufficiency

- Recurrent swelling of the lower calf and ankle.

- Chronic limb swelling.

- Telangiectasias (spider veins): intradermal venules of 1 mm or less in diameter.

- Reticular veins: dilated subdural veins of 1-4 mm.

- Varicose veins: palpable, distended veins of > 4 mm in diameter.

- Venous claudication: burning sensation, pain in legs during exercise due to venous congestion from chronic outflow obstruction.

- Stasis dermatitis: a "tanning" or brown discoloration of skin in the lower calf, ankle and foot. Chronic increase in capillary pressure results in leakage of fluid, fibrinogen and cells out of the capillaries. Hemosiderin is deposited in the tissue as the red cells break down. The skin in the "gaiter" area may be weakened and predisposed to bacterial infection.

- Venous stasis ulceration: leakage of fibrinogen from veins, as well as deficiencies in fibrinolysis, cause fibrin to build up around the vessels of the skin. This process prevents oxygen and nutrients from reaching the cells and contributes to a breakdown in tissue.2 Venous insufficiency may also cause white blood cells (leukocytes) to accumulate in small blood vessels and release inflammatory factors that further contribute to chronic wound formation.3 Venous ulcers are difficult to heal unless chronic venous pressure in reduced.

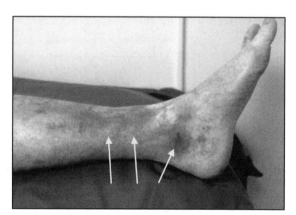

Venous stasis dermatitis

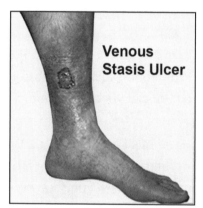

Venous ulcer

Additional information on this topic in the Imaging for Venous Insufficiency chapter.
References

1. Caggiati A, Bergan JJ, Gloviczki P, Eklof B, Allegra C, Partsch H. Nomenclature of the veins of the lower limb: Extensions, refinements, and clinical application. J Vasc Surg. 41 (4):719-724 2005

2. Brem H, Kirsner RS, Falanga V. Protocol for the successful treatment of venous ulcers Am. J. Surg. 188 (1A Suppl): 1-8. (2004)

3. Stanley AC, Lounsbury KM, Corrow K, et al. Pressure elevation slows the fibroblast response to wound healing. J. Vasc. Surg. 42 (3): 546-51, (2005)

CHAPTER 6: VENOUS DUPLEX IMAGING: LOWER EXTREMITIES

DEEP VENOUS THROMBOSIS (DVT): ETIOLOGY & RISK FACTORS

DVT annual USA estimates

- 1-10 million cases.

- 600,000 cases of pulmonary embolus (PE).

- 200,000 deaths from PE.

Etiology of DVT

In the mid 1800s, Rudolf Virchow postulated that venous thrombosis occurred when 3 conditions existed. This became known as the Virchow's triad.

1. Circulatory stasis.
2. Vein wall (intimal) injury.
3. Hypercoagulability state.

Risk factors for DVT

- Post-operative state
- Previous DVT
- Cancer- malignancy
- Trauma
- Pregnancy
- High-dose estrogen
- Immobility (long car or plane travel)
- Thrombophilia
- Bed-rest > 4 days

Symptoms of acute DVT

- Acute onset, persistent calf pain and/or tenderness (usually posterior or medial calf).

- Persistent calf or leg swelling.

- Symptoms that have persisted for longer than 2-3 weeks are usually not caused by DVT.

- Anterior leg symptoms are not associated with DVT.

- Phlegmasia Cerulea Dolens.

  ⇒ massive thigh and calf swelling.

  ⇒ cyanotic limb.

  ⇒ caused by iliofemoral thrombosis.

- The symptoms of DVT are not reliable in predicting the condition.[1]

Symptoms of superficial thrombophlebitis

- Local erythemia.

- Local tenderness/pain.

- Palpable subcutaneous "cord".

IMAGING SEGMENT #1: COMMON FEMORAL TO POPLITEAL VEIN

Transverse Imaging Technique

⇒   The exam is begun with the patient in a semi-Fowler's or a reverse Trendelenburg position with the head of bed elevated about 25-45 degrees.

⇒   The distal external iliac vein located just proximal to the inguinal ligament at the groin crease is identified and scanned in a transverse plane with a 5 or 7 MHz transducer.

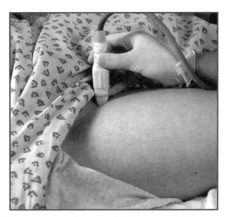

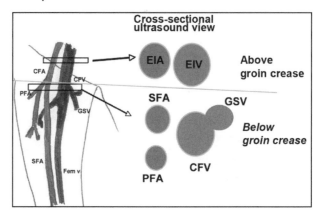

Correct probe position at groin crease.

Utrasound image with transducer superior to the groin crease, vein is medial. Just below the groin crease the EIA and EIV become the CFA and CFV respectively. The sapheno-femoral junction occurs at the location of the CFA bifurcation. However, anatomic variations do occur.

⇒   The veins are compressed and collapsed with moderate probe pressure, and then reopen when compression is released (Figure 6-3, below).

⇒   The vein segment beneath the transducer should be observed to completely coapt (collapse) and then reopen as probe pressure is released.

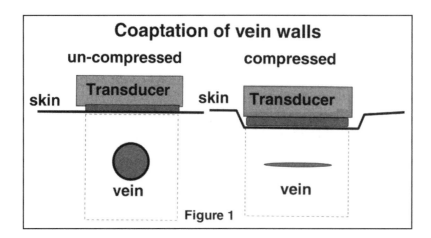

Figure 1

TIP: Try to keep the transducer perpendicular to the vein for optimum image quality (image below left). The probe position shown below (right) will produce a sub-optimal ultrasound image.

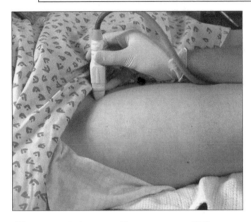

Correct transducer position.

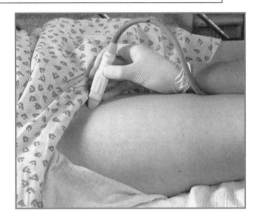

Don't tilt the probe!

⇒ Scan and compress the CFV, the femoral vein origin and the proximal segment of the deep femoral vein.

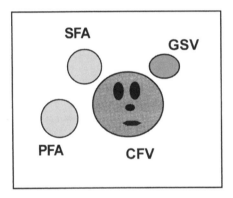

Anatomy seen slightly inferior to the groin crease. The SFA, CFV, and GSV transverse view sometimes resembles "Mickey Mouse ears".

⇒ Compress the proximal great saphenous vein (GSV) near the sapheno-femoral junction.   If symptomatic for superficial thrombophlebitis, follow the entire GSV.

NOTE: If the patient is symptomatic for superficial thrombophlebitis, evaluate the superficial system first. If positive, don't aggressively compress the deep veins with the transducer over the tender regions as this will cause a lot of discomfort. Use an alternative imaging plane, or rely on color Doppler to evaluate that specific region of the deep veins.

The image on the right demonstrates a thrombosed great saphenous vein in proximity to the sapheno-femoral junction (SFJ). If thrombus in found in the GSV, determine if the thrombus extends into the CFV at the sapheno-femoral junction.

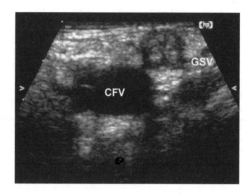

⇒   Compress every 2-4 centimeters along the length of the common femoral, femoral, popliteal, and calf veins.

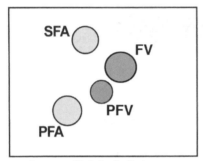

Image slightly inferior to sapheno-femoral junction.

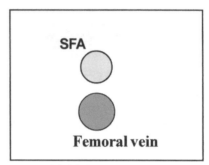

Mid thigh SFA and FV

⇒   At the level of the adductor canal the femoral vein may be difficult to compress due to the depth of the vessel and proximity to the adjacent femur. This segment of the vein may be compressed by placing your hand behind the leg (posterior distal thigh), level with the transducer, and pushed upward with your hand into the transducer to coapt the vein.

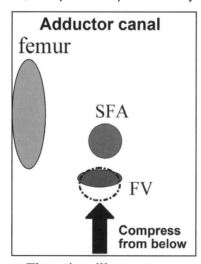

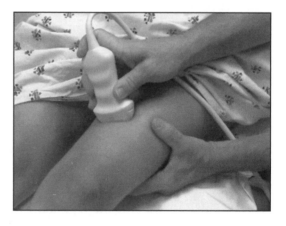

The vein will not compress with transducer pressure if the vein segment is below the femur, so press from posterior with your free hand.

⇒ Although a medial scan position is typically used at the distal thigh, try an anterior approach with the leg straightened. There is often an excellent acoustic window at this probe position for the FV in the adductor canal. See image below.

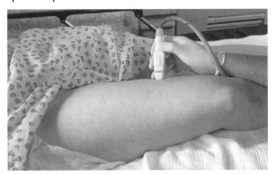

Medial scan position.

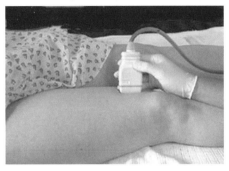

Anterior scan position at adductor canal.

⇒ The popliteal vein is evaluated from a posterior approach with the patient's knee rotated externally.

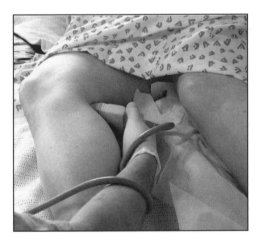

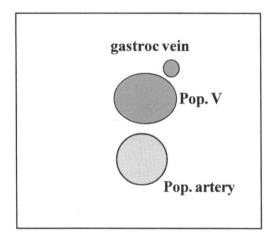

⇒ Care should be taken not to place the transducer directly over the biceps femoris tendon laterally or semitendinosus tendon medially in the popliteal fossa as this may prevent coaptation of the popliteal vein.

⇒ The distal popliteal vein, to the confluence of the anterior tibial and tibioperoneal trunk, should be carefully imaged using compression techniques.

⇒ If the distal popliteal vein is not clearly visualized (due to its course and oblique transverse scan plane), it can usually be imaged with color Doppler in longitudinal view.

⇒ The paired tibial veins of the calf are assessed in a similar fashion, see SEGMENT # 2, Below the Knee.

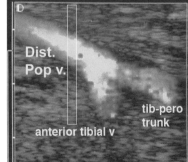

Figure pg. 95:5

See Color Plate #6: E.

Doppler Technique

Color Doppler may be used throughout the leg, but its best utility is in the femoral vein at the level of the adductor canal, the distal popliteal, and the calf veins. Spectral Doppler evaluation is essential for the proximal veins.

With the patient in supine position as above, place the transducer longitudinally over the vein of interest. Activate the spectral Doppler and adjust PRF and other parameters for low flow detection. The following venous flow characteristics are evaluated:

1. Spontaneity - flow that is present without augmentation maneuvers.

2. Respiratory phasicity - flow should increase and decrease with respiration.

> Augmentation is optional, and much less important than the presence or absence of respiratory phasicity. Augmentation is useful for calf vein flow evaluation, and for reflux assessment (see chapter on venous insufficiency testing), but it is not useful for the detection of DVT. Augmented flow can easily occur via collateral channels in the presence of DVT.

Spontaneous flow with respiratory phasicity should be apparent in all deep veins superior to the calf (see image on right), but may not be present in normal posterior tibial and peroneal veins. Absence of respiratory phasicity in the proximal leg veins is suggestive of obstruction superior to the transducer.

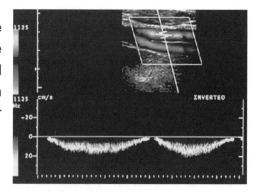

Spontaneous & phasic venous flow from a femoral vein.

Traditionally, the Doppler waveform has been displayed below baseline; a carry-over from the days of continuous-wave Doppler with a "pencil" probe, and before duplex ultrasound imaging This is not necessary with duplex ultrasound systems. Some Doppler systems are designed so that all "forward" (antegrade) flow, whether arterial or venous, is displayed above the baseline, and all "reverse" (retrograde) flow is displayed below the baseline.

Respiratory phasicity may not be present due to:
- Shallow breathers, (patients with pulmonary embolus-PE).
- Patients who are lying supine.
- Patients who have their arms raised and hands behind their head.
- Spinal cord injured patients due to reduced abdominal muscle tone.
- Proximal DVT or extrinsic venous compression.

<u>Spectral Doppler sample sites, proximal veins (color Doppler is optional):</u>
- Common femoral.
- Proximal and distal femoral vein in the thigh.
- Proximal deep femoral vein (profunda femoris vein).
- Popliteal vein distally, beyond the popliteal valve.

Steady, continuous, nonphasic flow unilaterally in the CFV warrants a scan of the iliac veins in the pelvis. This flow condition can occur with isolated iliac vein thrombosis (very uncommon) or with extrinsic compression of iliac veins by a mass (not uncommon).

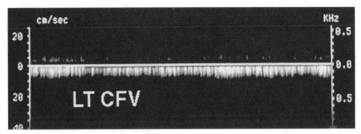

Abnormal, steady, continuous venous flow.

IMAGING SEGMENT #2: BELOW THE KNEE

Calf Vein Imaging

⇒ Calf vein imaging is an integral part of the venous duplex exam of the lower extremities. Patients referred for a venous scan often have symptoms in the calf region.

⇒ Many vascular laboratories do not scan the calf for the following dubious reasons:

1. Because isolated calf vein thrombosis is thought to be clinically unimportant. Pulmonary emboli may result from calf vein thrombus but they are not fatal and may not be symptomatic.

2. Calf veins are time-consuming.

3. More often, calf veins are not imaged because the technologist lacks the experience and confidence to evaluate them adequately.

⇒ Calf veins should be imaged if possible, particularly if the patient is symptomatic in this region.

⇒ Calf symptoms are the most common cause for referral.

⇒ Some calf clots are significant as they propagate into the larger proximal veins. It has been reported that this occurs in up to 32% of patients with isolated calf vein thrombosis.[2]

⇒ Duplex imaging of the calf can also determine other sources of calf pain.

∗ Dissected popliteal synovial cysts.

∗ Intramuscular hematoma.

 * Lymphedema.

 * Abscess.

Calf Anatomy

⇒ Posterior tibial veins (PTV) are paired and lie along the PT artery (posterior to the tibia).

⇒ Peroneal veins (PER) are paired and lie along the peroneal artery medial to the fibula.

⇒ Anterior tibial veins (ATV) are paired and lie along the anterior tibial artery anterior to the interosseous membrane and lateral to the tibia.

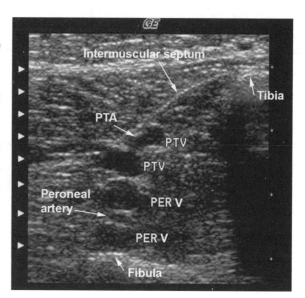

⇒ Tibioperoneal trunk (also known as the peroneal-tibial trunk) is formed by the confluence of the posterior tibial and the peroneal veins. It then joins the distal popliteal vein at the confluence of the anterotibial trunk.

Calf intramuscular veins

• Soleal veins or sinuses lie in the soleal muscle and drain into the PTV or PER veins.

• Gastrocnemius veins lie in the gastroc muscle and drain into the popliteal vein. They have an accompanying artery.

Superficial venous system

• Small saphenous vein lies subcutaneously in the posterior calf and joins the popliteal vein.

• Great saphenous vein courses medially and superficially in the calf. It has many superficial tributaries.

• Perforating veins connect the great saphenous vein or tributaries with the deep veins and are not readily apparent unless they are incompetent.

Scan Technique for Calf Veins

⇒ Patient in reverse Trendelenburg position, the higher the elevation of the upper body, the easier the visualization of calf veins.

⇒ Scan the distal popliteal vein to the level of the ATV confluence. The distal portion is best imaged in longitudinal view, with and without color Doppler.

Although on some patients it is possible to continue down the calf from the distal popliteal, this is a difficult segment in many patients. After the distal popliteal, proceed to the distal PTV's just proximal to the medial malleolus and work proximally.

Posterior Tibial Veins

⇒ Identify the PTV's and artery proximal to the medial malleolus, posterior to the tibia, and adjacent to the intermuscular septum in the transverse plane.

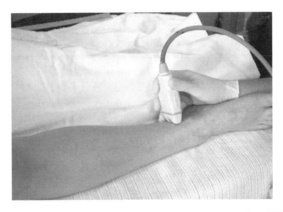

NOTE: If the veins do not compress, be certain that the transducer is not pressing against the tibia.

⇒ Using compression techniques, evaluate every few inches as you scan proximally to the confluence with the peroneal veins.

⇒ In longitudinal plane, evaluate the paired veins with color Doppler.

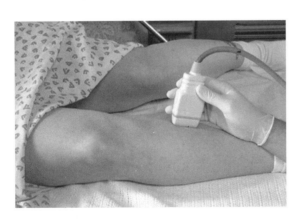
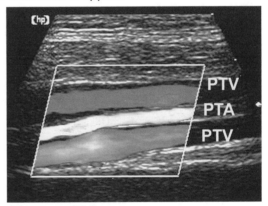

Figure pg. 99:3

See Color Plate #6: F.

⇒ Flow usually must be augmented by squeezing the leg or foot distal to the transducer.

⇒   Carefully evaluate regions that do not fill with color for the presence of thrombus.

Peroneals

⇒   From a medial side of the calf at mid-level, locate the peroneal veins and artery just above the fibula.

⇒   Use the same technique used for the PTVs: transverse compression, followed by color assessment in longitudinal plane.

⇒   Alternatively, these veins may be evaluated in transverse plane with color Doppler, but Doppler angles are nearly perpendicular, so the transducer must be angled either superior or inferior to achieve an angle less than 90 degrees.

⇒   Depending on the patient's body habitus, peroneals may also be seen from a posterior calf access and also anterio-laterally deep to the interosseous membrane.

Anterior Tibial Veins: DON'T BOTHER!

The incidence of isolated DVT in these veins is very low, if not nonexistent.[3] For this reason, many do not routinely scan these veins. Using an anterior lateral approach, they are located just anterior to the interosseous membrane in the "saddle" between the tibia and fibula.

Saphenous Veins

⇒   If symptomatic, the GSV & SSV veins and varicosities should be evaluated with compression techniques using a high frequency transducer (7 -14 MHz range).

Intramuscular Veins

⇒   These veins are easily seen when they are thrombosed, and if thrombosed they are often symptomatic, especially in ambulatory patients. Ask the patient to identify the region of pain/ tenderness and scan that location with a larger field of view. Compression techniques will ascertain patency.

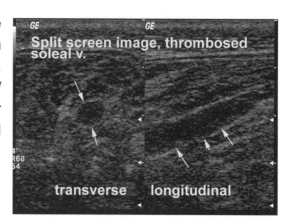

Split screen image, thrombosed soleal v.

transverse   longitudinal

HELPFUL HINT: Repositioning the leg often helps visualization of the tibial veins. Position the leg so that the lateral aspect of the calf is on the bed and medial side is up. Calf veins may also be evaluated with the leg dependent and hung over the edge of the bed.

Calf Imaging Caveats

♦ Color Doppler in longitudinal view works better than color in transverse plane.

♦ Extensive calf swelling is NOT due to only isolated tibial thrombosis; the popliteal vein or more proximal veins must be involved.

♦ Flow in calf veins is usually not spontaneous, you often must augment flow by squeezing the calf or ankle. Also, having the patient plantarflex will elicit a flow augmentation.

♦ If the patient is symptomatic (tenderness), look for muscular vein thrombosis.

♦ If you find calf, SSV, or gastroc vein thrombosis, look carefully for extension into the popliteal vein. Partially occlusive thrombus in the distal popliteal vein is sometimes difficult to visualize. Try to gently "jiggle" the region with the transducer and look for vertical movement of a hypoechoic floating thrombus.

INTERPRETATION

Criteria For Patency: All Veins

• Complete coaptability of the vein walls with the ultrasound transducer.

• Absence of visible intraluminal thrombus on B-mode image in transverse and longitudinal planes.

• Normal venous Doppler (conventional or color) signals of spontaneity and phasicity.

• Visualization of blood flow throughout the lumen with color Doppler.

Criteria For Venous Thrombosis

• Lack of complete compressibility of vein (beware: a normal femoral vein in adductor canal region may not compress). The split-screen image on the right demonstrates the appearance of the popliteal vein without, and with transducer compression. The vein does not compress in the right-side image.

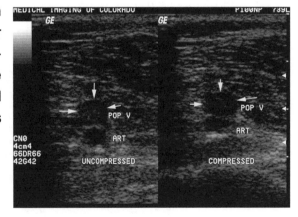

- Visualization of intraluminal thrombus with complete or partial obstruction of the vein lumen.

- Distention of the vein compared to the adjacent artery.

- Abnormal venous Doppler signals, i.e., continuous non-phasic flow, reduced or absent flow with distal augmentation, or no detectable signal.

- Continuous, non-phasic flow in CFV unilaterally, with phasic flow in contralateral CFV, suggests iliac vein outflow obstruction, i.e., DVT or extrinsic compression.

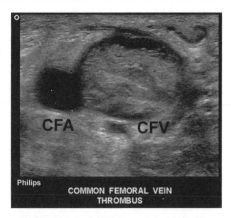

> NOTE: Free floating, partially attached thrombus should not be aggressively compressed.

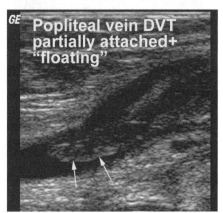

- Patients should be transported to physician's office or hospital, or to hospital bed by wheelchair or stretcher.

- Referring physician must be notified promptly of a positive result.

Chronic DVT

- Chronic DVT implies that the thrombus is at least several months old.

- Thrombus has increased echogenicity.

- Vein is contracted and is often the same size or smaller than the adjacent artery.

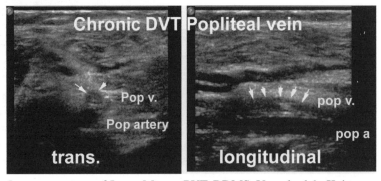

Images courtesy of James Moore, RVT, RDMS, Vascular lab, Kaiser Permanente, Irvine, CA

- In very old DVT, the vein may be so contracted that it may not be apparent in the ultrasound image. It may have similar echogenicity as the surrounding tissue.

- Large collateral veins are often present. In the image at the right, the distal popliteal vein is thrombosed. The gastrocnemius vein is dilated, as it's functioning as a collateral pathway for blood flow out of the lower leg.
  See Color Plate #7: A.

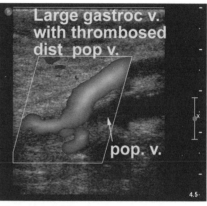

  This image courtesy of James Moore, RVT, RDMS, Vascular lab, Kaiser Permanente, Irvine, CA

Figure pg. 103:1

- Recannalization with partial lumen restoration.
  See Color Plate #7: B.

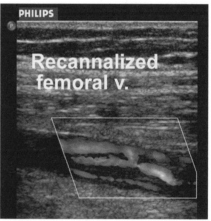

- Phleboliths, or calcium deposits within old thrombus, are sometimes observed.

Figure pg. 103:2

- Vein walls may be thickened, residual, fibrous bands are often seen following recannalization.

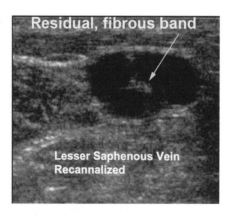

Acute versus Chronic DVT

If a patient is symptomatic for DVT and you find thrombus of uncertain chronicity, the thrombus should be considered acute unless it can be clearly demonstrated to be chronic.

Subacute versus Acute DVT

The differentiation of acute thrombus from sub-acute (4-12 weeks old) disease is often difficult. Patients who present with new symptoms a few weeks or months following anticoagulation therapy for deep venous thrombosis (DVT) are an enigma. Comparison with the previous ultrasound exam can be helpful. If the present study shows partial or complete resolution of the previously thrombosed vein, then the new symptoms are probably not due to new DVT. However, if the extent of the DVT is the same or greater, it remains uncertain whether this represents an acute process, or if the thrombus propagated during the early stages of the initial anticoagulation therapy. It has been shown that thrombus propagation can occur during intravenous heparin therapy.[4] For this reason, a baseline venous duplex exam is recommended at the time the patient is discharged. Remember that heparin and Coumadin (warfarin) do not directly dissolve or lyse blood clots.

Recent refinements in D-Dimer testing (a blood test) may provide a solution. A positive D-dimer indicates the presence of an abnormally high level of fibrin degradation and can indicate that there has been significant thrombus formation in the body. However, other conditions can cause a positive D-dimer result. A negative D-dimer test is perhaps more significant: it means that an acute thrombotic process is **not** occurring.

PRACTICAL "STUFF"

1. Difficult patients, huge legs. Even on large patients the CFV and popliteal veins can usually be imaged. Lensing et al., in a large study comparing compression ultrasound with venography found that if the CFV and popliteal veins are normal, (femoral veins were not imaged) it is very unlikely that acute DVT exists in the femoral veins.[5] Calf veins were not evaluated. Another study by Pezzullo et al.,[6] compared a limited ultrasound exam (compression of CFV and Popliteal veins only) with a full ultrasound study; the limited exam detected DVT in all seven positive cases.

2. A full scan of the proximal veins should be the standard method, but in technically difficult studies, a limited exam of the CFV and popliteal veins (compression and Doppler assessment) should suffice in ruling out DVT above the calf level.

3. Extrinsic compression of iliac vein versus isolated iliac DVT.

    ⇒ If no DVT is detected but flow is continuous in the external iliac or CFV, careful comparison must be made to the contralateral leg.

Abnormal flow pattern in the left CFV caused by extrinsic compression of the iliac vein by a pelvis mass.

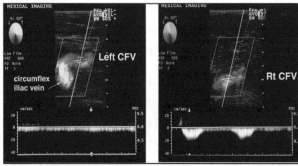

- Unilateral continuous flow may be due to:

  ⇒ Isolated iliac vein DVT (acute or chronic).

  ⇒ Extrinsic compression by a mass in the pelvis (more likely).

  ⇒ If unilateral continuous flow is detected, scan the pelvis and the iliac vein.

- Bilateral continuous flow can be due to:

  ⇒ Shallow breathing due to chest pain, PE, etc.

  ⇒ Patient supine position.

  ⇒ IVC obstruction (does patient have bilateral swelling?).

> **NOTE: It is recommended that the contralateral common femoral vein be imaged routinely in a unilateral exam. Compare waveforms to the symptomatic side.**

4. Use a worksheet (similar to the one below) to draw in regions of thrombosis.

  ⇒ In addition to videotape, digital clips, or hard copy, provide treating/referring and interpreting physician with a leg vein diagram. This diagram is very useful for detailing the extent and location of thrombus. It is also helpful for comparison in follow-up exams.

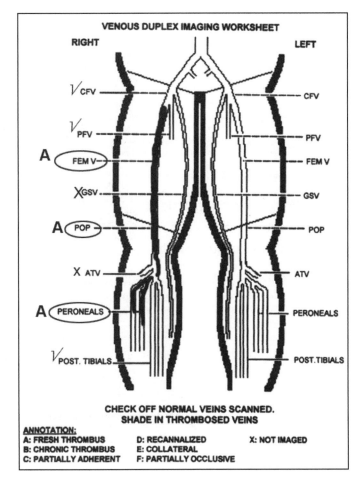

DIFFERENTIAL DIAGNOSIS OF CALF PAIN AND SWELLING

Once you've ruled out venous thrombosis, look for other sources of calf pain.

Baker's cyst, AKA, popliteal cyst, synovial cyst

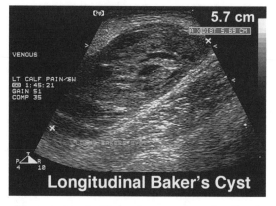

Hemorrhagic Baker's cyst, longitudinal

- The synovial lining and synovial fluid bulges into the popliteal space. Careful imaging can demonstrate a connection or communication with the joint space in the knee.

- Popliteal cysts may remain in the popliteal space, or:

   ⇒ Dissect into medial aspect of calf.

   ⇒ Rupture into calf.

   ⇒ Become hemorrhagic.

   ⇒ Should not be mistaken for popliteal artery aneurysm.

   ⇒ All of the above.

- Identify, and measure in three dimensions.

Hematoma, muscle tear

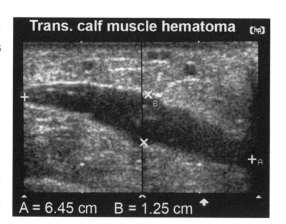

- Hematomas are often related in injury or trauma. A bleed can occur into the calf muscle groups causing pain and swelling.

- Hematomas:

   ⇒ Do not extend to the knee joint space.

   ⇒ May compress the popliteal vein.

   ⇒ If there is any doubt, should be imaged in dual or split screen format with comparisons to contralateral limb at the same location.

   ⇒ Hematomas may be exacerbated if the patient is taking aspirin.

Lymphedema

- This is a very common cause of lower leg and ankle swelling. It is caused by obstruction in the lymph channels, resulting in an excess of lymph fluid in the tissue, usually in the foot ankle and lower leg.

- Lymphedema:

   ⇒ Demonstrates pitting edema.

⇒ Has an "ant farm" appearance on US, with numerous subcutaneous fluid channels.

⇒ Swelling is often recurrent, reduced in the morning, more severe late in the day.

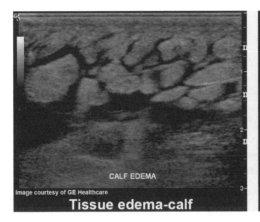

Tissue edema-calf

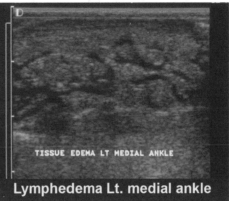

Lymphedema Lt. medial ankle

Lymph Nodes

⇒ Commonly seen in the groin region.

⇒ Kidney-shaped and can be swollen in the presence of systemic infection, malignancy, etc.

⇒ Should not be mistaken for a thrombosed GSV, nodes are not elongated.

⇒ Should be measured in three dimensions and reported.

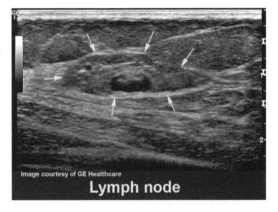

Lymph node

Cellulitis

⇒ An infection or inflammation of the soft or connective tissue in the calf.

⇒ The limb becomes red and sometimes "streaky", the skin becomes shiny and warm to touch.

⇒ This condition is not related to DVT and can be differentiated clinically from venous thrombosis.

Compression syndromes

The IVC lies to the right side of the aorta. The left common iliac vein courses underneath the right common iliac artery. In a certain subset of patients, including women who are in late pregnancy, there can be extrinsic compression of the left common iliac vein that results in iliac vein thrombosis. This is known as May-Thurner Syndrome.

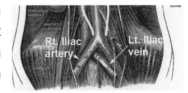

Other differential diagnoses

- Tumors: often have increased arterial flow noted with color Doppler.

- Abscess: look for swirling debris within.

- Arterio-venous fistulas: high venous flow and low arterial resistance (high velocity, low resistance flow).

Pitfalls and Pearls of Imaging

♦ A "heavy hand" on the transducer will compress veins inadvertently; if you cannot see the veins it's difficult to evaluate them ! Ease up.

♦ Any vein segment that does not compress should be carefully evaluated in longitudinal plane and with color Doppler. You must be certain that the transducer is not being pressed against an adjacent bone or tendon that prevents compression of the vein.

♦ The distal popliteal vein is difficult to image. You must examine this segment carefully and be certain that you evaluated the entire popliteal vein all the way to the anterior tibial vein confluence.

♦ Beware of bifed/duplicated femoral and popliteal veins; they're common. One may be patent and the other thrombosed.

♦ Popliteal or Baker's cyst may contain hemorrhage and look like a popliteal DVT. However, these cysts are not continuous with a vein segment, and do not lie along the course of the popliteal artery.

♦ Color Doppler may obscure partially adherent thrombus. The slice thickness of color Doppler beam may be wide and detect flow along the side of the thrombus. In the two-dimensional display of the CRT screen color may be displayed in place of (overwrite) the thrombus.

♦ Some patients may not exhibit respiratory variation in the Doppler display in the proximal veins. You must determine if this is a systemic phenomenon by evaluating the other leg. If this is a unilateral phenomenon and no DVT is detected in that leg, iliac vein thrombus or extrinsic compression of the iliac vein should be suspected.

Other Facts of Venous Imaging Life:

♦ You do not have to "angle correct" or adjust the angle correction cursor to the axis of flow (unless your system mandates that you do, e.g., some Philips and older Hewlett Packard systems), because there usually is no need to measure venous velocity. However, for improved Doppler sensitivity to low frequency shifts associated with low velocity, keep the spectral Doppler angle less than 70 degrees (in venous application).

◆ Normal venous flow can and may be displayed above or below spectral baseline. It is not "written in stone" that venous flow must always be presented below baseline.

◆ Orders for ARTERIAL AND VENOUS: It is not uncommon to receive "orders" to perform an arterial and venous exam on the same person on the same day. However, in the USA, most medical carriers for Medicare will not allow reimbursement for both of these exams unless, there are specific and clearly different indications for each exam. You should perform the exam appropriate for the symptoms. If the order for the exam does not match the symptoms, it is appropriate that you, or your medical director, contact the referring physician and verify the "correctness" of the order.

◆ In the event that you're required to perform a venous and an arterial exam on the same patient, perform the venous exam first to rule out DVT. Obtaining arterial limb blood pressures on someone that might have venous thrombosis could have dire consequences.

Comparison of venous thrombosis symptoms and arterial disease symptoms.

VENOUS	ARTERIAL
• acute onset of symptoms	• progressive symptoms
• limb swelling	• intermittent pain when walking
• persistent pain in thigh or calf	• foot/limb coolness
• local tenderness	• limb pallor
• palpable, subcutaneous "cord"	• rest pain in feet
• SOB, chest pain	• gangrene, tissue necrosis

VENOUS INSUFFICIENCY TESTING - DUPLEX IMAGING

Venous insufficiency is the clinical manifestation of incompetent venous valves in the deep, superficial, and/or perforating veins. Insufficiency can also be caused by chronic outflow obstruction caused by previous, unresolved DVT.

Vein incompetency is categorized by the etiology:

• PRIMARY INSUFFICIENCY is a congenital absence of valves.

• SECONDARY INSUFFICIENCY is due to damaged valves, and perhaps persistent outflow obstruction, from previous episode(s) of vein thrombosis.

Symptoms of insufficiency include:

⇒ Recurrent calf, ankle, or foot swelling.

⇒ Varicosities.

⇒ Venous claudication.

⇒ Stasis dermatitis.

⇒ Ulceration.

⇒ Chronic limb swelling.

Note that these symptoms are distinctly different from those of acute venous thrombosis.

• Venous insufficiency, also referred to as "venous incompetence" is characterized by reverse flow in either the deep, superficial, or perforating veins, or a combination of systems.

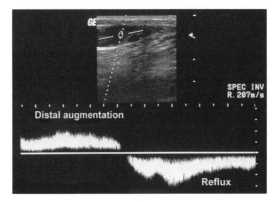

Techniques for evaluating venous insufficiency, and methods for preoperative assessment are covered in **CHAPTER 7**-Imaging for Insufficiency.

Symptoms of Acute DVT	Symptoms of Insufficiency
• Acute, persistent limb swelling	• Recurrent limb swelling
• Recent onset, persistent pain: calf, thigh	• Varicose veins
• Local tenderness	• Chronic Leg "heaviness", discomfort
• Limb warmth	• Stasis dermatitis
• Shortness of breath (? PE)	• Ulceration

PROTOCOL RECOMMENDATIONS

The combined examination of ruling out acute DVT, superficial thrombophlebitis, evaluating for insufficiency, and in many cases, providing additional information pre-operatively for vein ablation procedures has made the venous duplex exam complicated and lengthy. The following protocols are recommended to streamline the examination while providing all necessary information. Because symptoms of DVT are very different from those of insufficiency, these two conditions require different emphasis in protocols.

Venous Protocol #1: Rule out Deep Vein Thrombosis

⇒   Use methods described in this chapter. Scan for superficial thrombophlebitis if symptomatic.

⇒   Perform this protocol for patients with acute symptoms (SX within 2 weeks).

⇒   Don't evaluate for insufficiency or valvular incompetence: these are chronic symptoms.

Venous Protocol #2: Evaluation for Insufficiency.

⇒   Perform this exam for patients with non-acute symptoms of insufficiency.

⇒   Rule out DVT and chronic outflow obstruction (quickly) by scanning the CFV and popliteal veins only; use compression and Doppler methods.

⇒   Evaluate CFV, proximal femoral and popliteal veins for reflux.

⇒   Evaluate GSV for flow reflux, evaluate the small saphenous vein if large.

⇒   Identify incompetent perforating veins and where they connect to deep veins.

⇒   Don't scan calf veins except for perforator connection.

⇒   **See Chapter 7 for methods and detail.**

Venous Protocol #3: Pre-ablation protocol

⇒   Perform protocol # 2, and add the following procedures (as preferred by the referring physician).

⇒   Evaluate GSV for flow reflux, identify the highest level of incompetence.

⇒   Mark (map) the course of the GSV with an indelible marker (establish beforehand if this is needed).

⇒   "Mark" incompetent perforating veins (establish beforehand if this is needed). Ignore competent perforators.

⇒   Measure and record the GSV diameter at its widest spot.

⇒   Measure the depth of the GSV at its shallowest position.

⇒   Identify the source vein of large varicosities.

⇒   **See Chapter 7 for methods and detail.**

Venous Protocol #4: Vein Mapping for Arterial Bypass

⇒   Rule out femoral vein thrombosis (removing the saphenous vein is a contraindication if it's the main collateral channel in the presence of chronic femoral-popliteal DVT).

⇒   Determine suitability of the great saphenous vein

•   Is it continuous to the ankle?
•   Does it have residual thrombus?

- Is it a duplicated system?
- Any areas of abnormal narrowing or dilation (aneurysm)?

⇒   Measure the diameter in the proximal, mid, distal thigh, and mid & distal calf.

⇒   Mark the course of the GSV on the skin with an indelible marker.

More detail will be found in the chapter on bypass grafts.

REFERENCES

1. Barnes RW, Hoak JC. The fallibility of the clinical diagnosis of venous thrombosis. JAMA 234:605, 1975

2. Lohr JM, Kerr TM, Lutter KS, Cranley RD, Spirtoff K, Cranley JJ. Lower extremity calf thrombosis: To treat or not to treat? J Vasc Surg 1991;14: 618-623

3. Mattos MA, Melendres G, Sumner DS, Hood DB, Barkmeier LD, Hodgson KJ, Ramsey DE. Prevalence and distribution of calf vein thrombosis in patients with symptomatic deep venous thrombosis: A color-flow duplex study J Vasc Surg 1996;24:738-44

4. Krupski WC, Bass A, Dilley RB, Bernstein EF, Otis SM. Propagation of deep venous thrombosis identified by duplex ultrasonography. J Vasc Surg 1990; 12:467-75.

5. Lensing A, et al. Detection of deep venous thrombosis by real time B-mode ultrasonography. N Engl. J Med, 1989;320:342-345

6. Pezzullo, JA, et al. Symptomatic Deep Venous Thrombosis: Diagnosis with limited compression US". Radiology 198:67-90.1996

CHAPTER 7: IMAGING METHODS FOR VENOUS INSUFFICIENCY

VENOUS INSUFFICIENCY TESTING - DUPLEX IMAGING

Venous insufficiency is the clinical manifestation of incompetent venous valves in the deep, superficial, and/or perforating veins. This condition can also be caused by chronic outflow obstruction that results in increased venous intramural pressure.

Vein incompetency is categorized by the etiology:

- PRIMARY insufficiency is caused by a congenital absence of venous valves, or weakness in valve structure.

- SECONDARY insufficiency is due to valve damage from previous venous thrombosis. The thrombosed vein may become recannalized and be patent, but the valve leaflets don't work properly. Additionally, proximal veins may still be obstructed with outflow relying on collateral (smaller) vessels. During calf muscle contraction venous blood volume is ejected upward towards the heart, only to return downward through incompetent valves.

Symptoms of insufficiency include:

- Recurrent calf, ankle, or foot swelling.

- Varicosities.

- Venous claudication (heaviness and pain in thighs when walking, due to venous congestion).

- Stasis dermatitis.

- Ulceration.

- Chronic limb swelling.

It's important to differentiate symptoms of venous insufficiency from acute venous thrombosis. If the patient presents with symptoms of acute deep venous thrombosis, you must proceed with the protocols described in Chapter 6. If the patient has symptoms of insufficiency, proceed with the following protocols.

Patient Position

The patient should be in a steep reverse Trendelenburg, or semi-Fowler's position. If possible, position the patient or the exam cart so that the leg that you're examining is closest to you. This may require rotating the bed so that the patient's torso is behind you.

> TECHNICAL NOTE: Use venous presets on the ultrasound system, ie., low wall filters, low PRF scale for color and spectral Doppler, and longer sweep time on spectral Doppler (8 second sweep time). Also, optimize color and spectral Doppler steering direction and angle.

INSUFFICIENCY PROTOCOLS

Step #1. Rule out chronic venous outflow obstruction

Chronic outflow obstruction can contribute to venous insufficiency. Perform a quick assessment for this condition. In transverse scan plane determine patency with compression and coaptation methods, and evaluate the following veins:

- Common femoral vein (CFV).

- Proximal femoral vein.

- Popliteal vein.

> NOTE: Patients with outflow obstruction, whether acute or chronic, have increased intramural pressure in the distal veins. You may find that the veins distal to the obstruction will compress, but with some difficulty or resistance due to the increased pressure.

In longitudinal plane, evaluate flow in the distal popliteal vein with spectral Doppler. The presence of normal spontaneous flow with respiratory variation excludes the condition of chronic outflow obstruction in that limb. Steady, continuous flow without respiratory phasicity, is suspicious for outflow obstruction (or extrinsic compression of

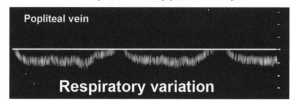

the iliac vein). If steady, continuous flow is present, evaluate the contralateral popliteal vein and compare. If this popliteal lacks respiratory change, check to see if the patient is a shallow breather. Otherwise, scan the proximal veins for chronic obstruction. This portion of the insufficiency exam should be done quickly. There is no need to scan the calf veins for outflow obstruction in this protocol.

Step #2. Determine if the deep veins are competent

Evaluate the following veins for reflux (transient reversed flow) with the patient in reverse Trendelenburg or semi-Fowler's position.

- CFV.

- Proximal femoral vein.

- Popliteal vein.

Note: it might be easier to start this step as a continuation of the popliteal vein assessment, before moving to the CFV.

Popliteal Vein for Reflux

- Position the spectral PW-Doppler sample volume in the distal popliteal vein. Activate the

Doppler, and optimize controls for low flow-velocity detection. Use a slow (8 second) sweep speed.

- Squeeze the calf to augment flow upward, and watch for reflux (downward flow) following augmentation. Allow a few moments for the veins to refill, then repeat the augmentation.

- In a competent venous segment, there will be no, or minimal, retrograde flow after augmentation, as well as a short valve closure time.

- Freeze the spectral sweep and record to demonstrate the normal response.

- If retrograde flow persists following augmentation, "freeze" the Doppler sweep and assess the reflux duration (time). This can be done with system calipers, or by comparing the duration to the time markers on the Doppler display. Popliteal reflux ≥ 1 second is abnormal; see table below.

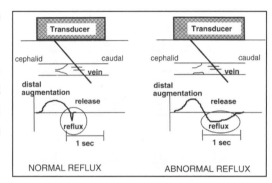

- An alternative method is to initially assess the vein segment with color Doppler (optimized for low flow-velocity). Spectral Doppler is not required if normal. If retrograde flow is noted with color, then spectral Doppler is activated and reflux time is measured. However, it's more difficult to document normalcy with this method.

Abnormal Reflux Times: [1]

Location	Time
Deep veins	≥ 1.0 second
GSV, SSV	≥ 0.5 seconds
Perforating veins	≥ 0.35 seconds
Longer durations observed in supine patients	
Above values apply for patient in a standing position.	

The image on the right demonstrates popliteal vein reflux following distal augmentation (calf squeeze). If the popliteal vein is normal (no reflux, or less than the above parameters), it is unlikely that venous insufficiency is caused by deep venous incompetence.

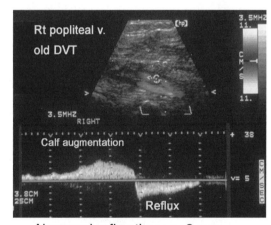

Abnormal reflux time: > 2 sec.

> **TECHNICAL NOTE**: Traditionally, normal venous flow has been displayed below the spectral baseline. Some ultrasound Doppler systems, however, are designed to display appropriate flow direction ABOVE baseline, and retrograde flow below. Knowing how your system displays flow direction is imperative in a venous insufficiency study.

Common Femoral Vein for Reflux

♦ In longitudinal plane, position the spectral Doppler sample volume in the CFV proximal to the sapheno-femoral junction (SFJ). Activate the Doppler, and optimize controls for low flow-velocity detection (low PRF scale), adjust spectral- baseline direction and establish appropriate Doppler steering. Record a few waveforms displayed during respiratory variation.

♦ Have the patient perform a Valsalva maneuver to check for reflux. This maneuver, if performed correctly, will increase venous intraluminal pressure in the vena cava, iliac and common femoral veins and test valve function in the CFV, FV and GSV. The following modification has been recommended by Steven Talbot as a "patient friendly" method.[2]

  • Place your free hand on patient's abdomen and ask the patient to stop breathing and to press upwards against your hand with their "stomach".

  • Have them start gradually, then strain harder.

  • Practice a couple of times before the real test.

  • Turn on the spectral (or color) Doppler, repeat the Valsalva maneuver and test for reflux in the CFV.

  • Flow should stop during the Valsalva "strain" if the vein segment is competent. After 2-3 seconds have the patient relax their abdomen; flow should then continue in a normal direction.

  • If the valves in this segment are incompetent flow will become retrograde (reversed) during the "strain", then continue antegrade with relaxation.

  • Freeze the image after the Valsalva test, measure reflux time (if any) and record image.

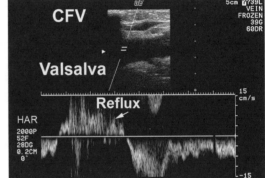

♦ Next, augment CFV flow by squeezing the thigh distal to the sample site, then look for reflux following augmentation. If reflux is found, measure the duration.

Proximal Femoral Vein for Reflux

♦ Place the Doppler sample volume in the FV just distal to the FV-PFV bifurcation. Use the Valsalva maneuver to elicit reflux or confirm competency.

♦ If reflux occurs in the CFV, but not the femoral vein, the flow is probably heading "south" through an incompetent terminal valve in the great saphenous vein.

It's uncommon for venous insufficiency to be due solely to deep vein valvular incompetence. Superficial vein and perforator vein incompetence is far more likely to be the cause of venous insufficiency. Occasionally, short segments of the deep system appear to be incompetent, but the reflux is due to flow going outwards in an incompetent perforating vein.

Distribution of valvular incompetence in venous stasis ulcers in 95 limbs.[3]

D only	2.1 %
P only	8.4 %
S only	16.8 %
P & D	4.2 %
S & D	11.6 %
S & P	19.0 %
S & P & D	31.6 %

D = deep veins, S = superficial veins, P = perforating veins

In this study, venous stasis ulcers occurred most frequently in patients with multiple system incompetence, i.e., superficial, perforating and deep systems, followed by superficial and perforating system incompetence.

Step #3. Determine if the superficial venous system is incompetent

Evaluate the following veins for reflux:

- Entire great saphenous vein (GSV).

- Small saphenous vein (SSV.)

- Perforating veins, if large.

Great Saphenous Vein Reflux

◆ Identify the GSV at the saphenofemoral junction (SFJ).

◆ Measure the diameter of the vein at the proximal, mid and distal levels.

⇒ GSV diameter exceeding 9 mm, 7.5 mm, and 5 mm at the SFJ, mid-thigh and calf respectively, is highly predictive of incompetence.[4]

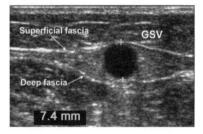

◆ The GSV lies within the fascial envelope, between a superficial and a deep fascial layer. The appearance of the GSV within these fascia layers is sometimes referred to as the "eye of Cleopatra".

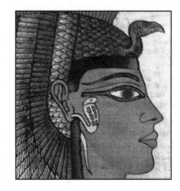

◆ In longitudinal plane, position the Doppler sample volume in the GSV just distal to the SFJ and the terminal valve. The GSV is assessed by the modified Valsalva method described above, and by squeezing the limb distally.

◆ Because the GSV does not drain muscle groups, flow during distal augmentation may be minimal. Press and squeeze along the course of the vein to "milk" flow upwards, and note reversed flow.

♦ Measure the time of any reflux detected. In the example on the right, reflux duration is 3.5 seconds.

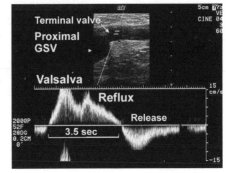

♦ If the terminal valve is incompetent, usually the entire GSV will be incompetent as well. The vein becomes dilated and the valves leaflets, although present, may not coapt or meet.

♦ If the terminal valve is competent, proceed distally down the GSV with color Doppler, augment flow periodically, and look for reflux. If reflux is observed with color Doppler, confirm and measure the reflux time with spectral Doppler.

♦ Try to determine the highest level of incompetence along the course of the GSV. In the diagram on the right, reflux occurs in mid GSV and distally. This "segmental incompetence" can occur due to incompetent tributaries or perforating veins.

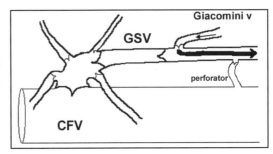

♦ Note the presence of duplicate GSVs, and/or accessory saphenous veins; evaluate these for competence as well.

Image courtesy of Olivier Pichot. MD
Atlas of Ultrasound Images, www.VNUS.com

> NOTE: Veins that join the GSV and appear to course through the SUPERFICIAL fascia are thin-walled tributary veins or accessory veins. These veins are prone to dilation and can become varicose veins. Veins that join the GSV and course through the DEEP facial plane are usually perforating veins. These connect with the deep veins, gastrocnemius veins and soleal veins.

Standing position versus reverse Trendelenburg

Some symptomatic patients with incompetent valves may not exhibit venous reflux while in supine or reverse Trendelenburg positions because the intraluminal hydrostatic pressure is low and the veins are not completely distended. When these patients are standing, the intraluminal pressure increases and the valve leaflets are forced apart contributing to valve dysfunction. Although this situation in uncommon, (most patients with symptomatic CVI have pronounced venous reflux in reverse Trendelenburg position), some clinicians recommend testing the deep and superficial venous system with the patient standing. The non-weight bearing leg is tested for reflux following distal augmentation. This can be accomplished with the help of a colleague (to squeeze the calf), or with a rapid cuff inflation and deflation device. The latter device standardizes the augmentation maneuver. Testing for reflux with the patient standing is awkward for the examiner, as it's difficult to view the ultrasound monitor and operate the system controls. If the patient exhibits abnormal reflux in the reverse Trendelenburg position, there is no reason to retest with the patient standing. However, there may be a benefit to having the patient stand while you mark the location of varicose veins.

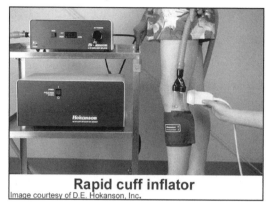

Rapid cuff inflator
Image courtesy of D.E. Hokanson, Inc.

It's the opinion of this author that testing in a standing position can be reserved for patients that have symptoms of chronic venous insufficiency, but do not exhibit venous reflux in the reverse Trendelenburg position.

Small Saphenous Vein (SSV) Reflux

The patient should be in a reverse Trendelenburg, or semi-Fowler's position with leg rotated to the side. If possible, position the patient or the exam cart so that the leg that you're examining is closest to you. Alternately, the patient should lie on their side.

♦ Use a high frequency transducer (7-12 MHz), as the SSV is very superficial.

♦ Identify the small saphenous vein (formerly known as the lesser saphenous vein) in transverse plane on the posterior calf at mid-calf level. (The small saphenous vein is aptly named, as it's often < 2 mm and difficult to image. Look for it between the two bellies of the gastrocnemius muscle.

♦ Follow its course; scan proximally to determine whether it joins the popliteal vein or whether it continues to the Giacomini vein (intersaphenous vein). Next, follow the SSV distally in the calf and determine whether it has any large tributaries or varicosities.

♦ In longitudinal plane, assess the SSV with color Doppler. Squeeze the calf to augment flow and look for reflux. If reflux occurs, activate the spectral Doppler, repeat the augmentation, and measure the reflux time duration.

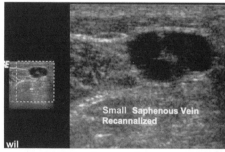 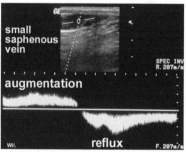

In the composite image above, the recannalized post-phlebitic small saphenous vein is dilated and has residual fibrous bands. Spectral Doppler demonstrates incompetence.

♦ If the SSV is small (less than 2 mm), flow may not be detectable unless there are large communicating tributaries, varicosities, or perforating veins. If the SSV is small, it's most likely competent.

PERFORATING VEINS

Step #4. Determine whether the perforating veins are incompetent.

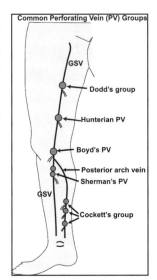

Common Perforating Vein (PV) Groups

Perforating veins (PV) have valves that direct flow from the superficial to the deep venous system. Although perforating veins exist in the thigh (Dodd's and Hunterian), the ones most commonly visualized with ultrasound are Cockett's perforators on the medial aspect of the calf. Competent perforating veins are usually difficult to see, whereas incompetent perforators are larger and therefore more obvious.

Incompetent perforating veins are a major contributor to the development of venous ulceration and varicose veins. The severity of CVI appears to be directly related to the number of incompetent perforator veins.[5]

Patient Position: The patient should be sitting with legs dependant off the side of the exam table or bed. If possible, raise the bed and sit on a low stool to have comfortable access to the lower leg. Alternatively, patients may be scanned while they're standing. This method may be necessary to identify thigh perforating veins (Dodd's perforating veins), but it's very awkward position for imaging the lower leg.

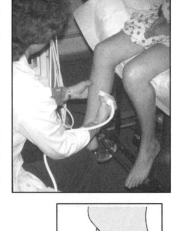

♦ Scan the calf in transverse plane from the tibial medial condyle to the medial malleolus. Carefully interrogate the echogenic deep fascia (1-2 cm below the skin lying in a horizontal plane) and look for perforators as they penetrate the deep fascial plane and dive away from the transducer.

♦ Shift the transducer one transducer width to the side and scan back up the calf. Repeat this procedure to scan the entire circumference of the calf.

♦ Although most incompetent PV will be found on the medial side of the calf, they can also be found on the lateral calf.

◆ If a perforator is identified, try to elongate or "open" the vein image with transducer rotation. Transducer orientation may be longitudinal, transverse or oblique.

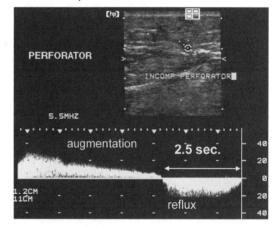

◆ Activate color Doppler (controls should be optimized for low flow velocity) and evaluate the perforator competence. Squeeze the limb distally and observe whether flow is present, and note direction of flow.

◆ Because of the tortuousity of some PVs, flow direction on color Doppler display can be confusing. However, within an incompetent perforating vein, bi-directional flow will occur, i.e., you'll observe flow in one direction when you augment, and then observe flow in the opposite direction after augmentation.

◆ Repeat the above step with proximal calf compression.

◆ If bidirectional flow is observed, activate the spectral Doppler and record reflux flow duration.

◆ Reflux time ≥ 0.35 seconds is consistent with perforator incompetence.[1]

> Incompetent Cockett's perforator with 2.5 second reflux duration. Initial augmentation flow is inward, with outward, reflux flow, following augmentation.

◆ If the perforator is incompetent, identify the deep vein connection.

> There is no need to document or record **normal** perforating veins.

Perforator size

Perforating vein incompetence has been associated with large perforator diameter. Labropoulos, et al., demonstrated that an ultrasound diameter of ≥ 3.9 mm in a perforator was a reliable predictor of reflux. A diameter of ≥ 3.0 mm had a positive predictive valve for reflux of 84.4%, but not all 3 mm PV were incompetent.[5] Other studies have demonstrated that size alone cannot completely distinguish competent and incompetent PVs, and that Doppler demonstrated reflux is the ultimate demonstration of incompetence.[6]

Some clinical labs will measure the diameter of incompetent PVs, but the "gold standard" is not size, but Doppler-demonstrated reflux.

Preoperative Protocol for Vein Ablation

Not all patients presenting for a venous insufficiency exam will require the following additional protocol, so it's essential that the referring physician communicate whether the additional information is required. If the patient is a surgical or vein ablation candidate, the previously-described protocol for insufficiency, with steps 1-4, should have been performed.

♦ Incompetent saphenous veins can be ablated with radio frequency or laser intraluminal devices, or with a sclerosing foam agent.

♦ Measure the diameter of the incompetent great saphenous vein at the SFJ, mid and distal thigh. This will be useful for the interventionalist in selecting the appropriate ablation catheter (size).

♦ Note whether the GSV is excessively superficial or deep. Measure the depth of the vein from the skin to the upper wall of the vein. A superficial saphenous vein may require additional tumescence during the ablation procedure to prevent heat from burning the skin.

♦ Identify the source or the origin of large varicosities. Varicose veins may appear in a location that is not adjacent to their source.

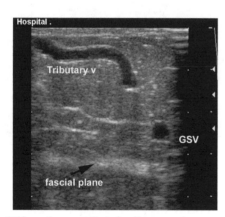

Dilated superficial tributary in the thigh: the source is the GSV.

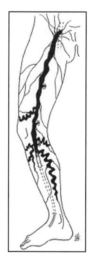

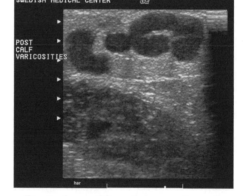

Posterior calf varicose veins: the source is the SSV

♦ If requested, "map" and mark the course of the incompetent GSV in the thigh from the SFJ to the proximal calf. If the SSV is incompetent, mark its course along the posterior calf.

Vein Mapping & Preparation

- Various marking devices are available commercially and facilitate this otherwise "messy" job.

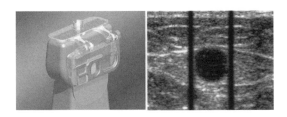

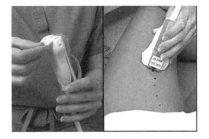

Skin marking device from Sonomark*   AIM transducer skin marker device**

- For a "home made" solution, mark the mid-point of the transducer. Apply a strip of clear tape on the side of the transducer. Make a small indelible mark on the tape adjacent to the middle of the length of the transducer face. Alternatively, place a thin piece of colored tape in the same location directly on the transducer casing; avoid marking the transducer itself (they're expensive!). This will serve as a reference mark for the center of the ultrasound image.

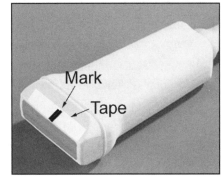

- Position the patient in reverse Trendelenburg.

- Clean the leg along the approximate course of the GSV with 70% alcohol.

- Place a thin layer of WARM acoustic gel along the course of the GSV.

- Identify the proximal *GSV* at the SFJ; position the vein in the center of the ultrasound field of view (don't use the Zoom function). This should correspond to the mark on the transducer casing tape. Use a plastic drinking straw to create an indentation on the skin over the vein (adjacent to the mark on the casing). A ballpoint pen, point retracted, may also be used. Gently press the straw or pen for a few seconds to create the indentation. Move the transducer distally a few centimeters and repeat. Mark the confluences of large tributaries as well.

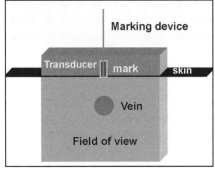

- After the GSV in the thigh has been indented, wipe off the gel and place an indelible

* SonoMark. www.sonomarking.com. MPM, Inc. 1775 Gunnison, Delta, CO 81416, 866-477-760

**AIM Medical Technologies. www.vascularmapping.com 866-511-5487

(Sanford Marker Deluxe works well) mark over the skin indentations.

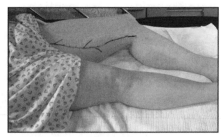

- Connect the dots with the marker to map the course of the GSV and major confluences; see image on right.

- Mark incompetent perforators using the above methods. Also, a diagram of incompetent PV location(s) can be of help to the surgeon or interventionalist.

REFERENCES

1. Labropoulos N, Tiongson J, Pryor L, et al. Definition of Venous Reflux in Lower Extremity Veins. J Vasc Surg. 2003; 38: 793-798.

2. Talbot SR. Diagnostic and Interpretative Challenges Encountered During Venous Duplex Studies. Vascular Ultrasound Today. 9(1):1-28, 2004

3. Hanrahan LM, Araki CT, et al. Distribution of valvular incompetence in p[atients with venous stasis ulceration. J Vasc Surg 1991;13:805-12

4. Engelhorn, Englehorn A, Salles-Cunha S, Picheth F, CastroN, Dabul N, Gomes C. Relationship between reflux and great saphenous vein diameter. J Vasc Technol, 21 (3):167-172,1997

5. Labropoulos N, Mansour MA, Kang SS, Gloviczki P, Baker WH. New Insights into Perforator Vein Incompetence. Eur J Vasc and Endovasc Surg. 1999;18, Issue 3, 228-234

6. Yamamoto N, Unno N, Mitsuoka H, Saito T, Miki K, Ishimaru K, Kaneko H, Nakamura S. Preoperative and intraoperative evaluation of diameter-reflux relationship of calf perforating veins in patients with primary varicose vein. J Vasc Surg 2002;36:1225-30.

Venous worksheets next page.

VENOUS INSUFFICIENCY WORKSHEET #1

Lab name and address here.

Page 1

Venous Insufficiency Ultrasound Exam Worksheet

Note: this worksheet is not for a DVT exam

Patient Name:_____ Gender: M ☐ F ☐   Date: _____

Patient ID :_____ Birthdate: ___/___/_____   Age_____

Ordering Physician_____Sonographer_____

Patient History and Symptoms: CPT code_____ ICD-9 code_____

HX of DVT	**Rt** ☐	**Lt** ☐	Recurrent swelling	**Rt** ☐	**Lt** ☐
Superf. thromphl.	**Rt** ☐	**Lt** ☐	Stasis dermatitis	**Rt** ☐	**Lt** ☐
Spider veins	**Rt** ☐	**Lt** ☐	Limb ulcer	**Rt** ☐	**Lt** ☐
Varicose veins	**Rt** ☐	**Lt** ☐	Other	**Rt** ☐	**Lt** ☐
Vein surgery	**Rt** ☐	**Lt** ☐	Description:_____

Reason for referral and exam?_____

DEEP VEINS

Evaluate deep venous system for chronic outflow obstruction and valvular incompetence.
Superficial venous system is on reverse side of this form.

RIGHT   **Sp= spontaneous, Ph= phasic, Pul= pulsatile, C= continuous, R=reflux**   **LEFT**

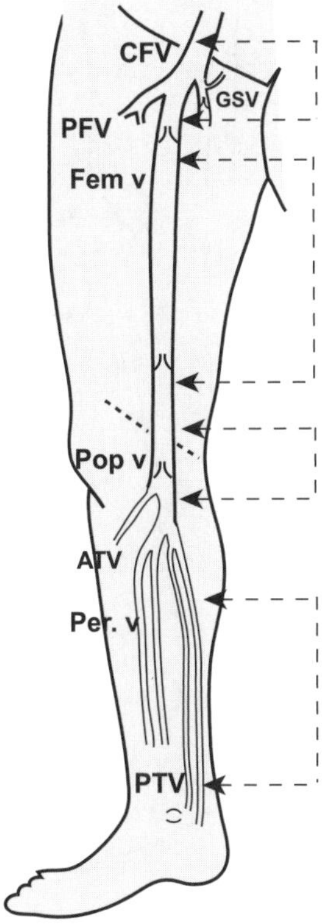

CFV
Sp ☐ , Ph ☐ , Pul☐ , C☐ , R☐
Patent: Y ☐ , N ☐ ,
Residual DVT ☐
Outflow Obstruct. ☐

Femoral v.
Sp☐ , Ph☐ , Pul☐ , C☐ , R☐
Patent: Y ☐ , N ☐ ,
Residual DVT ☐
Outflow Obstruct. ☐

Popliteal v.
Sp☐ , Ph ☐ , Pul ☐ , C☐ , R☐
Patent: Y ☐ , N ☐ ,
Residual DVT ☐
Outflow Obstruct. ☐

PTV- optional
Pul ☐ , C ☐ , R ☐ ,
Patent: Y ☐ , N ☐ ,
Residual DVT ☐

CFV
Sp☐ , Ph☐ , Pul☐ , C☐ , R☐
Patent: Y ☐ , N ☐ ,
Residual DVT ☐
Outflow Obstruct. ☐

Femoral v.
Sp ☐ , Ph☐ , Pul☐ , C☐ , R☐
Patent: Y ☐ , N ☐ ,
Residual DVT ☐
Outflow Obstruct. ☐

Popliteal v.
Sp ☐ , Ph ☐ , Pul ☐ , C☐ , R☐
Patent: Y ☐ , N ☐ ,
Residual DVT ☐
Outflow Obstruct. ☐

PTV- optional
Pul ☐ , C ☐ , R ☐ ,
Patent: Y ☐ , N ☐ ,
Residual DVT ☐

Right leg labels: CFV, PFV, GSV, Fem v, Pop v, ATV, Per. v, PTV

Left leg labels: CFV, PFV, GSV, Fem. v, Pop.v, ATV, Per. v, PTV

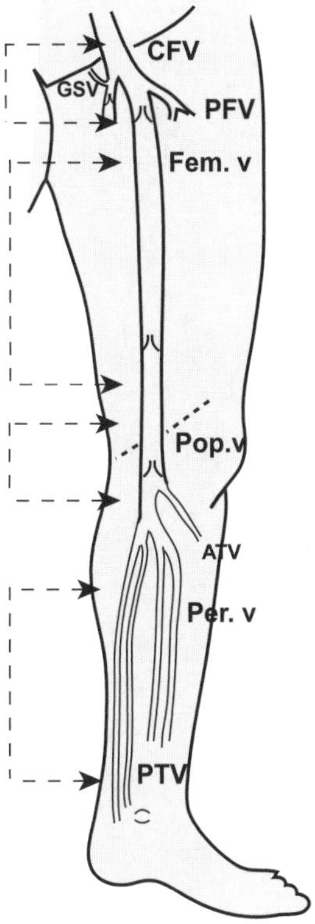

Comments:

(over for superficial veins)

From Techniques in Noninvasive Vascular Diagnosis, Summer Publishing, LLC

VENOUS INSUFFICIENCY WORKSHEET 2

Venous Insufficiency Worksheet- Superficial Veins

Worksheet instructions: This worksheet provides a rough diagram of superficial venous anatomy. Anatomy will vary from patient to patient.

1) Determine saphenous vein competence at various levels. Mark "C" for competent or mark "I" for incompetent.

2) Draw in duplicate saphenous veins or anatomic variations.

3) Draw in location of incompetent perforating veins, and mark "IP". Optional; measure the maximum diameter of incompetent perforating veins. Sketch in varicose veins and identify their origins.

4) Optional protocols-pre-ablation: 1) If GSVs or SSVs (small saphenous vein) are incompetent, measure vein diameter and note maximum size. 2) Measure depth of vein from the skin. Note minimum depth and location.

C = competent segment, I = incompetent segm., Ph= phasic, Pul=pulsatile, IPV = incomp. perforating vein SFJ= sapheno-femoral junction, GSV = great saphenous vein, SSV = small saphenous vein (SSV).

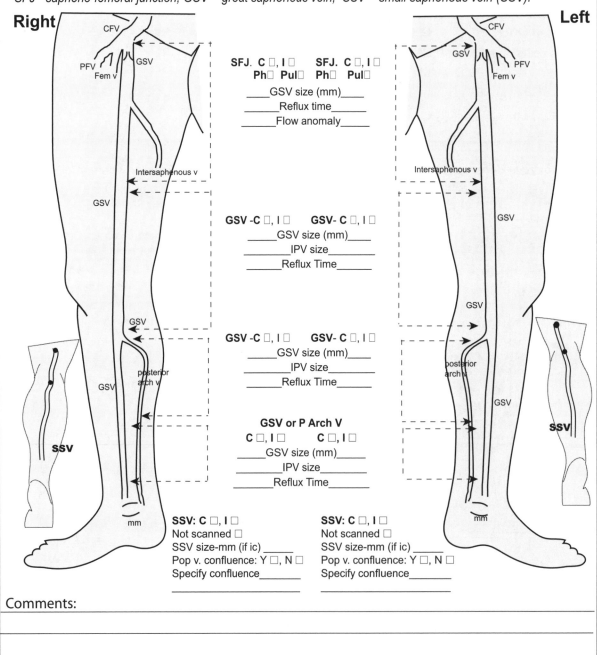

Right

Left

SFJ. C □, I □   SFJ. C □, I □
Ph□ Pul□   Ph□ Pul□
_____GSV size (mm)_____
_____Reflux time_____
_____Flow anomaly_____

GSV -C □, I □   GSV- C □, I □
_____GSV size (mm)_____
_____IPV size_____
_____Reflux Time_____

GSV -C □, I □   GSV- C □, I □
_____GSV size (mm)_____
_____IPV size_____
_____Reflux Time_____

GSV or P Arch V
C □, I □   C □, I □
_____GSV size (mm)_____
_____IPV size_____
_____Reflux Time_____

SSV: C □, I □
Not scanned □
SSV size-mm (if ic) _____
Pop v. confluence: Y □, N □
Specify confluence_____
_____

SSV: C □, I □
Not scanned □
SSV size-mm (if ic) _____
Pop v. confluence: Y □, N □
Specify confluence_____
_____

Comments:

CHAPTER 8: VENOUS IMAGING OF UPPER EXTREMITIES

INDICATIONS

Indications the for upper extremity vein evaluation include:

- Pain and swelling of the arm or neck.

- Pulmonary embolus.

- Dilated superficial veins of the arm and shoulder.

- Palpable subcutaneous "cord" in arm.

- Infusion difficulty with indwelling catheter.

- Pre-operative assessment for hemodialysis access placement.

- It is estimated that up to 28% of patients with indwelling subclavian lines incur venous thrombosis.[1]

The etiology of thrombosis includes:

- Intimal injury due to intraluminal catheter or pacemaker wires.

- Compression of the venous thoracic outlet (effort induced thrombosis).

- Extrinsic compression by a mass.

- Radiation-induced fibrosis.

- Venipuncture.

- IV drug abuse.

- Idiopathic.

VENOUS ANATOMY - UPPER

The upper extremity has a deep and a superficial venous system similar to the legs. The deep veins have an accompanying artery and the superficial veins do not.

Deep Venous Sysyem
- Radial, Ulnar, Interosseous
- Brachial
- Axillary
- Subclavian
- Internal Jugular
- Innominate
- Superior Vena Cava

Superficial Venous System
- Cephalic
- Basilic
- Median cubital

Other (central) Veins
- External jugular
- Anterior jugular
- Jugular arch vein
- Transverse scapular
- Inferior thyroid
- Internal mammary

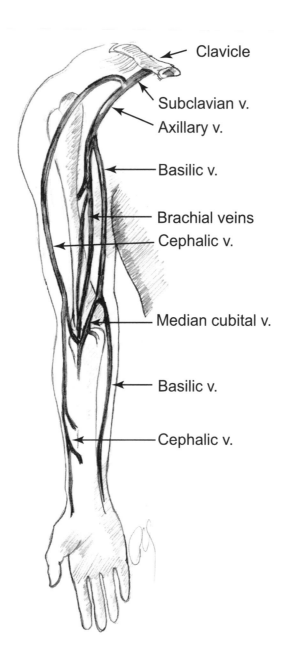

Clavicle

Subclavian v.

Axillary v.

Basilic v.

Brachial veins

Cephalic v.

Median cubital v.

Basilic v.

Cephalic v.

Venous Anatomy of the Arm

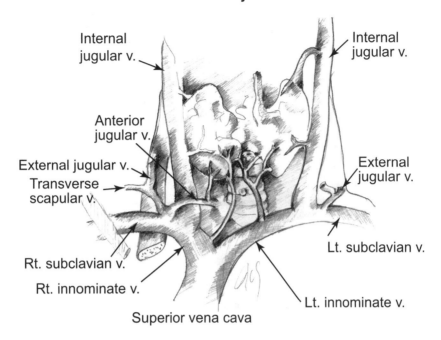

IMAGING METHODS

Because the innominate (brachiocephalic), subclavian and proximal axillary veins lie in proximity to the clavicle, they do not lend themselves to transducer compression techniques.

- Color and spectral Doppler analysis of venous flow patterns are used to assess the patency of these central veins.

- Compression techniques should be reserved for the easily-compressed deep and superficial veins in the arm.

- In all veins, use transverse and longitudinal views to look for echogenic, intraluminal thrombus. Also, observe the motion of the vein walls in response to breathing. Walls of a thrombosed vein tend not to move with respiration.

- Insonate the vein segment with color Doppler using appropriate angle and color scale.

- Record pulsed-Doppler spectra and note whether flow, if present, is continuous, pulsatile, and phasic with respiration.

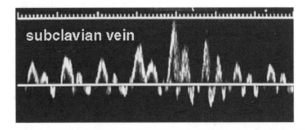

Normal distal subclavian vein flow with pulsatility and respiratory variation superimposed.

Supraclavicular region

- Patient is placed in a <u>supine</u> position with arm at side. ***Typical Doppler waveform characteristics will be affected if the patient is not supine.***

- Use a thin pillow under head and shoulders or remove the pillow altogether.

- If an indwelling subclavian catheter is in place, remove bandages or wound dressings from the shoulder region and cover the region with a sterile skin cover such as Tegaderm.

- If it is not possible to remove bandages, try to work around them and use sterile acoustic gel.

- Use a transducer with adequate penetration for the supraclavicular segment; 5 - 9 MHz linear array, curved array, or a phased array transducer with a small foot-print.

Internal Jugular Vein

- In transverse plane, identify the <u>internal jugular vein (IJV)</u> in the neck and follow its course to the confluence of the subclavian vein. Look for venous thrombus.

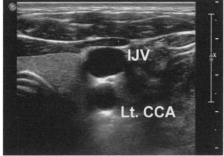

Transverse view of IJV; scan proximally to the subclavian vein confluence

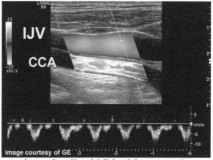

Longitudinal IJV with normal pulsatile flow pattern

- Carefully image the IJV in longitudinal plane for thrombus, then obtain and record spectral Doppler waveforms. Normal internal jugular vein flow should be strongly pulsatile, and flow direction should be towards the heart.

> Venous flow in the IJV, innominate, subclavian and axillary veins should demonstrate some respiratory phasicity and cardiac pulsatility (prominent). BEWARE: the pulsatility may be so pronounced in these veins that flow patterns resemble arterial flow; see previous image.

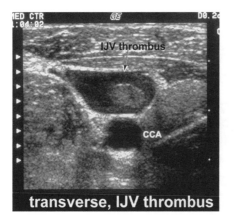

transverse, IJV thrombus

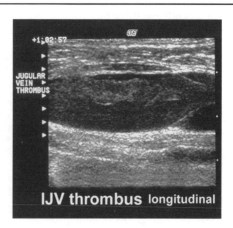

IJV thrombus longitudinal

- Always evaluate the IJV as part of the upper extremity venous exam.

- Beware of a prominent reverberation artifact that is often present within the IJV; this can look like a partially occlusive thrombus.

Subclavian Vein

- With the transducer parallel and along the cephalid border of the clavicle, identify the proximal <u>subclavian vein</u> emerging from beneath the clavicle, and follow its course to the IJV confluence.

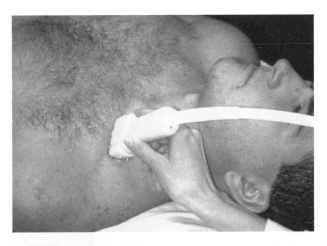

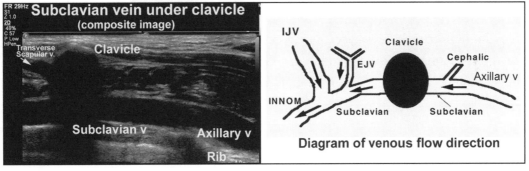

- Record flow pattern and note flow direction with the spectral Doppler.

> In longitudinal plane orient the transducer, or use image invert, so that "distal" (towards the hand) is to the right on the ultrasound image. Without a standardized image orientation, determining flow direction can be problematic.

- Use color Doppler to detect intraluminal filling defects that may be caused by partially occlusive thrombus.

- Scan in a medial direction along the subclavian and into the <u>innominate vein.</u> This vein is formed by the confluence of the subclavian and IJV. On some patients the innominate vein can be followed to the <u>superior vena cava (SVC)</u>, but usually only a small section of the innominate can be imaged.

- Identify the <u>external jugular vein (EJV)</u>; it joins the supraclavicular portion of the subclavian vein just before the IJV confluence. The EJV lies superficial to the subclavian vein and can be mistaken for the subclavian vein when the former is thrombosed. If flow is present in the EJV, it is important to observe the flow direction. Retrograde flow can occur in this vein in the presence of innominate obstruction.

Infraclavicular region

- Apply acoustic gel to the deltopectoral triangle region inferior to the clavicle and locate the distal subclavian artery and the adjacent <u>subclavian vein</u>. This segment lies between the clavicle and the first rib.

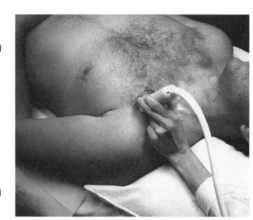

- With spectral Doppler, assess the distal subclavian vein and record waveforms.

- The cephalic vein joins the subclavian just distal to the clavicle. This can be evaluated with compression techniques.

- The vein segment distal to the cephalic confluence is the axillary vein. It courses distally to the confluence of the basilic and brachial veins.

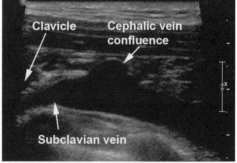

- Scan the <u>axillary vein</u> in transverse and long views.

- As with the supraclavicular region, pay close attention to waveform patterns and flow direction. Flow in the distal subclavian and axillary veins should be phasic and pulsatile.

NOTE: If the subclavian or axillary veins are not clearly seen, abduct the arm 90 degrees from the torso with the elbow bent ("pledge" position) and re-evaluate. Often the axillary vein is compressed by the first or second rib and this position resolves the compression. See below.

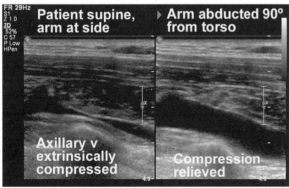

Dual screen image of axillary vein extrinsic compression and release with arm abduction

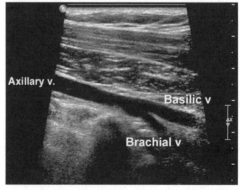

From an anterior scan approach, the basilic and brachial vein confluence in the axilla forming the axillary vein.

Arm, below axilla

Use compression techniques In the arm, similar to those used in the legs. This is the primary diagnostic method for the arm veins. Spontaneous flow may not be present in the arm veins, nor is there phasicity and/or pulsatility in many patients.

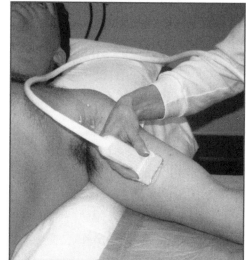

- Abduct the arm 90 degrees from the torso with the hand externally rotated. Support the arm on a pillow or on a shelf extension from the exam bed/table.

- In transverse view, just below the axillary fossa, identify and compress the <u>basilic</u> vein. Follow its course proximally to the axillary vein, and then distally to the forearm. Compressing and release the vein every few inches along its course.

- The smaller, paired <u>brachial veins</u> are found adjacent to the brachial artery and are often difficult to image due to their small size. Evaluate these with compression technique, but don't spend too much time evaluating these relatively unimportant veins.

TIP: When imaging the veins in the arm, start at the mid humerous level and work proximally, then distally. It's then easier to differentiate the basilic vein from the brachial veins, as the basilic vein is <u>not</u> adjacent to the artery at mid arm level. See example below.

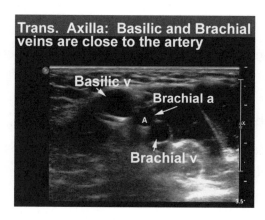

Trans. Axilla: Basilic and Brachial veins are close to the artery
Basilic v
Brachial a
A
Brachial v

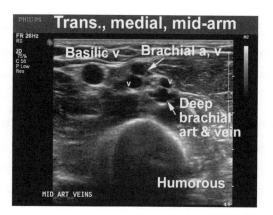

Trans., medial, mid-arm
Basilic v
Brachial a, v
v
v
Deep brachial art & vein
Humorous
MID ART VEINS

- On some patients the deep brachial veins and deep brachial artery may be visualized. The deep brachial artery will bifurcate from the main brachial artery.

- The <u>cephalic vein</u> is located superficially along the lateral aspect of the biceps muscle. It is often too small and superficial to image, unless it is thrombosed.

- If it's necessary to scan this vein (pre-op for hemodialysis access placement), sit the patient up to increase intraluminal pressure and to dilate the vein to make it easier to image.

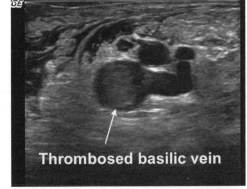

Thrombosed basilic vein

- When imaging the cephalic vein, use a "light touch" with the transducer to avoid inadvertent compression.

- Use compression methods along its course to the confluence of the axillary vein.

- Use a high frequency (7-12 MHz or higher) transducer to image this small vein.

- Identify the large tributary of the distal basilic vein in the antecubital fossa, the <u>median cubital vein,</u> and follow it to the cephalic vein.

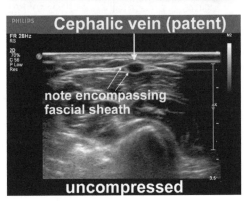

Cephalic vein (patent)

note encompassing fascial sheath

uncompressed

Forearm

- The veins of the forearm should be evaluated when the following indications exist, otherwise, skip them.

    √ Pre-op assessment for hemodialysis access placement, (scan the superficial veins only).

    √ Pre-op for vein harvest for arterial bypass (determine patency and size).

    √ Local, palpable cord; suspicion of superficial thrombophlebitis.

    √ Infusion difficulty with peripherally inserted central catheters (PICC lines).

- The basilic and cephalic veins are followed from more proximal segments and evaluated with compression techniques.

- The superficial veins may be too close to the transducer surface to image; if so, use a large "blob" of acoustic gel as a "transducer standoff".

Venous Thoracic Outlet Compression- Paget-Schroetter Syndrome.

- Repeated extrinsic compression of the subclavian and axillary vein can lead to thrombosis of these vessels. This phenomenon is called "effort thrombosis" or **Paget-Schroetter Syndrome.**

- Evaluate these veins as described above. If the veins are patent and the patient has symptoms of intermittent arm swelling during exercise, this could be a precursor to Paget-Schroetter syndrome.

- Re-evaluate the infraclavicular subclavian or axillary vein with the patient in the symptomatic position. Look for venous distention distal to the area of compression.

- Chronic thrombosis or extrinsic compression usually results in dilated, large superficial veins and extensive collaterals.

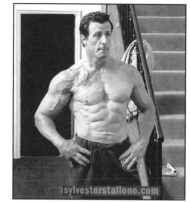

> Sylvester Stallone, on the right, with extensive superficial venous collaterals in the right arm, shoulder and neck, presumably from axillary/subclavian vein thrombosis.

- Use color and spectral Doppler to observe velocity increase from within the constricted vein segment at the site of compression. Return the limb to the asymptomatic position and reassess flow patterns distal to the point of compression.

Superior Vena Cava Syndrome

Venous inflow may be compromised with thrombosis or extrinsic compression in the superior vena cava (SVC) or right atrium. The symptoms include:

- Facial edema.

- Dilation of neck veins.

- Bilateral arm swelling.

Color duplex imaging may not directly identify the cause of obstruction, but can identify abnormal venous flow bilaterally. Evaluate the internal jugular veins, the subclavian veins, and the innominate veins (if possible), bilaterally, and carefully compare waveform morphologies.

Case study #1- "garden variety" upper extremity venous thrombosis

- 28 year-old female awoke with left arm pain and swelling.

- History of DVT in the right arm 2 years prior.

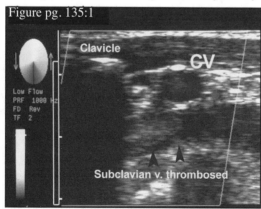

Thrombosed left distal subclavian, axillary, and cephalic veins.

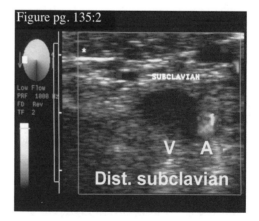

Transverse view of thrombosed distal subclavian vein.

See Color Plate #7: C-F, Plate #8: A-B.

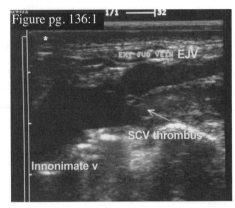

Tip of the proximal. subclavian vein thrombus, ending at the external jugular vein (EJV) confluence.

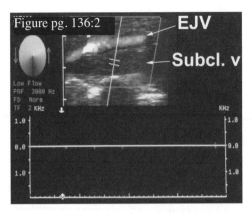

No flow in the proximal subclavian vein with color or spectral Doppler. Note color flow in the EJV.

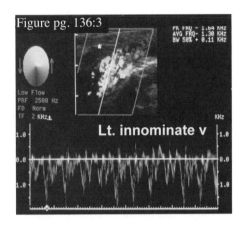

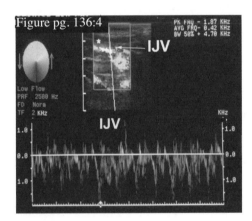

Normal, pulsatile flow with respiratory change in the left innominate and internal jugular veins (IJV). Flow direction is towards the heart and normal.

The left external jugular vein (EJV) has high flow to compensate for the thrombosed subclavian vein. This is a potential pitfall when evaluating the supraclavicular subclavian vein. i.e., misidentifying the EJV as a patent subclavian vein.

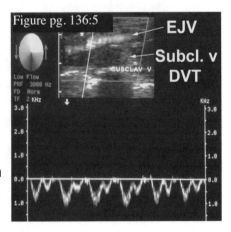

Findings:

⇒ Acute DVT of the entire subclavian vein and axillary vein to the confluence of the basilic and brachial veins. Also, the proximal cephalic vein was thrombosed.

⇒ Patient was hospitalized and treated with IV heparin.

Case study #2

- 52-year-old male presents with a recent history of left arm swelling.

- History of recent shoulder fracture.

- No known Hx of DVT.

> TECHNICAL NOTE: Flow direction with the old Hewlett Packard spectral Doppler system (now incorporated into some Philips systems) is established by aligning or pointing the Doppler cursor arrow in the direction that flow is supposed to be moving. Antegrade flow then is displayed above the baseline, and retrograde flow displayed below baseline.

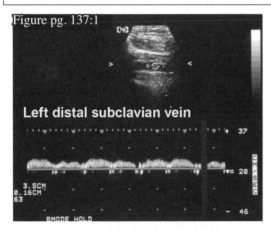

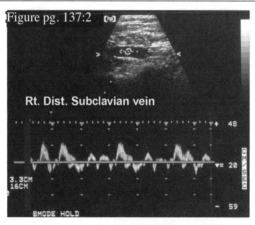

The left subclavian vein has pulsatile, antegrade flow, BUT, when compared to the right subclavian, it's not as pulsatile. Also, the right waveform demonstrated respiratory variation. Both sets of waveforms were obtained from the distal subclavian veins.

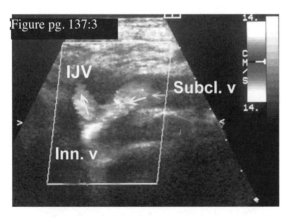

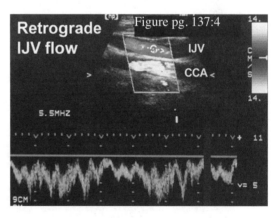

No flow was detected in the left innominate vein, but retrograde flow occurred in the IJV, i.e., the flow was going in the same direction as the CCA.

See Color Plate #8: C-E.

> TIP: To achieve better access to the subclavian and innominate veins under the clavicle, place a rolled-up towel under the shoulder to move the shoulder forward or upwards. This moves the clavicle away from the chest wall and creates an acoustic "window to the innominate vein.

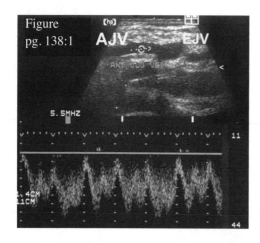

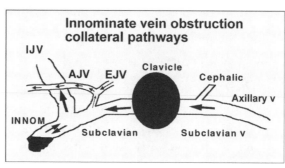

Diagram of collateral pathways in case study #2

The anterior jugular vein (AJV) usually drains into the EJV. This left AJV is dilated and has retrograde flow. This vein communicates with the contralateral AJV via the jugular arch vein; a common collateral pathway in the presence of innominate vein thrombosis.

Findings:

⇒   Obstruction of the left innominate vein, probably due to venous thrombosis.

⇒   Extensive collateral pathways with retrograde flow in the proximal IJV, inferior thyroid vein, external jugular vein and in the anterior jugular vein.

⇒   Due to well formed collateral pathways and good outflow in the left arm, the obstruction is most likely chronic.

This case illustrates the importance of a comparison to the contralateral subclavian vein flow. Also, careful attention to flow direction in the supraclavicular veins is essential in correctly diagnosing innominate vein obstruction.

Catheter-induced Thrombosis

Peripherally-inserted central catheters (PICC) lines can also be evaluated for thrombus formation. To optimize the image, orient the transducer perpendicular to the catheter.

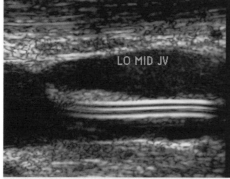

Multi-lumen PICC line in IJV with thrombus on catheter

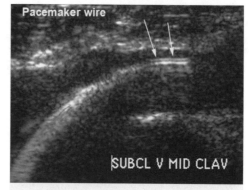

Pacemaker wire in subclavian vein

Images courtesy of Wayne Leonhardt, RDMS, RVT

UPPER EXTREMITY VENOUS INTERPRETATION

Normal

1. All veins central to the axillary vein, including the IJV, demonstrate cardiac pulsatility, superimposed respiratory phasicity, and central flow direction.

2. Color Doppler demonstrates complete intraluminal venous filling.

3. No intraluminal thrombus is seen.

4. Subclavian vein flows are symmetrical with the contralateral venous segment.

5. Veins below the axilla are easily compressed and coapted with transducer pressure, and demonstrate complete filling with color when augmented distally.

Abnormal

Collateral pathways develop very quickly in the upper extremity venous system. Knowledge of normal anatomy is essential in not mistaking a dilated collateral vessel for the "real McCoy".

1. In the proximal veins, absence of spontaneous flow and/or absence of cardiac pulsatility.

2. Absence of flow, or a filling defect in veins above the axilla.

3. Persistent <u>retrograde</u> flow in the internal or external jugular veins suggests obstruction in the innominate vein.

4. Retrograde flow in the anterior jugular vein and jugular arch suggests innominate obstruction.

5. Lack of coaptation of any vein below the axilla, confirmed by the absence of flow with color or spectral Doppler, indicates intraluminal thrombus.

6. The presence of echogenic material within the vein that moves in response to light transducer pressure may indicate a partially obstructive clot.

Accuracy and Limitations:

The reported accuracy of color duplex imaging in identifying venous thrombosis in the upper extremities depends on the location of the obstruction. If the thrombus resides in the subclavian-axillary segment, some studies have reported perfect correlation with venography.[2]

In study populations that include a higher incidence of SVC, innominate and proximal subclavian thrombosis, the reported accuracy is less. These studies, however, have shown respectable sensitivity (78 - 81%) and specificity (92 - 90%) for proximal thrombosis and obstruction.[3,4] The false negative findings in most cases were due to SVC obstruction, partially occlusive innominate-subclavian thrombosis, or short segment occlusion under the clavicle.

False positive results for venous thrombosis included extrinsic compression due to a mass, and intraluminal reflective artifact.

Technical Tip Summary:

- Arrange the screen anatomy so that the hand is to the right on the field of view, for both the right and the left arms. This makes it easier to discern flow direction. The exception is the right subclavian; if this segment is imaged with correct carotid orientation, screen anatomy may be reversed. Once you get to the clavicle, rotate the transducer or use image invert to standardize image orientation.

- The axillary vein is often extrinsically compressed along the chest wall. If it is not apparent adjacent to the artery, abduct the arm away from the body and re-evaluate.

- If possible, use a transducer with a small "footprint" for the proximal veins. A 5 MHz sector transducer or curved array may allow better access to the supraclavicular 'window'.

- If proximal access is limited, try to bring the patients shoulder forward (rolled-up towel placed under the shoulder) to bring the clavicle away from the chest wall. This often improves access to the proximal subclavian and IJV.

- For evaluating arm and forearm veins, position the patient so the arm is close to you and lay the abducted arm on a pillow placed in your lap.

- It's important to compare Doppler flow patterns in the contralateral subclavian vein in comparable anatomic locations. Asymmetry may indicate more proximal obstruction on the suspicious side.

- A common pitfall: In the presence of subclavian vein thrombosis, adjacent veins may become quite large. A tributary of the external jugular vein, the transverse scapula vein, courses superficial to the subclavian vein near the clavicle and can be mistaken for the subclavian vein. This vessel, however, courses over the clavicle, not beneath as the subclavian vein does.

REFERENCES

1. Horattas MC, Wright DJ, Fenton AH et al. Changing concepts of deep venous thrombosis of the upper extremity- report of a series and review of literature. Surgery 1988; 104:561-67

2. Froehlich JB, Zide RS, Persson AV. Diagnosis of upper extremity deep venous thrombosis using color Doppler Imaging system. J Vasc Technol 15(5): 251-53, 1991

3. Nack TL, Needleman L. Comparison of duplex ultrasound and contrast venography for the evaluation of upper extremity venous disease. J Vasc Technol16 (2): 69-73, 1992

4. Knudson,GL, et al. Color Doppler sonographic imaging in the assessment of upper extremity deep venous thrombosis. AJR:154:399-403, February 1990

CHAPTER 9: ARTERIAL HEMODYNAMICS, ANATOMY, AND PHYSIOLOGY

Blood flow is controlled by a number of physical principles that are common to the flow of electrical current, river flow (hydrodynamics) and gas flow.

FLUID DYNAMICS AND PHYSICAL PRINCIPLES

Energy Levels

In order for flow to occur there must be an energy gradient, or a state of high energy to low energy. Fluid energy gradient is reflected as a pressure gradient. In a closed circuit, blood, air or gas will flow from high pressure to low pressure.

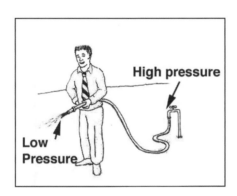

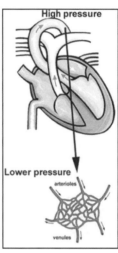

The highest pressure in the arterial system is in the left ventricle and thoracic aorta during systole. The intra-arterial pressure in the distal vascular bed is lower during left ventricular contraction, so blood flows towards the vascular beds.

The Doppler waveform below, from a popliteal artery, demonstrates a forward and reverse flow component. Explain how this reverse component can occur in terms of pressure gradients.

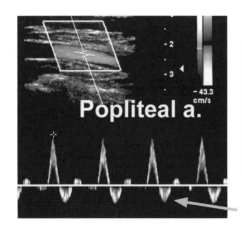

The intra-arterial pressure in systole is higher proximally (closer to the heart) than distal pressure. In diastole proximal arterial pressure decreases, but the distal arterial pressure is higher due to peripheral resistance in the distal vascular beds. The pressure gradient reverses, and blood flows back towards the heart momentarily.

Reverse flow towards heart.

Laminar Flow

Laminar flow is streamline or pathline flow that occurs when a fluid flows in parallel layers with no disruption between the layers, (picture a highway with cars traveling in discrete, parallel lanes).

Friction and Parabolic Flow

One factor that affects flow rate is friction. Friction is the property of a fluid or gas that resists flow. It exists between adjacent layers of fluid or a wall. In a blood vessel with steady flow, as well as in river flow, the resistance of movement of one fluid layer against another creates a parabolic flow pattern in which the center-stream layers move faster than layers closer to the wall or the shoreline. The flow layer in contact with the wall (or shoreline) may not be moving forward at all.

In the image below of a long, straight river, friction between water layers results in laminar flow and a parabolic flow curve: layers of flow tend to course parallel to one another (laminar), and layers in the middle of the river travel faster than outer layers.

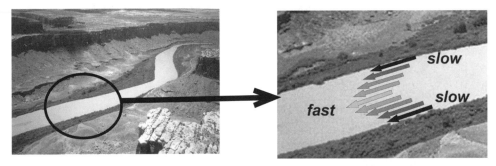

In the diagram below, the outside layers have greater surface area than the central layers. The result is a parabolic, conical shape to the flow profile.

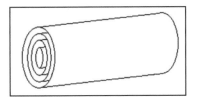 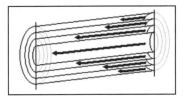 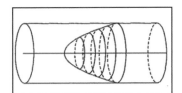

Friction is related to the diameter or radius of a vessel: the smaller the radius, the greater the friction. With a small diameter vessel, proportionally more fluid area is in contact with the walls thus increasing friction and decreasing flow.

> Remember:
> diameter (d) = radius (r) x 2
> area (A) = πr^2 $\pi = 3.14$
> circumference (C) = π d

Spectral Display of Plug Flow and Parabolic Flow

Flow is pulsatile in an artery and the parabolic flow curve changes during the cardiac cycle. "Plug flow" occurs during blood flow acceleration (in systole), and at the origin or entrance of a vessel. In plug flow, most of the blood cells are traveling at or near the same velocity. If we place a Doppler sample volume in a vessel with plug flow, the spectral "width" will be narrow, as almost all of the blood cells are being pushed at the same velocity. At end-systole and throughout diastole, blood flow returns to a parabolic flow pattern in which there is a larger variation in the speeds of the reflective red blood cells traveling through the sample gate. If we

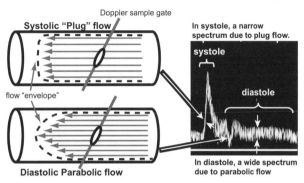

elongate the sample gate we'll sample more "lanes of traffic" in the vessel and the spectral display will be broadened. Conversely, a small sample gate will result in less spectral broadening.

Helical Flow and Flow Separation

In areas of bifurcations, and most notably, in the carotid artery bifurcation, a "disturbed" flow pattern, including helical flow may exist. Reverse flow occurs in the area of the bulb opposite the septum of the external carotid artery. In color Doppler, this appears as eddy flow. The boundary layer between the forward flow and the eddy flow is called flow separation.

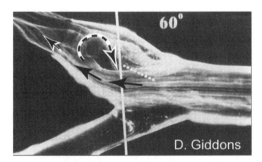

A glass model of a carotid bulb with smoke demonstration of the helical flow pattern

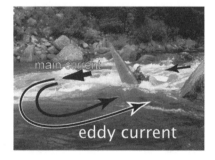

This kayaker is playing in the flow separation region of the river, The downstream current pushes the nose down, and the eddy current pushes the rear upward.

Viscosity

Viscosity describes a fluid's "thickness", and its internal resistance to flow. A river that contains suspended mud will be more viscous that a river flowing with clear water.

- Viscosity is affected by the temperature of the fluid. It is inversely proportional: the higher the temperature, the lower the viscosity.

- The higher the viscosity, the higher the resistance to flow.

- Water has low viscosity compared to blood.

- The viscosity of blood is directly related to hematocrit: the higher the hematocrit, the higher the viscosity.

- Viscosity is often represented by the greek letter "η" (ETA).

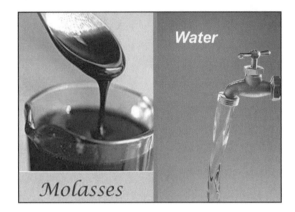

Molasses is more viscous than water, and is more resistant to flow.

Turbulence

As flow streams increase in velocity, a point is reached when laminar flow is disrupted. Flow becomes chaotic with small eddies and cross-currents.

The flow speed at which turbulence occurs depends on:
⇒   Density of the fluid.

⇒   Viscosity.

⇒   Diameter of the vessel.

The Reynold's Number (Re) is used to describe when turbulence is likely to occur.

$$Re = \frac{average\ flow\ \times\ density\ \times\ tube\ diameter}{viscosity}$$

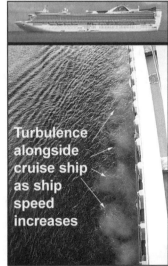

⇒   Turbulence occurs when the Reynold's number meets or exceeds approximately 2000.

⇒   In blood, density and viscosity are fairly constant, so velocity and vessel diameter are the most influential factors for turbulence.

⇒   An increase in flow speed increases the Reynold's number.

⇒   An increase in vessel radius increases the Reynold's number.

⇒   Turbulence also occurs distal to a stenosis in a vessel.

⇒   On spectral Doppler, turbulence is demonstrated as a broadening of the spectral waveform and a filling of the spectral envelope.

Inertia

The property that causes a fluid or object to resist a change in direction or speed.

Newton's first law of motion:

An object will not change its velocity spontaneously.

> **Inertia**: an object in motion tends to remain in motion, (so long as it is not acted upon by an external force).

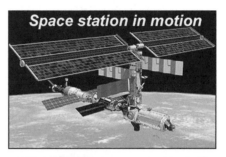

Space station in motion

> **Inertia**: an object at rest tends to remain at rest, (so long as it is not acted upon by an external force).

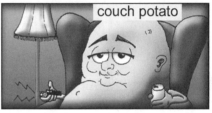

couch potato

Pressure, Flow, Resistance-Poiseuille's Law

The relationship between pressure, flow and resistance was neatly defined by Jean Leonard Poiseuille in the mid 1800's and has become known as Poiseuille's Law. This law of hemodynamics applies to flow in an incompressible vessel with uniform liquid viscosity through a cylindrical tube of constant diameter.

Poiseuille's law describes the relationship between flow, pressure gradient, viscosity, and length and radius of a tube.

Q = flow
ΔP = pressure gradient
π = pi (3.14)
r^4 = radius of vessel, 4th power
η = viscosity
L = length

Because vessel radius, length, and viscosity represent resistance (R), Poiseuille's law can be simplified as:

$$Q = \frac{P}{R} \qquad \text{Or} \quad Q \times R = P$$

⇒   Flow (Q) = pressure (P) divided by resistance (R). Another expression of the equation is:

⇒   Flow (Q) X resistance (R) = pressure (P).

Poiseuille's law comes into play in lower arterial hemodynamics during exercise. Vasodilation occurs in the arterioles (radius increases) during exercise and peripheral resistance (R) decreases. The muscle groups require more blood volume to sustain activity and flow (Q) increases. If the person exercising is normal (devoid of peripheral arterial disease), systolic pressure in the legs and ankles remains about the same during exercise as at rest.

$$Q \uparrow \text{(increases)} \times R \downarrow \text{(decreases)} = \text{distal } P \text{ (no change)}$$

An often-used analogy of this equation is Ohm's law of electrical resistance.

⇒   E (energy) = I (current) x R (resistance)

⇒   Q (flow) =   P (pressure) x R

Flow Volume Effect on Stenosis

A second aspect of Poiseuille's law concerns the hemodynamic effect of flow volume change over a region of stenosis. In a carotid artery, for example, the hemodynamic effect of a stenosis (60% diameter for example) remains fairly constant. A pressure gradient from prestenotic arterial pressure to post stenotic pressure may exist, and this probably doesn't vary unless the lesion becomes more severe. Although fluctuations occur in carotid flow volume through the day, these changes are minor.

For a similar stenosis in the lower extremities, things are quite different. Increased flow volume during exercise causes a dramatic increase in the pressure gradient over the stenosis. The diagram below illustrates a low flow and a high flow scenario over the same stenosis.

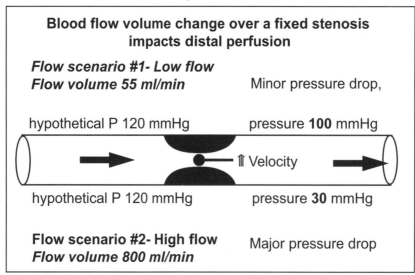

Blood flow volume change over a fixed stenosis impacts distal perfusion

Flow scenario #1- Low flow
Flow volume 55 ml/min   Minor pressure drop,

hypothetical P 120 mmHg   pressure 100 mmHg

⟰ Velocity

hypothetical P 120 mmHg   pressure 30 mmHg

Flow scenario #2- High flow   Major pressure drop
Flow volume 800 ml/min

In the words of Poiseuille: "For a fixed vessel stenosis with a constant resistance, the pressure gradient through the stenosis is thus proportional to the flow through the stenosis. Small pressure gradients across a stenosis become larger with increased flow volume."

Bernoulli's Law gets us off the ground!

The total energy at one location must equal all the total energy of another location.

⇒ Total energy = potential energy + kinetic energy.

⇒ Potential energy is stored or resting energy.

⇒ Kinetic energy is energy of motion and work.

One of the manifestations of the Bernoulli effect allows airplanes to fly. The pressure of a fluid, liquid or gas decreases as the speed of the fluid increases. Within the same fluid or gas, high speed flow is associated with low pressure.

Conversely, low-speed flow is associated with high pressure.

Airflow over a wing must travel farther and faster (due to wing profile) than the airflow under the wing. The faster airflow results in a lower pressure over the wing, and "lift" is produced.

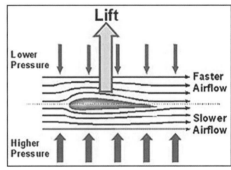

Bernoulli's law also explains the behavior of fluid (and gas) traveling through a narrowing or stenosis. As stated above, when flow increases in speed a pressure drop will occur.
A stenosis of approximately 75% area reduction, (or (50% diameter if the narrowing is circumferential) is known to cause a velocity increase. The Bernoulli effect is demonstrated in the figure below.

Flow velocity within the stenosis (V_2) increases compared to the velocity before the narrowing (V_1). The intra-arterial pressure decreases at the point of narrowing (P_2) compared to pressure before the stenosis (P_1).

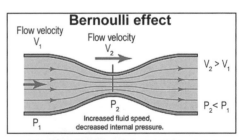

By measuring either the velocity or the increase in velocity we can estimate percent of arterial stenosis.

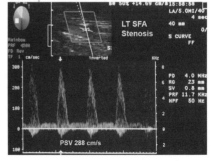

Hydrostatic Pressure

The weight of the column of blood affects distal arterial and venous pressure when sitting or standing. For each 12 inches (30.5 cm) of vertical distance below the heart, there is 22 mmHg of HP. For a person of 5' 10" in height (178 cm), the hydrostatic pressure at the ankle level is approximately 92 mmHg. This is in addition to the systolic blood pressure in the arterial system in the ankles. Ankle blood pressure determination should always be performed with the patient in a supine position to eliminate the effects of hydrostatic pressure.

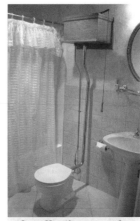

An effective use of hydostatic pressure!

ARTERIAL ANATOMY OF THE LOWER EXTREMITIES

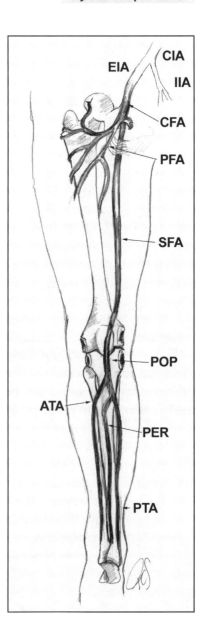

- Abdominal Aorta (AA)

- Common Iliac a. (CIA)

- Internal iliac a. (Hypogastric A) (IIA) - feeds pelvis, buttock area

- External iliac a. (EIA)

- Common femoral a. (CFA)

- Profunda femoris a. (deep femoral) (PFA)

- Superficial femoral a. (SFA) - conduit of blood to lower leg

- Popliteal a. (POP)

  ✳ Geniculate a.

  ✳ Gastrocnemius a.

- Tibial Arteries

  ✳ Anterior tibial a. (ATA) - continues as the Dorsalis pedis a. (DPA) on the dorsum of the foot

  ✳ Peroneal a.

  ✳ Posterior tibial a. (PTA)

- Microcirculation

  ✳ Arterioles

  ✳ Capillaries

Intima

- The intima, or inner most layer, consists of one layer of endothelial cells supported by an internal elastic lamina.

- Endothelium is a single cell layer that lines the inner surface of the artery and is in contact with the intraluminal moving blood. It provides the following functions:

    1. **Permeability** - it provides a barrier between blood and the artery wall that allows molecule and nutrient exchange between blood plasma and the wall.

    2. **Antithrombogenic** - it prevents platelets and monocytes (circulating white blood cells) from adhering to the artery wall.

    3. **Vasoreactivity** - endothelial cells release endothelin and prostacyclin which cause the artery wall (in the arterioles) to vasoconstrict and vasodilate, respectively.

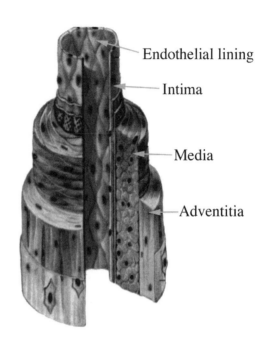

Media

- The middle layer of the arterial wall consists primarily of smooth muscle cells, and allows rhythmic changes in the arterial size that occurs during cardiac cycle.

- Collagen is also found in this area of the wall structure.

- The external elastic membrane lies between the media and the adventitia.

Adventitia

- The outer layer of the artery wall contains connective tissue and collagen, and the vasa vasorum; tiny blood vessels that supply the artery wall.

Capillaries

The smallest vessels in the circulatory tree are the capillaries. Small <u>arterioles</u> lead into the single-cell wall capillary beds, and <u>venules</u> carry blood back into the venous drainage system. The exchange of nutrients, gasses and metabolic waste occurs in the capillary beds.

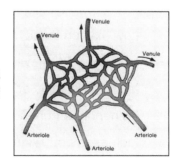

A HEMODYNAMIC PRIMER

Lower Extremity Normal Blood Flow

Cardiac output, intraluminal wall resistance, arterial wall compliance, and the dynamics of arteriolar vasoconstriction and vasodilation in the distal vascular beds control blood flow in the lower extremities. Arterioles are small arteries that lead into thin walled capillaries. Exchange of CO_2, O_2, and metabolic nutrients and waste takes place in these capillary beds.

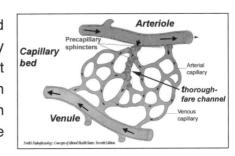

In the <u>basal or resting state</u>, the arterioles are vasoconstricted as the demand for blood volume is low. Due to pre-capillary sphincters, arteriovenous shunting occurs in channels that bypass the capillary beds. Only 20-25% of capillaries are open in the skeletal muscles at rest. The arteriolar vasoconstriction contributes immensely to the high resistance found in the arterial system below the renal arteries.

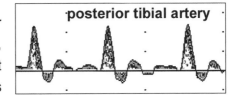

The effect of this resistance on blood flow is seen in the Doppler waveform. Blood flows forward towards the feet in systole, back towards the heart in early diastole, then towards the feet again prior to the next systolic contraction. The display of this normal flow pattern is known as the <u>triphasic</u> or multiphasic waveform.

Lower extremity resting (low demand) perfusion summary:

⇒ Vasoconstriction in distal arterioles.

⇒ Arteriovenous shunting in muscle capillary beds.

⇒ Not much blood flow to skeletal muscles.

⇒ Large blood volume exists in viscera and cerebral distributions.

⇒ High resistance in flow from aorta to arterioles.

<u>During exercise</u> muscles need increased levels of oxygen and metabolites. The circulatory system also needs to remove metabolic waste, carbon dioxide (CO) and lactic acid. Vasodilation occurs as a product of local, nervous and hormonal regulatory mechanisms. The "triggers" to vasodilation (relaxation of smooth muscle cells in the arteriole wall) include.

⇒ Low oxygen tension in tissue.

⇒ Increased CO_2 levels in tissue.

⇒ Increase in lactic acid.

⇒ Epinephrine from adrenal medulla.

⇒ Increased potassium ions.

⇒ Endothelium-mediated nitric oxide (NO) causes smooth muscle cells to relax.

<u>During heavy exercise</u>:

⇒   Heart rate and cardiac output increases.

⇒   Blood is shunted from the viscera to skeletal muscles.

⇒   Capillary A-V shunts close.

⇒   100% of capillaries open.

⇒   Dermal vasoconstriction.

In normal individuals a substantial increase in blood volume in peripheral arteries occurs during this exercise period and volumes may increase significantly over resting states. Arterial Doppler waveforms will exhibit low resistance waveforms.

Flow volumes were obtained from a popliteal artery at rest and compared to flow volumes after 3 minutes of treadmill exercise. Resting volume was 55 cc/min, (1cc/min = 1ml/min) and following exercise 914 cc/min, nearly a 20 fold increase in volume.

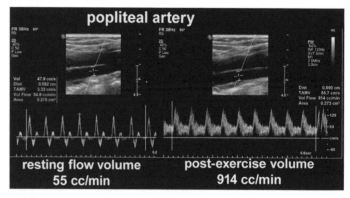

Peripheral resistance dramatically decreases during this time and blood flows in an antegrade direction throughout the cardiac cycle. Distal intraluminal pressure is maintained during vasodilation due to the increase in volume. Remember Poiseuille's Law:

$$Q \uparrow \text{(increases)} \times R \downarrow \text{(decreases)} = \text{distal } P \text{ (no change)}$$

Vasodilatation in the lower vascular beds occurs quickly with the onset of exercise. The images below were obtained from a popliteal artery with CW Doppler before and after just 5 toe raises.

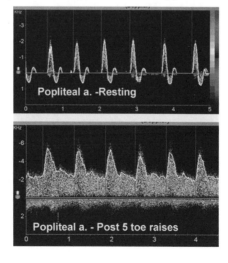

Arterial Occlusive Disease

In patients with arterial occlusive disease, adequate distal perfusion may exist at rest when there is low demand. During the high demand of exercise, vasodilation occurs in response to the same smooth muscle cell relaxation "triggers" as in normal individuals. However, the expected (and required) increase in blood volume to the skeletal muscles does not occur, or it is insufficient. Two scenarios contribute to inadequate volume:

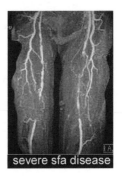

severe sfa disease

1. In the presence of occluded major arteries, the small-diameter collateral vessels cannot expand nor dilate and are limited in what volume they can carry.

2. In the presence of stenoses, Poiseuille's Law plays a part. Increase in blood flow volume over a stenosis causes a large pressure gradient across the narrowing. Small pressure gradients across a stenosis become larger with increased flow volume.

The required increase in flow volume doesn't occur. With vasodilated vessels, low resistance and decreased volume, an interstitial and intra-arterial pressure drop occurs. The skeletal muscles cannot obtain the necessary oxygen and metabolites to sustain exercise.

$$Q \text{ (no increase or decrease) } \times R \downarrow \text{(decreases)} = \text{ distal } P \downarrow \text{(decreases)}$$

If peripheral resistance decreases (due to vasodilation) and flow volume doesn't increase (or decreases), then distal pressure will drop. The figure on the right is a typical post-exercise ankle pressure graph demonstrating bilateral ankle pressure decrease after exercise, with slow recovery.

Patients may experience pain, fatigue, or cramping in the calf, thigh or buttock with exercise and this is known as <u>intermittent</u> claudication. Classically, the disability is progressive and is relieved by rest, or cessation of exercise.

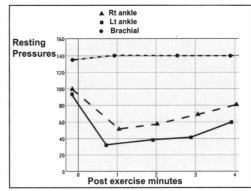

Vascular claudication usually takes place within the first few minutes of exercise and commonly limits the patient's walking distance to a city block or two, depending on the severity of disease and the extent of collateralization.

In the presence of mild to moderate arterial occlusive disease in large arteries, peripheral resistance may remain unchanged, but in more severe disease states the arterioles will <u>vasodilate at rest</u> and resistance will decrease. This can result in a Doppler waveform distal to the disease site in which flow is antegrade throughout the cardiac cycle and lacks the characteristic reversal in diastole. This arterial pattern can be seen proximal to lesions in many, but not all, patients with well-developed collateral pathways. The rise time is usually within normal limits.

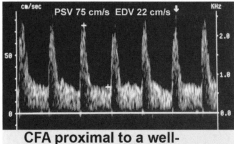

CFA proximal to a well-collateralized SFA occlusion.

If severe proximal disease is present, the Doppler waveform may be monophasic with a delayed rise time. As in the figure above, flow occurs throughout diastole due to distal arteriole vasodilation. An understanding of normal and abnormal Doppler waveform morphology helps us to locate the region of the occlusive disease.

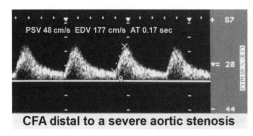

CFA distal to a severe aortic stenosis

Vasoreactivity also occurs in response to temperature, emotion (blushing), certain chemical reactions, and ischemia.

ATHEROSCLEROSIS

Risk Factors

* familial-generic component

* cholesteral >240 mg/dl

* hypertension

* diabetes mellitus

* severe obesity

* elevated triglycerides

* hypercholesterolemia

* LDL >160 mg/dl

* tobacco abuse

* depressed fibrinolytic system

* increased oxidation of LDLs

Arterial Symptoms of Peripheral Arterial Disease (PAD)

Mild arterial disease:

- Asymptomatic.

- May have decreased pedal pulses, or abdominal bruit.

- With exercise, mild decrease in ankle pressure.

- Athero disease may be seen with ultrasound, but it doesn't reduce blood flow.

Moderate disease: Claudication
- Asymptomatic at rest.

- With exercise, a significant decrease in ankle pressure.

- Intermittent claudication: pain, fatigue or cramping in the calf, thigh or buttock with exercise. Symptoms are relieved by rest. Claudication is brought about by a transient ischemic event in the muscles.

- This is the most common symptom of peripheral arterial disease.

Severe disease:
- "Night pain" in the feet or toes: ischemic pain brought about by the patient being supine; usually relieved by sitting up or standing (leg dependant).

- Ischemic rest pain in feet and toes (persistent).

- Non-healing wounds on feet/toes.

- Ulceration on lower leg or feet.

- Tissue necrosis, gangrene.

- Severe PAD requires surgical intervention to revascularize the limb. Alternatively, limb amputation is required.

Arterial Pathologies

⇒ Atherosclerosis.

⇒ Thrombosis (spontaneous thrombosis is uncommon, unless severe flow restrictive lesions are present).

⇒ Thromboemboli (often originating from aneurysms).

⇒ "Blue toe" syndrome: acute onset, painful cyanotic regions on toes or foot, caused by thromboemboli; also known as "trash foot".

⇒ Small vessel "fixed" occlusive disease: Buerger's disease (aka thromboangiitis obliterans)

⇒ Digit vasospastic disorder: Raynaud's syndrome.

⇒ Pulsatile masses: aneurysms, pseudoaneurysms.

⇒ Arteritis, giant cell arteritis: an inflammatory process of the arterial wall affecting medium and large arteries.

⇒ Entrapment syndromes: structures that extrinsically pinch or constrict arterial flow.

- Popliteal artery entrapment: claudication-like symptoms.

- Nutcracker syndrome: renal vein entrapment syndrome.

- Median arcuate syndrome: compression of the celiac axis.

- SMA syndrome: compression of the superior mesenteric artery.

- Thoracic outlet syndrome: compression of the subclavian or axillary artery.

Atherosclerotic Process

In the normal artery, platelets, red blood cells (RBC), leukocytes (white blood cells), low density lipoproteins (LDL), high density lipoproteins (HDL) (3:1 ratio) circulate freely in the blood. A monocyte is a type of leukocyte that ingests bacteria or invading organisms. A lymphocyte is another type of white blood cell. Lymphocytes have a number of roles in the immune system, including the production of antibodies and other substances that fight infection and diseases. The vasa vasorum are small arteries supplying blood flow to the arterial wall.

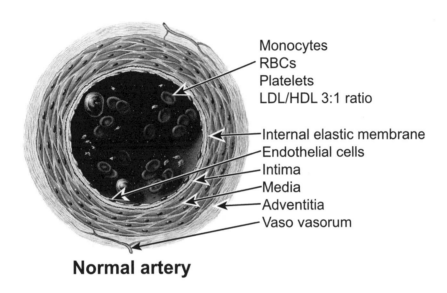

Monocytes
RBCs
Platelets
LDL/HDL 3:1 ratio

Internal elastic membrane
Endothelial cells
Intima
Media
Adventitia
Vaso vasorum

Normal artery

1.   Early Atherosclerosis: Injury

- Endothelial injury.

- Deposition of LDL into intima.

- Recruitment of lymphocytes, monocytes (types of white blood cells).

Early Atherosclerosis. Wall injury occurs due to increase in LDL, hypercholesterolemia and other risk factors. There is a change in the "slipperiness" of endothelial wall; monocytes and platelets become "sticky" and adhere to the endothelial surface. Endothelial cells transport excess blood lipids through to the sub-endothelial space, which then accumulate in the intima. Also, leukocytes migrate through the endothelial layer. This process is most likely to occur at branch points and bifurcations.

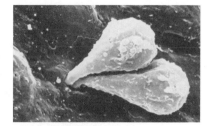

Electron microscope image of leucocyte migration from the blood stream through the endothelium and into the subendothelial space.

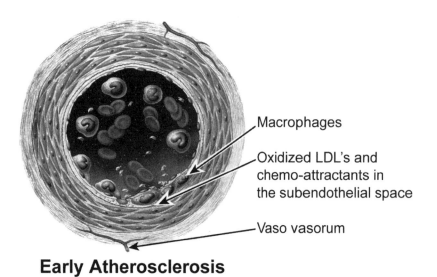

Macrophages

Oxidized LDL's and chemo-attractants in the subendothelial space

Vaso vasorum

Early Atherosclerosis

2.   Inflammatory response

- Monocytes in intima become macrophages.

- Macrophages ingest lipids, lipoproteins.

- Macrophages become foam cells.

- Fatty streak.

Lipids in the subintimal space can become oxidized forming free oxygen radicals. These are toxic byproducts that can attract monocytes from the blood. Macrophages take up lipids and lipoproteins then become foam cells. T-lymphocytes join macrophages, suggesting an immune response. Macrophages can synthesize growth factors, which cause smooth muscle cell growth and migration into the intima.

3.   Atheromatous Thickening: Plaque formation

- Migration/proliferation of smooth muscle cells from media.
- Neovasculature supplies plaque, feeds LDL and macrophages.
- Fibromuscular cap formation.

Smooth muscle cells (SMC) migrate and proliferate to "wall off" foam cells (lipid-laden macrophages). SMC produce fibrous (collagen) and non-fibrous connective tissue. A fibrous muscular cap (SMC and collagen) forms over the plaque. Although early plaque pushes into arterial wall and doesn't bulge into lumen, later development increases bulk and the plaque will protrude into artery lumen. Shear forces on the protruding plaque may further damage the endothelial lining.

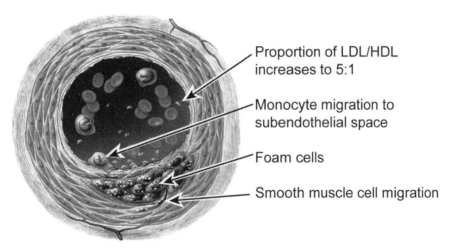

Proportion of LDL/HDL increases to 5:1

Monocyte migration to subendothelial space

Foam cells

Smooth muscle cell migration

Plaque formation

4.   Late changes: advanced atherosclerosis

- Cell necrosis.

- Scar tissue formation (fibrosis).

- Macrophage lysis.

- Intraplaque hemorrhage.

- Rupture of fibrous cap.

Necrosis occurs in the center of plaque and macrophages may lyse. Angiogenesis occurs as the vasa vasora extend into the plaque providing nutrients and removing cellular metabolic waste. Platelets can stimulate further smooth muscle cell proliferation. Vasa vasorum may rupture releasing blood into the necrotic core. The fibrous cap becomes thin as the plaque grows.

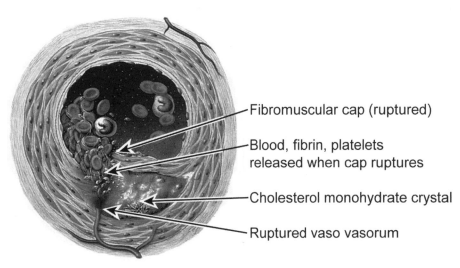

Fibromuscular cap (ruptured)

Blood, fibrin, platelets
released when cap ruptures

Cholesterol monohydrate crystal

Ruptured vaso vasorum

Advanced Atherosclerosis

Plaque in advanced stages may contain cholesterol crystals, scar tissue, necrotic material and calcium. Material within the necrotic core is very thrombogenic. Plaque rupture may occur, thrombi may break off and embolize. Lesions with necrotic core and fibrous cap are most likely to rupture.

Atherogenesis is a continuing, dynamic process. Some macrophages will migrate back out of the plaque and into the blood with material it has "ingested". These are transported to the liver, spleen, or lymph nodes.

CHAPTER 10: PHYSIOLOGIC ARTERIAL TESTING: LOWER EXTREMITIES

Indirect physiologic testing of the lower extremities is performed to detect hemodynamically significant arterial occlusive disease, i.e., disease severe enough to reduce arterial pressure and perfusion distally, whether at rest or during exercise. Stenoses which may cause focal velocity increase but which do not impact downstream perfusion are not readily detected with these methods.

THE GOALS OF LOWER EXTREMITY PHYSIOLOGIC TESTING

1. To determine if there is objective evidence for arterial disease.

2. To determine if the arterial disease is causing the patient's symptoms.

3. In patients with combined neuropathy and arterial obstruction, physiologic testing may be the only <u>objective</u> way to determine which condition is causing the patient's symptoms.[1]   In addition, segmental limb pressures are useful in predicting whether sufficient perfusion exists to heal ulceration and wounds.[2]

4. To assess increasing or decreasing limb perfusion during serial follow-up exams.

   • If intervention is not performed, the effect of conservative management (cessation of smoking, regular exercise, reduction in cholesterol levels, etc.) can be assessed in resting and post exercise states.

The advantages of indirect physiologic testing include:

⇒   It's simple to perform and requires only a short learning curve.

⇒   The testing time is short, ranging from 20 - 45 minutes for a complete bilateral exam.

⇒   It's accurate for hemodynamically significant disease.

⇒   It provides objective, quantitative physiologic information.

⇒   The instrumentation is relatively inexpensive compared to ultrasound systems.

Normal test results at rest and following exercise or post reactive hyperemia rule out hemodynamically significant arterial occlusive disease (> 60% diameter stenosis). These methods have high sensitivity and specificity for the presence of symptomatic atherosclerotic disease.

Limitations include the inability to identify the precise location of disease. Diagnoses tend to be generalized in regard to the region (aortoiliac, femoro-popliteal, popliteal-tibial) and to disease severity (mild, moderate, severe). Physiologic testing will not detect minor levels of diffuse atherosclerotic disease.

Indirect physiologic test methods include:

- Pulse Volume Recordings or Volume Pulse Recording (PVR or VPR).

- Doppler analog waveform analysis or Doppler spectral analysis.

- Segmental Limb Pressures (SLP) and calculated Ankle-Brachial Indices (ABI) and Toe Brachial Indices (TBI).

- Exercise stress test (or post-reactive hyperemia).

Diagnostic laboratories may perform all of the above tests, or may use a specific combination, e.g., SLP, PVR, and exercise stress test, or they may substitute Doppler waveforms for PVRs.

The traditional approach has been modified in some facilities to include only bilateral ankle and brachial pressure measurements, ankle to brachial indices, and Doppler or PVR waveforms obtained at the ankle level. This modified protocol will be described later in the chapter.

PATIENT HISTORY

Prior to any arterial testing, it is important to obtain a good patient history, including a complete description of the current symptoms.

Pertinent questions should include:

- Do you have leg pain when you walk, and if so, is it in both legs?

- Which leg is the worse?

- In what part of the leg is the pain (calf, thigh, buttock, or hip)?

- Is the pain progressive and does it stop you from walking?

- How many blocks can you walk before you cannot go on?

- Does the pain go away when you stop walking?

- Have you ever had a bypass graft or arterial operation, and if so, what type?

Risk factors should be noted:

- Is the patient a smoker, and if so, how many packs are smoked per day and for how many years?

- Does the patient have diabetes mellitus (DM) and does he/she take insulin?

- Has the patient ever had a stroke (CVA), transient ischemic attack (TIA), or myocardial infarction (MI)?

- Is there a family history of CVA, or MI?

- Does the patient have hypertension (HT)?

- Does the patient have hyperlipidemia (high cholesterol levels)?

Palpation of pulses- optional.

Although palpation of peripheral pulses has traditionally been part of the physical examination, it is subjective information. Limb pressure measurements are more objective and reliable that pulse palpation.

If limb pulses are obtained, they are rated in the following manner. Some institutions use a 5 gradation method, but 4 levels will be described here:

0   = no pulse.

1+ = weak pulse.

2+ = normal pulse.

3+ = very strong pulse or aneurysmal pulses (this is when you can observe your hand moving up and down with each pulsation).

Pulses may be obtained at the following sites:

- Groin - distal EIA or CFA.
- Popliteal fossa - Popliteal artery.
- Ankle - DPA & PTA.

> NOTE: Pedal pulses may not be palpated if ankle pressures are below 100 mmHg; Popliteal pulses in many normals are not palpated due to artery depth; CFA pulses are important in the diagnosis of inflow disease versus infrainguinal disease.

Physical Signs of Disease

Observe the physical signs of disease that may be present:

⇒ Pallor, pain, paresis, pulselessness.

⇒ Coldness.

⇒ Dependent rubor.

⇒   Cyanotic toes.

⇒   Ulceration.

⇒   Non-healing wound.

⇒   Blue toe syndrome- a symptom of embolization

In recent years the level of awareness of what symptoms indicate a venous examination versus an arterial exam has decreased. The federal agency governing Medicare, the CMS, has stated, "the provider of the service is ultimately responsible for the appropriateness of the examination". The technologist/sonographer must be aware of what constitutes appropriate indications for venous and arterial symptoms. If the indications do not match the ordered examination, the order should be confirmed with the ordering physician. In many states, reimbursement for an arterial and venous exam performed on the same patient for the same indication is not allowed.

Do not perform an arterial exam on someone suspected of having acute deep venous thrombosis. If an arterial exam is necessary, an ankle to brachial index exam should suffice.

SEGMENTAL SYSTOLIC LIMB PRESSURES

This technique compares limb blood pressures to systemic pressures obtained in the arms. Systolic pressure in each limb segment should be equal to or greater than arm pressure in normal patients. A significant pressure drop between contiguous segments signals the presence of occlusive disease in that region.

Procedure:
1. Patient Preparation

• All segmental and brachial pressures are measured with the patient supine and in a warm room. The patient should be supine for 5-10 minutes prior to obtaining pressures to insure a basal state.

• Introduce yourself, and explain the examination to the patient.

• Apply pressure cuffs to the arms and legs during this period.

Three–cuff versus Four–cuff method

• There are two methods for full segmental pressure testing: the three-cuff method and the four-cuff methods.

• These methods will be described below.

- The *three-cuff* method uses one large (17 cm air bladder) thigh cuff, plus calf and ankle cuffs.

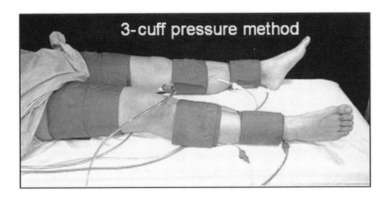

- The *four-cuff* method uses two smaller thigh cuffs (12 cm), as well as 2 cuffs below the knee. Most automated segmental systems employ the 4-cuff method. The four-cuff method is reported to be better at differentiating inflow disease from femoral artery disease.[4]

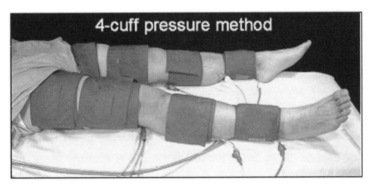

2. Pressure Cuff Application

Apply blood pressure cuffs to each of the following locations while the patient is in supine position (patients head may be slightly elevated for comfort). The cuffs should be appropriately sized (see below) and be applied very snugly, such that fingers should slide between cuff and limb with difficulty. All cuff sizes refer to the cuff air bladder width.

⇒ Upper arms (10 or 12 cm), bladders should be positioned over the brachial artery.

⇒ Upper thighs (12 cm).

⇒ Lower thighs, or above knee (12 cm).

⇒ Proximal calf (AKA, below knee, 10 or 12 cm).

⇒ Ankles (10 or 12 cm).

⇒ Optional: metatarsal (6–8 cm), great toe (2.0–2.5 cm).

Helpful hints on cuff application

- The AHA has recommended that the arterial cuff bladder size be 20% wider than limb diameter, or 40% of the limb circumference, for accurate pressure determination. In patients with large arms, use a 12 cm cuff; for pediatrics use a smaller 8 cm cuff.

- Do not let the patient lift their leg in an attempt to assist you when applying leg cuffs; as soon as they relax their muscles, the cuff becomes loose.

- In the legs, start the cuff wrap with the bladder on the posterior -medial aspect of the limb, bring the cuff one full wrap, then pull upward and across to tighten the wrap, trying not to get your hand caught in the folds of the cuff!

- Place the high (proximal) thigh cuff as proximal as possible.

- Cuffs may be placed over thin clothing, pajamas etc., it will not affect pressures or PVRs.

- Place the calf (below knee) cuff below the bony structures of the knee, otherwise, excessively high pressures may be recorded.

- Plastic wrap placed over a wound or ulcer will keep pressure cuff clean.

3. Obtain Bilateral Arm Pressures

- Place a continuous-wave (CW) Doppler over the radial (preferred method) or the brachial artery and locate the strongest signal by sweeping across the entire artery, then back to the center. Hold the Doppler probe close to the crystal end and support the transducer on the skin so that the Doppler beam does not drift off the vessel while taking the pressure (see examples on next page).

- Inflate the cuff manually, or with auto-inflation device, until the signal is obliterated, continue increasing pressure for an additional 15 or 20 mmHg. Slowly bleed the pressure down until the signal returns, and mark or note the return pressure from the pressure manometer or digital display. Now rapidly deflate the cuff pressure to zero. If possible, allow a few "beats" to be recorded after the return pulse to verify that it is not random noise, then deflate the cuff. Use system calipers to select the pressure as appropriate for your system design. This is the systolic pressure. (Diastolic pressure can only be obtained with a stethoscope). Repeat pressure if any ambiguity or inconsistency occurs.

- Obtain systolic pressure in each arm. Use the higher of the two arm pressures for subsequent leg comparisons and for calculating indices.

- ***Do not take a pressure in an arm with a shunt or dialysis access graft***.

- Alternative methods:

  ⇒ Photoplethysmography (PPG) on the index fingers.

  ⇒ Stethoscope held over the brachial artery (only use this if diastolic blood pressure measurement is needed).

⇒ Pressures may be obtained bilaterally if PPG sensors are used with automated systems. Attach the sensors to the index fingers bilaterally and adjust scale or gain to display good waveform amplitude. Inflate cuffs to obliterate PPG waveforms and bleed down until both PPG signals return. Care must be taken not to mistake random PPG noise for a returning pulse. Covering the PPG sensors with a dark cloth will help reduce room light interference.

4. Obtain Blood Pressures in the Legs

<u>Ankle Level</u>

- Use a CW Doppler held over the dorsalis pedis artery (DPA) and the posterior tibial artery (PTA) . Obtain pressures from both DPA and PTA. Pressures may also be obtained with PPG transducers located on the great toes.

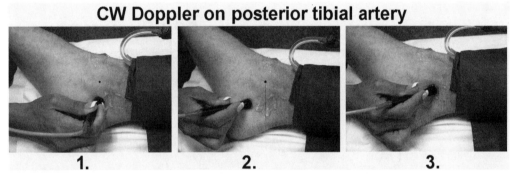

CW Doppler on posterior tibial artery

1.   2.   3.

Image **#1**: the Doppler probe is positioned over the artery at a 90° angle; this is not good.

Image **#2**: The Doppler probe is positioned to far distal to the medial malleolus (note dot on the ankle marking the center of the MM). This is the location of the smaller plantar arteries. Try to keep the probe forward of the line on the image.

Image **#3**: Probe is in a good position over the PTA with a good angle (45-60°) and pointed parallel to the long axis of the artery.

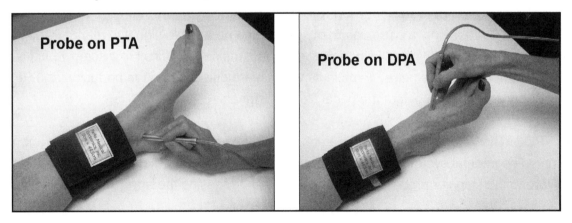

Probe on PTA

Probe on DPA

Note fingers and hand are resting on the foot to support the probe and prevent probe slipping.

- Pressures from both pedal arteries should be obtained in a subset of patients with tibial artery disease, suspected thromboembolus or those who have undergone femoral to tibial bypass procedures. Otherwise, a single vessel pressure from each ankle is sufficient (however, reimbursement guidelines may require both pressures). If pressures are obtained from both pedal vessels, use the higher pressure for ABI, and for post-exercise pressure comparison. Some labs routinely obtain a PTA and DPA pressure, this is OK, but it's time consuming.

- Cuffs should be inflated manually or with an autoinflator pump to approximately 20 mmHg above the occlusive pressure, and then bled down slowly until the distal Doppler signal or PPG tracing returns. Note the "opening" pressure on the manometer. This is the systolic pressure for that cuff segment.

- Pressures commonly need to be repeated to resolve ambiguity or inconsistency with other segment pressures.

Segmental pressures using PPG Sensors

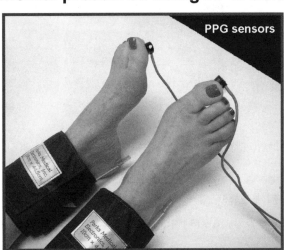

Doppler versus PPG pressure method for ABI and segmental pressures.

PPG CONS: There is only a visual return of a pulse and no audible signal to mark systole. The waveforms can be contaminated with "noise" or artifact making it difficult to discern which is the true returning pressure pulse. In patients with severe disease, the toe perfusion and PPG pulses disappear (flatline) before the pedal Doppler signals.

PPG PROS: The PPG method allows bilateral, simultaneous pressures to be obtained (on many automated segmental systems). Some of the pitfalls of the Doppler method are eliminated, i.e., allowing the Doppler probe to slip off the artery, and pressing the artery closed with probe pressure.

DOPPLER CONS: Beginners often have difficulty locating the PTA and/or DPA. They also allow the probe to slip off the pedal signal when the pressure is suprasystolic. If the probe is then moved back over the artery, the returning Doppler signal may be misinterpreted as the returning systolic blood flow. Novices can also inadvertently occlude the artery with probe pressure. Most systems do not have bilateral Doppler capability.

DOPPLER PROS: A Doppler signal can be seen **and** heard during pressure acquisition. A pedal Doppler signal can usually be detected even if the toe PPG pulse is undetectable. *In patients suspected of having arterial occlusive disease, **Doppler technique** is preferred over PPG as it is more sensitive than PPG in low flow and pressure situations.*

5. Calculate Ankle To Brachial Index (ABI)

- Divide each ankle pressure by the higher of the two brachial pressures to calculate an ankle-brachial index. This is also known as the Ankle to Arm Index (AAI). If pressures were obtained from both the DPA and PTA, report the higher of the two ABIs.

> NOTE: If the ABI is unequivocally normal bilaterally, there is no need to obtain additional segmental limb pressures (at calf and thigh levels).

6. Obtain Other Segmental Pressures

Calf Level

- Inflate the calf cuff (s) while monitoring blood flow at the ankle, as above, with PPG or Doppler, and obtain systolic pressures. The measured pressure at each cuff level is the pressure in the artery segment under the cuff.

Thigh Level

- Instruct the patient that this pressure measurement may be uncomfortable and caution him/her not to move their leg during the test.

- Quickly inflate the thigh cuff to suprasystolic levels and then bleed back down.

- Short Cut: If the ankle and calf pressures are normal (normal ABI), **skip the thigh pressure measurements**, as they'll be normal as well.

- Many patients cannot tolerate the discomfort and pain of thigh pressure, especially if they're hypertensive and the cuff must be inflated to very high level. If thigh pressures are necessary, they should be performed quickly and precisely. Get it right the first time!

- With both the single, large cuff (three-cuff technique) and the 12 cm cuff (four-cuff technique), the cuffs should be wrapped tightly, and positioned as high as possible on the thigh. (Don't let the patient lift his leg to help, as this will result in a loose cuff once the thigh muscles are relaxed). The low thigh cuff (4-cuff technique) should be positioned against the upper cuff, and should not extend over the knee. If two cuffs will not fit on the thigh, use one 12 cm cuff positioned high on the thigh.

- Inflate cuffs to at least 20 mmHg above systolic pressure, pause for a moment, then bleed pressure down and record systolic pressures as above. The high-thigh cuff (12 cm size) usually must be inflated to 40 mmHg above the arm pressure.

- The four-cuff method provides a high thigh and a low thigh measurement and is often useful in differentiating inflow disease from superficial femoral artery disease. Because the high thigh cuff is narrow compared to limb girth, **a pressure artifact** usually exists that elevates the pressure value 20 - 30 mmHg above systemic pressure.

> TIP: A common error in obtaining Doppler pressures occurs when the PTA or DPA is inadvertently compressed by excessive Doppler probe pressure. This can result in a falsely low pressure. This error is less likely to occur with the PTA and experienced technologists prefer this vessel for segmental pressure assessment.

7. Toe Pressures

- Toe pressures are useful in evaluating small vessel disease and in diabetic patients with calcified, incompressible large vessels. Toe pressures are difficult to obtain in patients with small vessel disease, as perfusion may be severely compromised. In most circumstances, however, toe pressures are an optional test when ankle pressures are normal.

- Pressures are obtained by placing a small (1.9 or 2.5 cm) digital cuff on the great toe and recording systolic pressure with a PPG transducer positioned distally on the toe.

- Inflate the cuff and bleed back down slowly until the PPG pulsatile trace returns. This is the toe systolic pressure.

- Pressures can be obtained with Doppler as well, but it's more difficult as the digit arterial signal is hard to locate. It's also difficult to obtain pressures on the 4 smaller toes, and they're probably inaccurate due to the size of the toe compared to the cuff size.

- A Toe/Brachial Index may be calculated by dividing each toe pressure by the higher brachial pressure. There is wide variation of TBI values in the literature, but a TBI of less than 0.60 is considered abnormal.[9]

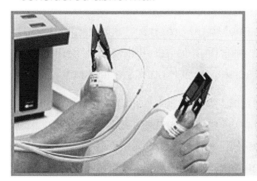
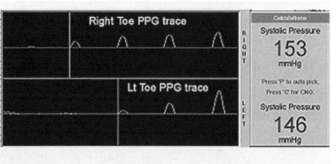

TBI > 0.75 = Normal   TBI < 0.60 = Abnormal

Segmental Limb Pressure Interpretation

Arm pressures:

A gradient of 20 mmHg or more between brachial pressures indicates subclavian stenosis/ occlusion on the side of the lower pressure. This finding should be confirmed with pulse volume recording, Doppler waveform analysis, or duplex imaging.

Resting Ankle Brachial index (ABI)*:

> 0.90 = normal

< 0.90 = abnormal, stress testing is appropriate

< 0.8 = probable claudication

< 0.5 = multi-level disease, or long segment occlusion

< 0.3 = ischemic rest pain - severe disease

> NOTE: If brachial systolic pressure is below 100 mmHg or above 200 mmHg, ankle pressures may be 25% lower than brachial pressure in an otherwise normal patient.[3]

* Values are a general correlation and vary with individuals.

If ABIs are unequivocally normal, there is no need to continue with full segmental pressures. If ABIs are abnormal, then consider segmental pressure decreases to determine the region of disease. Alternatively, some laboratories rely on segmental waveforms, instead of segmental pressures, to determine the level of disease.

If ABIs are abnormal, but Doppler or PVRs appear normal, recheck brachial pressure as it may have decreased prior to obtaining ankle pressures.

Segmental Three-Cuff Technique:
Normal:

⇒   All segmental pressures, including the thigh pressure, should be equal to or slightly greater than the brachial pressure.

Abnormal:

⇒   A 30 mmHg or greater drop in pressure generally is considered positive for hemodynamically significant stenosis (> 60% diameter) in the segment (s) leading into the cuff or under the cuff (as long as the more proximal cuff pressure is not artifactually elevated, and the ABI is abnormal).

⇒   A normal thigh pressure usually rules out significant aortoiliac disease. An abnormal thigh pressure can be due to aortoiliac disease, or femoral artery disease.

<u>Segmental Four-Cuff Technique</u>:
Normal:

⇒   A high-thigh pressure should be at least 20 mmHg above brachial pressure due to the "high-thigh cuff artifact" effect.

⇒   However, variations in the girth of the thigh relative to the fixed cuff size often eliminate the cuff artifact. If the thigh is relatively small, the thigh pressure may be equal to or near brachial pressure in a otherwise normal individual.

Abnormal:

⇒   A thigh pressure that is less than the arm pressure is abnormal and suggests inflow disease.

⇒   A pressure gradient of 30 mmHg or more between the high thigh and low thigh is suggestive of superficial femoral disease.

⇒   Studies have shown that a normal high-thigh pressure rules out significant aortoiliac (A-I) disease, and an abnormal high-thigh pressure will predict significant aortoiliac disease.[4]

⇒   *Other studies, however, have shown that a low high-thigh value can be due to superficial femoral artery disease and not necessarily A-I obstruction. The negative predictive value is high, but the positive predictive valve for A-I disease is low. [5, 6]*

⇒   The low thigh, calf, and ankle pressures are interpreted as in the 3-cuff technique.

> **NOTE: Segmental pressure gradients, in the presence of a NORMAL ABI, should not be interpreted as evidence for occlusive disease. If the ABI is normal, segmental pressure differences are "moot" for that limb.**

As with all indirect methods, SLPs cannot distinguish stenosis from total occlusion and are not specific in determining the exact location of disease.

Other Criteria:
Ankle pressures can quantify the severity of ischemia. A pressure of 50 mmHg or less is often associated with ischemic rest pain. In non-diabetics, foot lesions are unlikely to heal if ankle pressure is less than 50 mmHg.[2]

The "Bane" of Pressure Measurements: Calcified Arteries
Calcific medial sclerosis is a significant limitation for segmental arterial pressure assessment in the legs. Cuff pressure cannot obliterate the distal arterial pulse so that pressure recordings are unobtainable, or are erroneously high. This condition can occur in patients with diabetes, end-stage renal disease and those on long-term corticosteroid therapy.

You can rely on a low pressure recording, but not a high one. In the presence of calcific medial sclerosis and incompressible vessels, limb perfusion must be assessed with other methods, e.g., PVR, Doppler waveform analysis, or toe pressures.

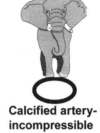

Calcified artery-incompressible

In general, the ankle cuff should be inflated to a pressure 30-40 mmHg above brachial pressure and "bled down". In hypertensive patients, the increased inflation pressure required to stop flow should not be misinterpreted as calcified vessels.

Other clues to calcified arteries include:

- An ABI exceeding 1.35.[8]

- High closing pressure (cessation of Doppler signal during inflation) with low opening pressure.

As with all indirect methods, SLPs cannot distinguish stenosis from total occlusion and are not specific in determining the exact location of disease.

PULSE VOLUME RECORDING (PVR), VOLUME PULSE RECORDING (VPR)

Segmental air plethysmography (pleth is mog grau phie), or Pulse Volume Recording, is used to measure the change in limb volume related to each cardiac cycle. Pulse Volume Recording is referred to as PVR. Parks Medical Electronics uses the term Volume Pulse Recording, or VPR. (The abbreviations PVR and VPR will be used interchangeably in this section). As blood is forced into the leg in systole, the girth of the limb increases and air in the segmental pressure cuff is temporarily displaced. This pulsating change in cuff air volume is recorded on the plethysmograph, a pressure transducer that's connected to a strip chart recorder, or recorded digitally. Modern systems can store PVR data for printout at the completion of the exam.

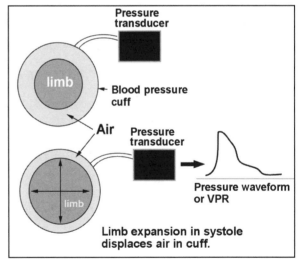

Procedure

- With the patient in a supine position with the heal of the foot placed upon a pillow or pad, apply appropriately sized blood pressure cuffs snugly to the thigh, calf, ankle, and if indicated, the metatarsal, and the great toes, bilaterally. These can be the same cuffs used for segmental pressure measurements.

- Cuffs are sequentially connected to the plethysmograph and inflated to a specific air pressure (60 ± 5 mmHg).

- Instruct the patient to be still and not to talk during the test to minimize motion artifact in the tracing.

- PVR waveforms are then recorded for each limb segment.

- Set the PVR gain or scale to optimize the waveform amplitude. The metatarsal and great toe PVRs usually require a higher gain setting as the tissue volume contained within these cuffs is obviously less than other cuff segments.

> TIP: Many elderly patients have a slight tremor in their limbs and this adversely affects the PVR at the calf, ankle, and metatarsal sites. If motion artifact is present in the waveform, have the patient perform a few plantarflexions, followed by a few moments of relaxation, then re-record the PVRs.

Interpretation

⇒ Pulse waveform analysis is a qualitative assessment of pulse contour and amplitude.

⇒ Pulse volume waveforms reflect the volume of blood coming into that cuff segment; so an abnormal PVR at the thigh would indicate aortoiliac disease, or more rarely, profunda femoris stenosis. Volume changes in the thigh cuff are predominately affected by perfusion in the deep femoral system.

⇒ If the thigh PVR is normal but the calf is abnormal, the occlusive disease will be in the superficial femoral and/or popliteal segments.

⇒ Proximal disease will affect the contour of all PVRs distally.

⇒ Calf PVR amplitude may be higher than the thigh and ankle. This is due to variations in limb girth and cuff size and air volume within the cuff.

⇒ Normal thigh and calf PVR with abnormal ankle recording suggests tibial disease.

⇒ This technique provides a subjective assessment of overall limb perfusion. PVRs are not affected by calcified artery walls and are easier to perform than CW Doppler waveform analysis.

A normal PVR waveform has a sharp upslope and a prominent reflected wave, also called the dicrotic notch, in late systole and early diastole.

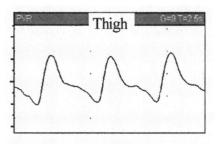

Mild disease will cause the waveform to broaden and the reflected wave will not be present. There is also a slight loss of amplitude.

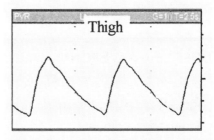

A moderately abnormal PVR has a rounded peak, no reflected wave and a pronounced decrease in amplitude.

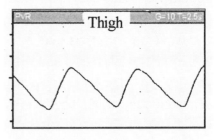

A severely abnormal PVR is of low amplitude, or even "flatline".

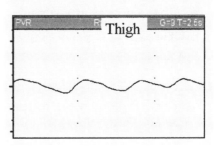

In the presence of severe proximal inflow disease, PVR accuracy in predicting <u>distal</u> disease is reduced. This method does, however, require good patient cooperation: limb motion or tremor adversely affect waveform contour. Waveform assessment is subjective and not quantitative, but does provide information of "global" limb perfusion, including the effect of collateralization. This procedure is easy to perform and has a short learning curve.

PVR Amplitude

Although attempts have been made to quantitate PVR amplitude, a number of variables influence the reproducibility of this effort. The tightness of the cuff wrap, the volume of air in the cuff, differences in limb circumference and changes in cardiac output all detract from precise quantitation. Originally, amplitude was measured in millimeters of strip chart grid. This method required a fixed gain or scale. If the gain was changed the PVR waveform height would be altered, but the grid scale remained unchanged! PVR amplitude measurement using mmHg of pressure change is preferred to the grid method, as it is independent of the display scale. The volume measurement method, in which air displacement within the cuff is measured in cubic centimeters, is available on many systems, but the accuracy and reproducibility are questionable.

DOPPLER WAVEFORM ANALYSIS

Continuous-wave (CW), bi-directional Doppler waveforms are obtained and recorded segmentally along the major arteries in each leg. Waveforms are subjectively assessed and compared to adjacent and contralateral sites for abnormality that would indicate the presence of hemodynamically significant disease.

CW waveform analysis may be performed using either a zero-crossing detector analog Doppler, or a more sophisticated spectrum analyzer. The former provides a single line trace of average velocity, while the latter offers full spectral capability and is less prone to "averaging" by simultaneous venous flow in the beam path.

Procedure

- With the patient in a supine position and in a basal state at rest, a CW Doppler probe is positioned at a 45-60 degree angle over the common femoral artery (CFA) just below the inguinal ligament, and pointed cephalad.

- Eliminate any intruding venous signals by relocating the probe, or have the patient hold their breath. Try to achieve the strongest arterial signal possible by scanning across the artery and finding the center.

- Doppler waveforms are recorded digitally, or the old-fashion way, on the strip chart recorder. Use appropriate gain, and maximize waveform height with scale controls optimize waveform amplitude.

In addition to the CFA site, obtain sample waveforms at the following locations:

- Proximal and distal superficial femoral artery

- Popliteal artery

- Posterior tibial

- Dorsalis Pedis artery

For the pedal vessels use a high frequency transducer, 8 or 10 MHz.

Repeat the procedure on the contralateral limb.

Interpretation:

Waveform morphology is assessed for three characteristics:
(1) pulsatility, (2) systolic forward flow, (3) early diastolic reverse flow

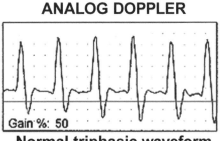

ANALOG DOPPLER

Gain %: 50

Normal triphasic waveform

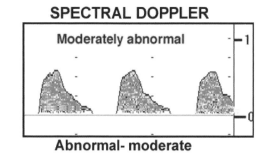

SPECTRAL DOPPLER

8MHz   Rt. Sup. Femoral   3.5s
Triphasic

Normal triphasic waveform

A normal waveform should be triphasic with a sharp systolic upslope, an immediate drop of waveform below baseline, then a small blip of amplitude before the next systolic rise.

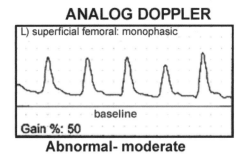

ANALOG DOPPLER

L) superficial femoral: monophasic

baseline
Gain %: 50

Abnormal- moderate

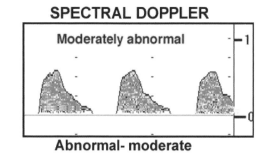

SPECTRAL DOPPLER

Moderately abnormal

Abnormal- moderate

Moderately abnormal waveform exhibits a loss of triphasic morphology, reduced amplitude and a "rounding" of the peak.

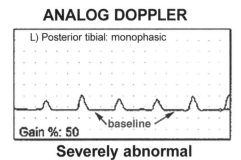

ANALOG DOPPLER

L) Posterior tibial: monophasic

baseline
Gain %: 50

Severely abnormal

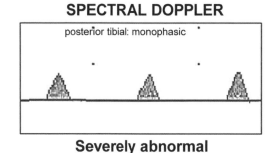

SPECTRAL DOPPLER

posterior tibial: monophasic

Severely abnormal

A severely abnormal waveform demonstrates no triphasic pattern, loss of amplitude and delayed upstroke to peak.

- This technique requires skill and experience.
- The recorded waveform must be free of artifact.
- The Doppler signal may be attenuated by obesity, scar tissue, hematoma, or calcified plaque within the artery.

- Waveform analysis is not quantitative for assessing the severity of disease.

- Abnormality between segments suggests the presence of disease in that region.

- If a venous signal is present along with the arterial signal, the waveform will be an average of venous and arterial signals and will not be representative of arterial flow. The venous signal must be eliminated; reposition the probe, or have patient hold their breath to acquire a "clean" waveform.

DOPPLER WAVEFORM DEFINITION PROBLEMS

Three spectral waveforms (below) obtained from lower extremity arteries illustrate the nomenclature problem. Some clinicians would use the term "biphasic" to describe A + B above, and use monophasic for waveform "C". But A + B represent two very different flow patterns. Others would call B + C monophasic; again, this single descriptor is not adequate to describe these two different flow patterns.

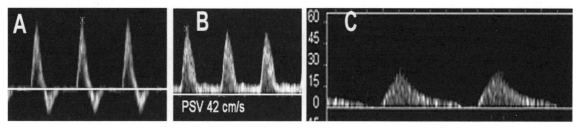

NOTE: The term "biphasic" originally was used to describe the sound of a Doppler signal that lacked 3 component sounds (triphasic). Because there is considerable confusion regarding what constitutes a "biphasic" waveform, the term should be abandoned and not used to describe Doppler waveform morphology; use multi-phasic, atypical, and monophasic.

EXERCISE STRESS TESTING

- This test is important for differentiating true vascular claudication from pseudo-claudication, i.e., true ischemic muscle pain with exercise, from the pain caused by neurospinal compression, osteoarthritis, or some other non-vascular cause.

- The exercise stress test is performed on all patients that complain of pain when walking, with the exception of those that have contraindications.

- Resting blood flow over a stenotic lesion may be sufficient to maintain normal or near normal distal pressure. When flow is augmented over the stenosis, as in exercise or reactive hyperemia, distal pressure may drop revealing the presence of disease. It is appropriate to exercise those with claudication symptoms despite a normal resting exam.

- If the patient's symptoms occur at rest (non-claudication symptoms) and the resting examination is negative, there is no need to exercise the patient.

Contraindications for treadmill exercise

- Questionable cardiac status, known cardio-vascular disease.
- Severe pulmonary disease.
- Inability to ambulate at treadmill speed.
- Ischemic rest pain.
- Ischemic limb ulceration.

> NOTE: This test does not equate to the rigors of a cardiac stress test and the risk of cardiac complications is small. It is appropriate, however, that a written protocol be established and followed in regards to exercise contraindications, methods, and response to cardiac emergency. EKG monitoring should be used if available.

Procedure

- Following resting segmental pressures, or ABIs, the patient is screened for contraindications. If patient has no contraindications and is a candidate, proceed.

- Explain the test to patient, ask that they walk for 5 minutes or until the pain stops them from walking. Request that they tell you of the onset, location and severity of pain, if any. Remind them to report any chest pain, shortness of breath, or severe fatigue.

- Set treadmill speed to 1.5 or 2.0 mph at a 10% grade, depending on the patient's age and mobility.

- Standard walking time is for 5 minutes or until pain or other factors (angina, SOB, fatigue, etc.) prevent further walking. The patient must be carefully observed for distress during exercise and the technologist must not leave the room.

- Claudication symptoms are noted, as well as the location, severity, and the total walking time.

- Immediately following exercise, return the patient to the exam bed and quickly obtain bilateral ankle pressures from either the PTA or DPA. Use the pedal artery that had the higher resting pressure. There is no need to obtain pressures from both arteries on one foot. Obtain the brachial systolic pressure from the arm with the higher resting pressure.

- PVR or Doppler waveforms may also be recorded at the ankles following pressures to confirm pressure values, e.g., if you get a low pressure but the PVR is normal, retake the pressure. Post-exercise PVRs or Doppler waveforms may be useful in patients in whom pressures cannot be obtained due to calcified vessels. Pre and Post PVRs can be subjectively assessed for disease severity.

- Calculate post exercise ABIs.

- Some laboratories record ankle pressures (or ABIs) at one or two-minute intervals for ten minutes following exercise, or until ankle pressures return to baseline levels. A prolonged recovery time may suggest multilevel disease, or poor collateralization.   In the example below, both ankles demonstrate significant post-exercise pressure decrease with slow recovery time.

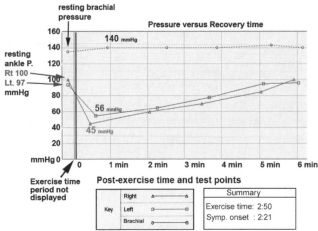

Example of post exercise graph

If the post-exercise pressures are normal and no pressure drop has occurred at the ankles, there is no need to continue serial pressure measurements.

It's the opinion of this author that serial pressure acquisition following exercise is a waste of time. A single post exercise ABI is sufficient to determine the severity of disease. Color duplex imaging is a better methods to determine the extend of disease and whether there are multiple segments involved.   *However,* changes in CPT guidelines for 2011 indicate that ABIs should be obtained at "timed intervals" following treadmill exercise.

Interpretation

- Some normal patients may experience a very mild, transient drop in ankle pressure following exercise, while others will maintain a normal ankle/brachial index.

- Those with arterial occlusive disease will experience a pressure drop of varying degree, depending on the severity of disease and the amount of collateral blood flow.

- A substantial decrease in ABI signals the presence of disease.

- An immediate post exercise ankle pressure of 60 mmHg or less confirms a vascular cause for claudication. A vascular etiology for pain is unlikely if immediate post-exercise ankle pressures are well above 60 mmHg. Vascular claudication pain is a transient "ischemic" pain.

- Post exercise pressures must be obtained as soon as possible following cessation of exercise. Ankle pressures will rise following exercise and a delay may result in erroneously high measurements.

POST OCCLUSIVE REACTIVE HYPEREMIA

This test may be substituted for treadmill stress test in patients that are unable to ambulate due to questionable cardiac status or other reasons. It mimics the physiologic response to exercise by causing vasodilatation in the vascular beds of the skin and muscle, which are temporarily deprived of blood flow. When the occlusive thigh "tourniquet pressure" is removed, blood flow volume into the leg increases. If significant stenosis or occlusion is present, the distal pressures will drop.

Procedure

- Obtain a resting ABI as described above.

- Apply a blood pressure cuff to the thigh of the limb being evaluated and inflate to 20 mmHg above thigh pressure.

- Maintain this pressure for 3-5 minutes then release the thigh pressure and obtain an ankle pressure in a fashion similar to post exercise stress testing.

Interpretation

- Normal patients will experience little, if any, drop in ankle pressure.

- An ankle pressure decrease of 20 mmHg suggests the presence of arterial occlusive disease.

- This test can help identify arterial disease that may not be obvious with resting ABIs, particularly in cases of borderline normalcy.

Limitations

- This procedure is not well tolerated in many patients because of the severe pain caused by the occlusive thigh pressure. You should try this on your thigh, as it can be VERY painful.

- Although the test is appropriate for uncovering "hidden" occlusive disease, it is not good for differentiating true vascular claudication from pseudo-claudication. The thigh cuff must be inflated quickly to reduce discomfort.

- Some labs place the tourniquet on the calf instead of the thigh to reduce discomfort. This is appropriate as long as the disease is below the CFA and restricted to the fem-pop-tibial segment.

- **Exercise in the form of Toe Raises is more "patient-friendly" than reactive hyperemia.**

TOE RAISES

Toes raises (active plantar flexions, also called "heel raises") have been advocated as a useful alternative to PORH as a form of stress exercise.[7] Baseline ankle and arm pressures are obtained with the patient supine.

Procedure

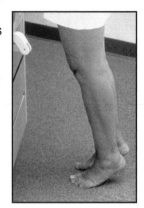

- The patient stands and extends both feet fully, then relaxes and returns the feet flat to the floor at one second intervals.

- The "toe raises" are repeated up to 50 times, or until the patient cannot continue.

- The onset of pain and the number of toe raises are recorded. Immediately after exercise, ankle/arm pressures are obtained.

- Compared to the resting values, a pressure drop of > 20 mmHg or a decrease in ABI of 20% constitutes an abnormal exam.[7]

Although this exercise test eliminates the need for a cumbersome treadmill and may have lower risk of cardiac complications, it does not reproduce the patient's symptoms of ischemic claudication, nor does it invoke the same muscle groups used when walking. Although the patient may have mild vascular disease and demonstrate a slight drop in pressure after toe raises, the calf pain may be solely due to fatigue. It is important to correlate claudication symptoms with a significant pressure drop to confirm a vascular etiology for the pain. The patient most likely did not present with symptoms of leg pain occurring during toe raises! This test is a good substitute for reactive hyperemia, but is a poor substitute for treadmill exercise in patients with intermittent claudication.

PHYSIOLOGIC CASE STUDIES

Several case studies are presented below for interpretation practice. The graphics in each exam have been enhanced to provide better "readability", increased font size, etc. Exam content has not been altered. Whenever possible, pertinent clinical information has been provided, as well as correlative information.

Try to make your own diagnosis prior to reading the explanation in "discussion" following each case study. There is a tendency to "over-read" physiologic studies, so remember the objectives:

1) Is the objective evidence for arterial occlusive disease?
2) Is the disease, if present, causing the patient's symptoms?
3) How severe is the disease ?
4) What is the region of disease: aortoiliac, femoral -popliteal, or popliteal-tibial?

INTERPRETATION TIPS:

Step #1: Look at the ABIs first.

Step #2: Confirm that ankle waveforms correlate with ankle pressures. If the ankle pressures are normal, the ankle waveforms should also be normal. If pressures are low, waveforms should be abnormal.

Step #3: Determine the disease location (inflow versus infrainguinal), by assessing thigh PVRs (or CFA waveforms), and thigh pressures.

Step #4: Determine multi-level versus single level disease.

Step #5: Determine severity and if disease is related to the patient's condition.

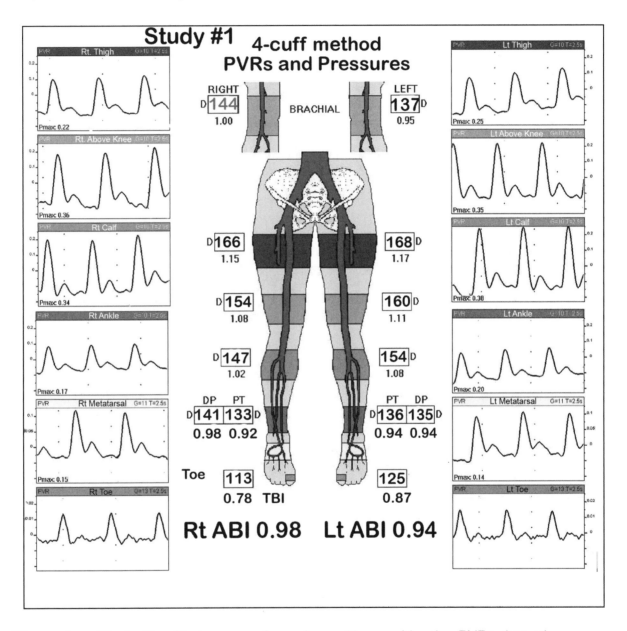

Discussion: Study #1a. Study was performed on a 48 year old male. PVRs showed pronounced reflective waves (dicrotic notchs), probably due to good arterial wall elasticity. (The reflective waves are reduced in elderly patients, or in those with poor compliance). ABIs were normal.

Normal Doppler Exam from the same patient

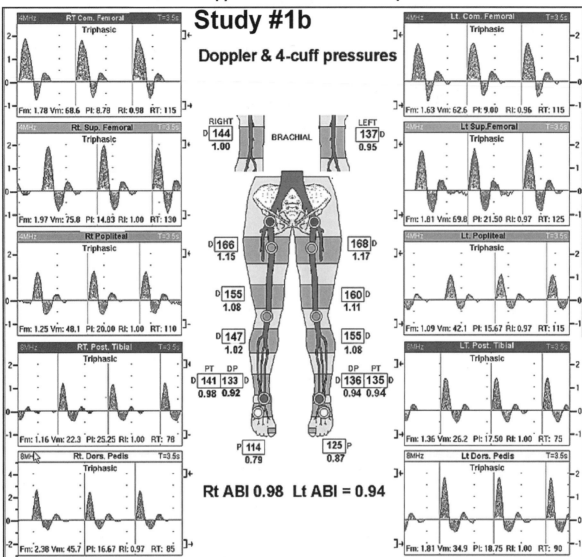

Study #1b

Doppler & 4-cuff pressures

Rt ABI 0.98 Lt ABI = 0.94

Discussion: Study # 1b. Doppler waveforms (spectral) are multi-phasic at all sites. ABIs are normal bilaterally.

NORMAL EXAM

Patient: J. Doe

- 53-year-old male presented with progressive history of left buttock, thigh and calf claudication which limited walking to 2 blocks.
- Hx of smoking 1-2 ppd, recently quit.
- Hx of HT and angina. HX of coronary angioplasty.

Study #2a

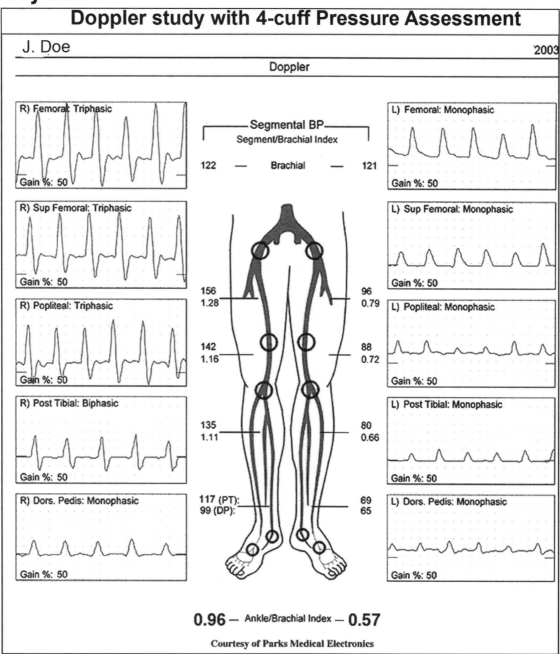

Doppler study with 4-cuff Pressure Assessment

J. Doe   2003

Doppler

R) Femoral: Triphasic
Gain %: 50

R) Sup Femoral: Triphasic
Gain %: 50

R) Popliteal: Triphasic
Gain %: 50

R) Post Tibial: Biphasic
Gain %: 50

R) Dors. Pedis: Monophasic
Gain %: 50

L) Femoral: Monophasic
Gain %: 50

L) Sup Femoral: Monophasic
Gain %: 50

L) Popliteal: Monophasic
Gain %: 50

L) Post Tibial: Monophasic
Gain %: 50

L) Dors. Pedis: Monophasic
Gain %: 50

Segmental BP
Segment/Brachial Index

122 — Brachial — 121

156   1.28   96   0.79

142   1.16   88   0.72

135   1.11   80   0.66

117 (PT):   69
99 (DP):   65

0.96 — Ankle/Brachial Index — **0.57**

Courtesy of Parks Medical Electronics

- Discussion: Study #2a. J. Doe - Doppler and pressure portion of study

- ABI is normal on right 0.96 and abnormal on left 0.57.

- Doppler waveforms are normal on right side demonstrating triphasic pattern. However, the right dorsalis pedis waveform is somewhat abnormal and the pressure is reduced. This may indicate tibial disease in the anterior tibial or DPA, or it may be due to a small, atrophic DPA, a common finding.

- Doppler waveforms are abnormal at the left common femoral artery and abnormal flow patterns persist at all distal sites.

Study #2b

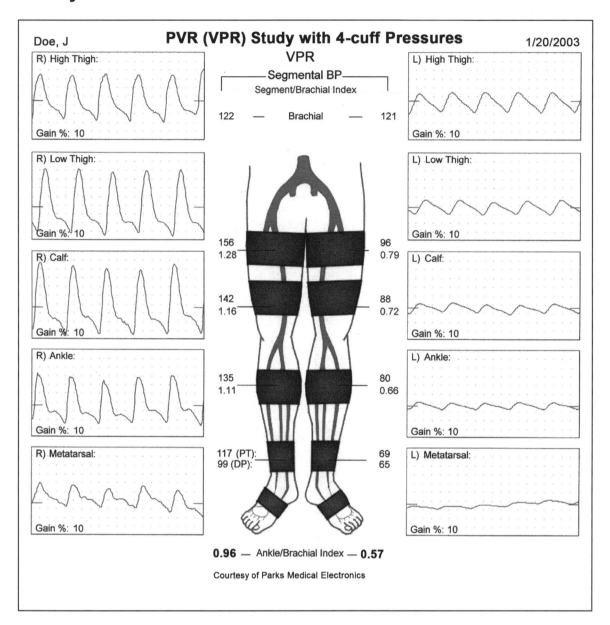

Discussion: Study# 2b-J. Doe - Pulse Volume Recording and Pressures

- Volume pulse recordings, VPR, (some manufacturer refers to pulse volume recording as VPR) are normal on right side demonstrating good amplitude and reflected waves at all sites.

- VPR on the left is abnormal in the upper thigh with loss of amplitude (compared to the contralateral side) and absence of a reflected wave. An abnormal VPR at the high thigh usually indicates inflow disease. VPR abnormality persists at all distal locations.

- Segmental pressures are normal on right (upper thigh with "high-thigh cuff artifact").

- ABI and segmental pressures are abnormal on left. High-thigh pressure of 96 mmHg, compared to brachial pressure and contralateral normal thigh, indicates inflow disease on left.

- There is no significant (>20 mmHg) pressure drop distal to the upper thigh; this suggests no further disease.

- The patient was not exercised due angina and the probability (based on a low, left ankle pressure) that the inflow disease was causing the vascular claudication.

Summary

Right leg is probably normal (with question of tibial disease in right DPA). Doppler waveforms, VPRs and segmental pressures all indicate severe aortoiliac disease on left side.

Patient:GH Study #3

- This 82-year-old female presented with an ulcer on her left lateral ankle. Pulses: right CFA 2$^+$, right Pop 2$^+$, right DPA 1$^+$, right PTA 2$^+$; left CFA 2$^+$, pulses below were absent.

- No history of smoking, MI or DM. History of hypertension.

Study #3

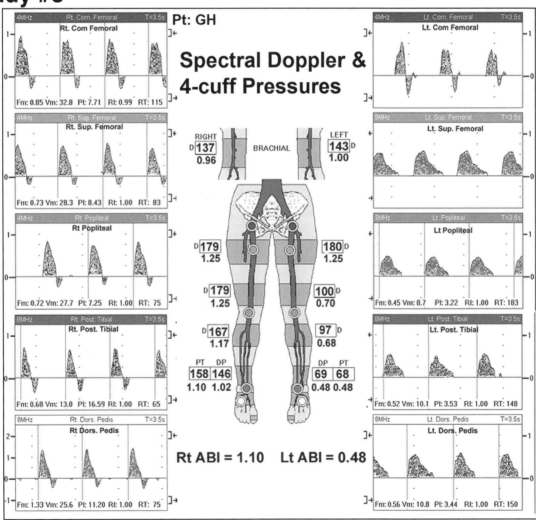

Discussion: Study #3. Patient GH

- ABI on right side is normal. Doppler waveforms are multi-phasic at all sites and are normal. The Doppler waveforms do not exhibit the third (triphasic) component in the diastolic portion of the cardiac cycle, but this often seen in otherwise normal patients. This may result from the Doppler probe angle being too high, or if wall compliance is poor.

- The left ABI is abnormal (0.48) and is in the range of multi-level disease or long segment occlusion. The left CFA Doppler wave is similar to right and is multiphasic. The SFA, POP and tibial waves are monophasic and abnormal.

- High-thigh pressures are normal bilaterally (both have the high-thigh cuff artifact). A significant pressure drop occurs at the left low thigh cuff.

- An additional pressure drop occurs at the ankle, but there is no degradation of the waveforms so the significance is questionable.

- Patient was unable to exercise.

Impression:

⇒   No significant inflow disease.

⇒   Moderate to severe left femoro-popliteal disease, with question of tibial involvement.

⇒   Resting study in right leg is normal.

Patient: BM Study #4

- A 90-year-old female presented with gangrenous toes in right foot.

- Pertinent medical history was unavailable.

- Pulses right leg all 0, left leg 1+ at CFA, 0 at sites below.

Study #4

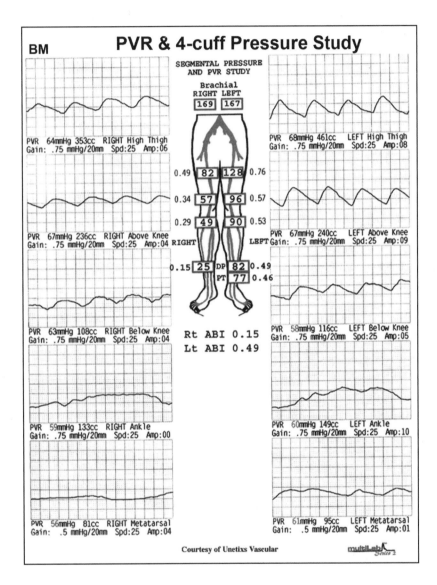

PVR & 4-cuff Pressure Study

BM

SEGMENTAL PRESSURE
AND PVR STUDY

Brachial
RIGHT LEFT
169   167

PVR 64mmHg 353cc RIGHT High Thigh
Gain: .75 mmHg/20mm Spd:25 Amp:06

0.49 82 128 0.76

0.34 57 96 0.57

0.29 49 90 0.53

PVR 67mmHg 236cc RIGHT Above Knee
Gain: .75 mmHg/20mm Spd:25 Amp:04 RIGHT

0.15 25 DP 82 0.49
        PT 77 0.46

PVR 63mmHg 108cc RIGHT Below Knee
Gain: .75 mmHg/20mm Spd:25 Amp:04

Rt ABI 0.15
Lt ABI 0.49

PVR 59mmHg 133cc RIGHT Ankle
Gain: .75 mmHg/20mm Spd:25 Amp:00

PVR 56mmHg 81cc RIGHT Metatarsal
Gain: .5 mmHg/20mm Spd:25 Amp:04

PVR 68mmHg 461cc LEFT High Thigh
Gain: .75 mmHg/20mm Spd:25 Amp:08

PVR 67mmHg 240cc LEFT Above Knee
LEFT Gain: .75 mmHg/20mm Spd:25 Amp:09

PVR 58mmHg 116cc LEFT Below Knee
Gain: .75 mmHg/20mm Spd:25 Amp:05

PVR 60mmHg 149cc LEFT Ankle
Gain: .75 mmHg/20mm Spd:25 Amp:10

PVR 61mmHg 95cc LEFT Metatarsal
Gain: .5 mmHg/20mm Spd:25 Amp:01

Courtesy of Unetixs Vascular

multilabs
Series 2

Discussion: Study #4. Patient BM-

- ABIs are abnormal bilaterally (right 0.15, left 0.49), and in the ischemic range on the right.

- PVRs are abnormal at both upper thighs, indicating bilateral inflow disease right > left.

- There is a decrease in PVR amplitude between the upper and lower thigh on the right, and a similar decrease at the calf level on the left. This suggests bilateral SFA disease. (Although

PVRs are often unreliable for concomitant disease assessment distal to severe inflow disease, a decrease in amplitude at the calf cuff compared to the upper or lower thigh PVR suggests additional disease).

- Segmental pressures are abnormal at the upper thigh bilaterally, right > left. This alone could be due to SFA disease or inflow disease (abnormal high thigh pressure has only a 42% positive predictive value for iliac disease [5]) but it is consistent with abnormal inflow PVRs.

- Significant pressure decrease at the low thigh on the right, and calf on the left is consistent with SFA or popliteal disease. A 25 mmHg pressure drop at the right ankle suggests tibial involvement as well.

Patient BM, Impression:

⇒   Severe ischemia right leg, severe aortoiliac disease, (probable iliac occlusion), with severe femoral-popliteal disease. Cannot rule out tibial involvement.

⇒   Left side: moderate aortoiliac and femoral-popliteal disease.

Patient: Betty, Study #5

In September of 2001, this 78-year-old female presented with recent onset right hip and leg pain soon after she started to walk. She was limited to walking 1 block. There was no history of MI, CVA, DM, HT, vascular surgeries or smoking. She had been an active walker prior to the recent onset of discomfort.

- Previous history includes a rapid onset of bilateral, intermittent calf claudication in 1993. Indirect physiologic studies revealed bilateral superficial femoral artery disease. Her resting ABI on the right was 0.67 and 0.63 on the left. Following a treadmill exercise test she experienced a significant ankle pressure drop bilaterally to confirm a vascular etiology for her claudication. Duplex scanning revealed bilateral SFA stenoses. The findings were unusual in that the disease had a very atypical appearance. The arteries were narrowed, with a smooth lumen, and concentric thickening. It did not have the appearance of atherosclerotic disease. The board-certified vascular surgeon with whom she consulted thought her disease was a form of arteritis related to polymyalgia rheumatica. She was treated with steroids and an active walking program. Her symptoms improved over the course of several months to a point that she was not limited by claudication.

- The study below is from 2001.

Study #5

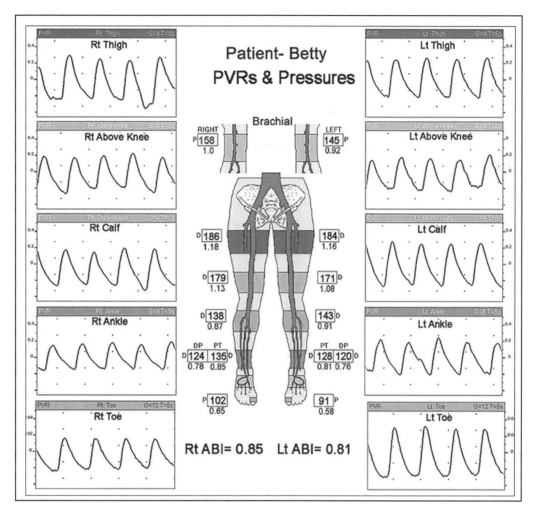

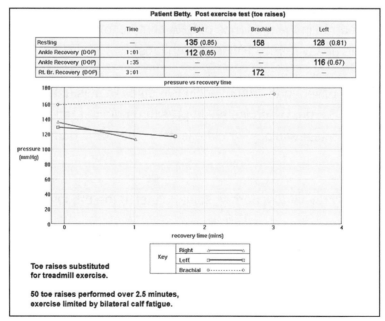

Discussion: Study #5. Patient Betty.

<u>Resting study</u>

- Four-cuff pressure and PVR method used.

- ABIs are abnormal bilaterally (0.85 on right, 0.81 on left). The highest pressure value was used for the reported ABI.

- The upper thigh pressures are 30 mmHg above the arm pressure (high-thigh cuff pressure artifact) and are normal. This rules out significant inflow disease.

- Although there appears to be a slight pressure drop between upper thigh and above knee cuffs, the drop between the above knee and calf cuffs is significant bilaterally.

- The pressure decrease at the ankles is within 20 mmHg of the calf pressures, so this is not significant.

- PVRs appear to be mildly abnormal at all sites.

- The resting study would suggest mild to moderate femoral–popliteal disease, bilaterally.

<u>Exercise Stress test.</u>   The patient was unable to walk on the treadmill due to pain in right hip when standing. Toe raises were performed as a substitute for treadmill with a reasonably good effort. Ankle pressures immediately following the 2.5 minute exercise period were decreased bilaterally, with the right ankle at 112 mmHg and the left at 116 mmHg, down from 135 mmHg and 128 mmHg respectively. Serial pressures were not obtained.

<u>Color duplex imaging</u> of the common femoral, profunda femoral, superficial femoral (SFA) and popliteal arteries bilaterally demonstrated proximal SFA stenoses of both legs. Proximal right SFA PSV was 66 cm/s and at stenosis, 597 cm/s. Proximal left SFA 70 cm/s and 272 cm/s at stenosis. Noted were atypically large profunda femoral arteries, often seen when good collateralization has occurred in the presence of SFA obstruction.
This may account for the nearly normal PVRs in both legs.

<u>Summary:</u>   Although this patient has arterial occlusive disease, it is unlikely that this is the source of her symptoms. Her post exercise ankle pressures did not reflect an ischemic condition necessary to explain a vascular etiology for claudication. Her ABIs had, in fact, improved since 1993.

Computerized tomography revealed a narrow spinal canal at the L-5 level.

This case demonstrates the importance of physiologic testing in assessing the ***effect*** of disease on overall limb perfusion.

Patient: JD- Study #6

- This 76-year-old male presented with 1 year history of right ankle, knee and hip pain when walking, relieved by rest. History of osteoarthritis in feet.

- History of hypertension, hyperlipidemia, MI, and smoking (quit 5 years ago).

Study #6

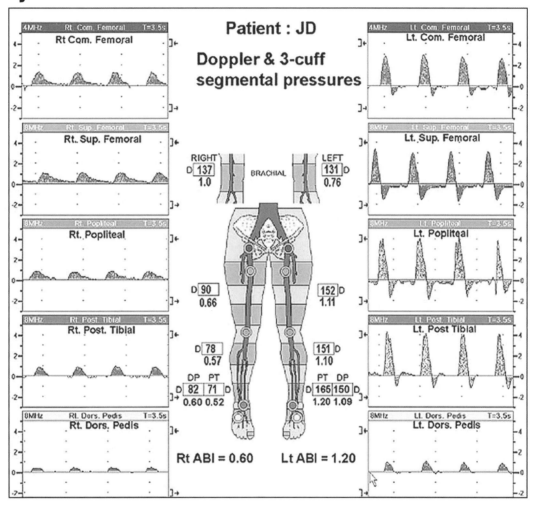

Discussion: Study #6. Patient JD

- Three-cuff pressure test with Doppler spectral analysis.

- Abnormal, monophasic CW Doppler waveform at the right CFA suggests significant inflow disease.

- Doppler waveforms are persistently abnormal distally.

- Abnormal ABI on right, normal on left.

- Left thigh pressure is low without additional significant drop to calf.

- Left side Doppler waveforms and pressures are normal.

Impression: significant aortoiliac disease on right; normal study on left leg.

Patient McG ----No history available. Study #7
Study #7

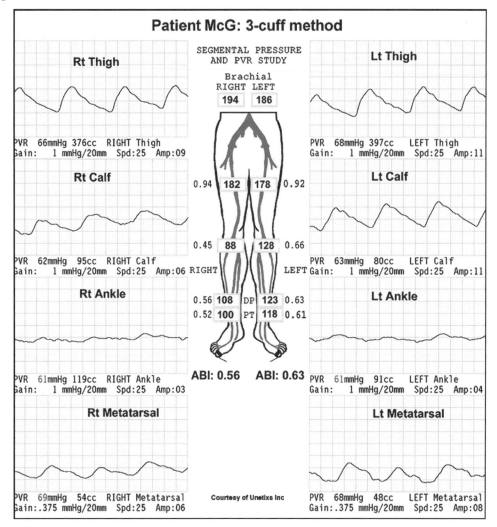

Patient McG: 3-cuff method

SEGMENTAL PRESSURE AND PVR STUDY

Rt Thigh

PVR 66mmHg 376cc RIGHT Thigh
Gain: 1 mmHg/20mm Spd:25 Amp:09

Rt Calf

PVR 62mmHg 95cc RIGHT Calf
Gain: 1 mmHg/20mm Spd:25 Amp:06

Rt Ankle

PVR 61mmHg 119cc RIGHT Ankle
Gain: 1 mmHg/20mm Spd:25 Amp:03

Rt Metatarsal

PVR 69mmHg 54cc RIGHT Metatarsal
Gain:.375 mmHg/20mm Spd:25 Amp:06

Brachial
RIGHT LEFT
194   186

0.94   182   178   0.92

0.45   88   128   0.66

RIGHT   LEFT

0.56 108 DP 123 0.63
0.52 100 PT 118 0.61

ABI: 0.56   ABI: 0.63

Courtesy of Unetixs Inc

Lt Thigh

PVR 68mmHg 397cc LEFT Thigh
Gain: 1 mmHg/20mm Spd:25 Amp:11

Lt Calf

PVR 63mmHg 80cc LEFT Calf
Gain: 1 mmHg/20mm Spd:25 Amp:11

Lt Ankle

PVR 61mmHg 91cc LEFT Ankle
Gain: 1 mmHg/20mm Spd:25 Amp:04

Lt Metatarsal

PVR 68mmHg 48cc LEFT Metatarsal
Gain:.375 mmHg/20mm Spd:25 Amp:08

Discussion: Study #7. Patient McG

- PVRs at both thighs are marginally normal (there are no distinct reflective waves).

- Thigh pressures are normal (for 3-cuff technique) bilaterally. Normal PVRs, and in this case normal pressures, rule out significant inflow disease.

- PVR waveforms are abnormal at the calf level bilaterally, right greater than left. (Typically in a three-cuff method using a 17 cm thigh cuff, the calf PVR amplitude is higher than the thigh PVR in normal perfusion).

- A significant pressure drop occurred at both calves.

- Ankle PVRs are abnormal.

- Metatarsal PVRs are high in amplitude than the ankles due to a difference in PVR gain.

Note: There are a few technical glitches in this study. The ankle PVRs and the pressures do not agree. The PVRs are almost flatline and the pressures are over 100 mmHg. The technologist should have repeated the pressures and PVRs at the ankle level.

Patient: R. S. Study #8

- A 53-year-old male presented with history of stable, bilateral intermittent hip, buttock and thigh claudication limiting walking to 3 blocks.

- Hx of angina, HT, smoking 1-2 ppd.

- CABG 3/23/2000.

- Pulses CFA 1+, POP 0, PTA 1+, DPA 1+, bilaterally.

Study #8

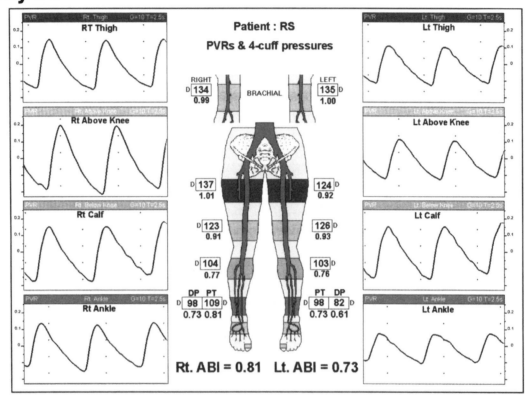

Rt. ABI = 0.81   Lt. ABI = 0.73

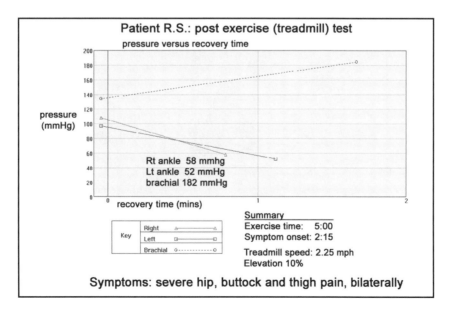

Patient R.S.: post exercise (treadmill) test

Rt ankle 58 mmhg
Lt ankle 52 mmHg
brachial 182 mmHg

Summary
Exercise time: 5:00
Symptom onset: 2:15

Treadmill speed: 2.25 mph
Elevation 10%

Symptoms: severe hip, buttock and thigh pain, bilaterally

Discussion: R.S Study #8

• ABIs are abnormal bilaterally.

• PVRs are borderline abnormal on the right upper thigh, with mildly abnormal waveform on the left upper thigh. Distal PVRs are mildly abnormal and similar to thigh waveforms.

• Upper thigh pressures are abnormal (they should be 20- 30 mmHg above brachial pressure).

• There is a borderline significant pressure drop at the calf level bilaterally; this may suggest femoro-popliteal disease, but there is no significant change in PVR morphology.

Post exercise:

• Patient walked for 5 minutes but experienced severe hip, buttock and thigh pain bilaterally.

• Ankle pressures were 58 mmHg (ABI 0.32), and 52 mmHg (ABI 0.29) in right and left ankles respectively.

Impression: Moderate aortoiliac disease bilaterally resulting in vascular claudication. Question of mild femoro-popliteal disease bilaterally.

Color Duplex Imaging revealed bilaterally severe common iliac artery stenoses.

===

Patient: JF. Study #9.

• A 34-year-old male presented with acute onset right calf claudication.

• No symptoms in left leg.

• Study date 6/16/99.

• Hx of Aorto-Rt. common femoral bypass 3/98.

• Right pulses CFA, POP, DPA, PTA all 0,   Left pulses all 2+

Study #9

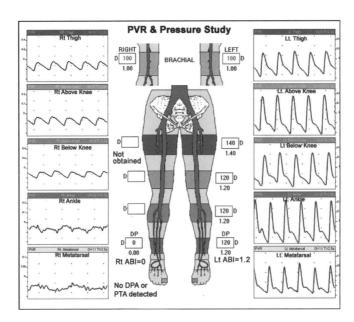

Discussion: Study #9 Patient JF.

- Normal PVRs and ABI on left side.

- Unable to obtain pressures in right leg (no flow detectable by Doppler in either pedal arteries).

- Abnormal PVR at left upper thigh indicates severe inflow disease. The fact that he has a graft on the right side suggests graft occlusion.

- Angiography revealed a thrombosed aorto-femoral graft. Patient underwent a successful thrombectomy.

Patient KC. PVR and 4-cuff segmental pressure. Study #10

No History available.

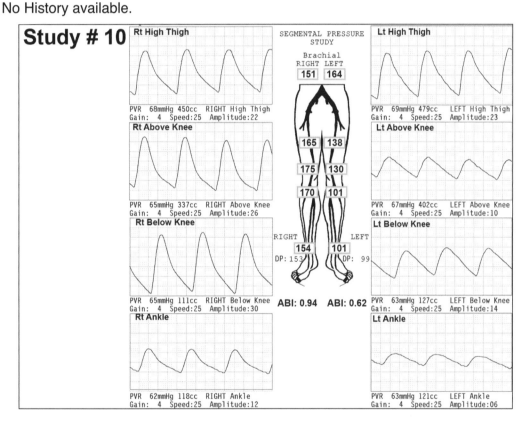

Discussion: Study #10, Patient KC   Patient was not exercised.

Right Leg: Normal ABI: 0.94

- Rt. thigh pressure is equal to the highest brachial pressure, (some normal individuals do not exhibit the "high-thigh" cuff artifact). There is an insignificant pressure decrease between the calf and ankle.

- PVR waveforms at high thigh through the ankle are normal with the dicrotic notch or the reflected wave.

Left Leg: Abnormal ABI: 0.62

- Lt. upper thigh pressure is low compared to the contralateral segment and to the brachial pressure. There is an additional pressure decrease between the low thigh and calf. An abnormal thigh pressure can be due to either inflow disease or femoral artery disease.

- The PVR is normal at the upper thigh. This suggests that inflow is normal: the upper thigh PVR reflects perfusion into the deep femoral artery system. The PVRs below this level are abnormal

Impression: Moderate to severe femoro-popliteal disease left leg.

ABBREVIATED, EFFICIENT ARTERIAL PROTOCOLS

Objective #1 of physiologic testing: Is there objective evidence for peripheral arterial disease?

⇒   Perform Single Level Physiologic study (CPT code 93922).

⇒   Perform exercise in appropriate (claudicating) patients, or borderline normals.

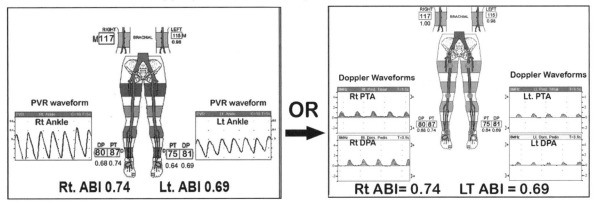

⇒   If ankle PVRs are non-diagnostic due to motion artifact, acquire Doppler waveforms from the pedal arteries.

- Patient has peripheral arterial disease bilaterally; slightly greater on the left.

- It's moderate.

- Exercise stress testing at this point would confirm that PAD is causing claudication.

◆   *This information has been provided in a 15 minute examination.*

Questions NOT answered in this abbreviated exam:

- Disease Level - Inflow or infrainguinal (is this important?).

- Single level or multilevel disease (is this important?).

- Is the disease causing the claudication? (Probably).

To answer these questions, extend exam to a "segmental" exam.

⇒   The addition of multiple level PVRs or Doppler waveforms indicates the disease level.

⇒   Abnormal upper thigh PVRs (and abnormal CFA Doppler waveforms) indicate that this patient has inflow disease, or aortoiliac disease, bilaterally.

♦   This information was provided with an additional 5-10 minutes of exam time. Total exam time to this point 20-30 minutes.

Would segmental pressures help here?

*   **NO!** Thigh pressures are painful for many patients, and because there is confusion about high thigh pressure interpretation (some patients have the "high-thigh cuff artifact", and some don't), the best method to assess inflow is with thigh PVR (easier than Doppler) or Doppler waveforms.

*   A low thigh pressure can be due to femoral disease <u>or</u> aortoiliac disease.

*   The additional time and effort had not provided any additional useful information in this case.

*   A multi-level physiologic segmental study is designated as CPT code 93923.

Questions NOT answered in this exam at this point:

*   Is the vascular inflow disease causing the patient's claudication ?

*   How do we answer this clinical question?

⇒ Assumption (low resting ankle pressures).

⇒ Perform exercise stress test.

Post treadmill exercise procedure.

⇒ Measure post-exercise ankle pressures, if they're below 60 mmHg, it's a vascular cause for claudication.

Exam efficiency:

♦ ABI with ankle waveforms: total exam time =10-15 minutes.

♦ ABI with addition of segmental PVRs: total time 20-25 minutes.

♦ Doppler segmental waveforms instead of PVRs: total time 30-35 minutes.

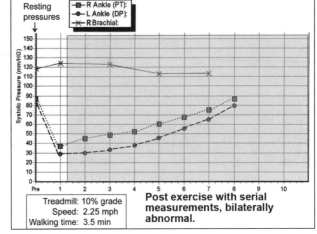

Post exercise with serial measurements, bilaterally abnormal.

♦ ABI, segmental PVRs, and stress test: total time 35-45 minutes.

♦ Proceed to Imaging methods knowing disease level and severity.

REFERENCES

1. Rutherford, RB, Lowenstein DH, Klein MF. Combining segmental systolic pressures and plethysmography to diagnose occlusive disease of the legs. Am J Surg 138:211-218, 1979

2. Raines J K, Darling R C, Bluth J., et al. Vascular laboratory criteria for the management of peripheral vascular disease of the lower extremities. Surgery 79:21, 1976

3. Belcaro et al, Noninvasive Diagnostic Techniques in Vascular Disease. E. Bernstein , editor, third edition P 507 Mosby, St. Louis

4. Heintz SE, Bone GE, Slaymaker EE, Hayes AC, Barnes RW: Value of arterial pressure measurements in the proximal and distal part of the thigh in arterial occlusive disease. Surg Gynocol Obstet:146:337-43,1978

5. Kupper CA, et al. Spectral Analysis of the Femoral Artery for Identification of Iliac Artery Lesions... Bruit 8: 157-63 June 1984

6. Flanigan DP et al. Utility of wide and narrow blood pressure cuffs in the hemodynamic assessment of aortoiliac disease.Surg 92: 16-20, 1982

7. Harris LM, Koerner NA, Curl GR, Ricotta JJ. Active pedal plantarflexion: a hemodynamic measurement of claudication. J Vasc Technol 19(3): 115-118,1995

8. Carter SA. Clinical measurement of systolic pressure in limbs with arterial occlusive disease JAMA 1969;207:1869-1874

9. Bridges RA, Barnes RW. Segmental limb pressures. In: Kempczinski RF and Yao SJS. Practical Noninvasive Vascular Diagnosis. Yearbook Medical pp 79-93.

CHAPTER 11: COLOR DUPLEX IMAGING: LOWER EXTREMITY ARTERIES

INTRODUCTION

Color duplex imaging (CDI) of the arterial tree, when used as an adjunct to indirect methods, can provide valuable anatomic and hemodynamic information. CDI in the hands of experienced operators can:

*   Identify the exact anatomical location of arterial occlusive disease.

*   Differentiate stenosis from total occlusion.

*   Define the length of occlusion.

*   Identify aneurysms.

*   Identify pseudoaneurysms (high pressure extravasation of blood out of an artery and into the surrounding tissue).

*   Identify Arteriovenous malformations (AVM), A-V fistulas, and venous malformations (VM).

CDI is also used to evaluate femoro-popliteal or femoro-tibial bypass grafts. It has been shown to be more sensitive than ABIs in surveillance for progression of occlusive lesions or thrombus formation within the graft. This will be addressed in a later chapter.

> NOTE: Color duplex imaging should not be performed to rule out arterial occlusion or stenosis in native arteries. It is not a good screening test for the presence of arterial occlusive disease because it is labor intensive and time consuming. A difficult, bilateral lower extremity duplex study can easily take 2 hours. It should be used as an adjunct to the aforementioned physiologic tests.

FEMORAL - POPLITEAL ARTERIAL SEGMENT

The common femoral, superficial femoral, and popliteal arteries are the most common segments for arterial occlusive disease in the lower extremities, and these arteries are amenable to color duplex imaging.

Procedure

*   The patient should be in a supine position and head slightly elevated.

*   Identify the common femoral artery (CFA) and CFV in transverse plane at the inguinal ligament. The vein lies medial to the artery at this level.

- Rotate the transducer to the longitudinal plane such that the right side of the image is in a caudal direction.

- Image the distal external iliac artery (EIA) and the common femoral artery (CFA) with color Doppler. Optimize color Doppler for correct steering angle, PRF scale, wall filter and gain.

- Observe any flow disturbances with color Doppler.

> NOTE: Normal flow in the legs is triphasic, and the color Doppler frame rate must be optimizes for speed to observe this transient reverse flow within the cardiac cycle. If frame rates are too slow, the color assigned to the retro flow will get mixed in with the antegrade flow colors. This can have the appearance of disturbed, turbulent flow.

- Obtain and record a spectral waveform from the EIA and measure peak systolic velocity.

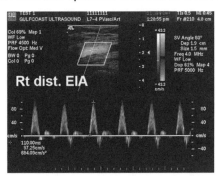
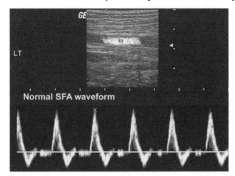

- Obtain an acceleration time (AKA, Rise time) if your system has the capability. A waveform of low amplitude, delayed rise-time (> 144 msec, or 0.14 sec), or turbulence suggests iliac disease.

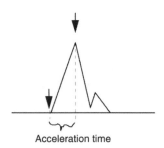

Acceleration time

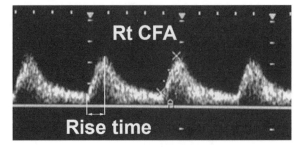

- Evaluate the distal CFA and bifurcation of the CFA into the superficial femoral (SFA) and profunda femoris arteries (PFA) with color Doppler.

- Obtain spectral waveforms from origins of the SFA and PFA.

- Continue down the leg with color Doppler (now steered in a caudal direction) and carefully assess the entire SFA.

- Look for atherosclerotic disease along the walls, and any change in the color Doppler color saturation that might indicate increased velocity.

- Use pulsed Doppler spectral analysis to "map" stenotic areas that are seen with color Doppler. Measure velocity before the stenosis, at maximum stenosis, and also document post - stenotic turbulence.

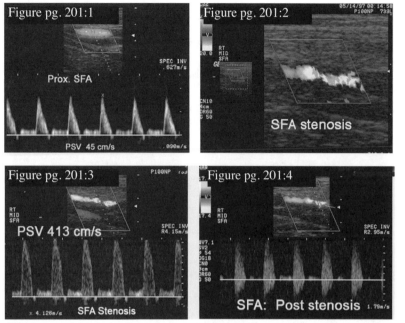

Figure pg. 201:1-4 **See Color Plates #8: F-G, and Plate #9: A-B.**

- If there is no detectable flow in an artery segment, identify collateral runoff proximally, follow the segment distally using the vein as a guide, and identify the region of inflow or reconstitution. In this manner the length of the occlusion may be estimated.

- The distal SFA at the adductor canal is more difficult to evaluate and is frequently the site of disease. Use both the anterior window above the medial aspect of the knee, and the posterior view with the transducer behind the knee to interrogate this region.

- Obtain spectral waveforms from the mid and distal SFA.

POPLITEAL ARTERY

The popliteal artery is studied from behind the knee with the leg rotated externally, or alternatively, with the patient in a prone position. Be sure to scan both proximally to overlap the distal SFA. This region is a very common site for atherosclerotic occlusive disease. Also, scan to the distal segment of the popliteal and obtain a spectral waveform as close to the anterior tibial branch as possible.

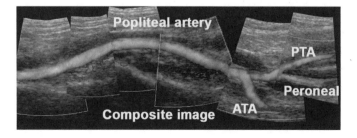

Interpretation Criteria

• In the distal external iliac artery (or CFA), an acceleration time (AT) of >144 msec suggests significant iliac disease (>75% diameter reduction).[1]

• Velocity acceleration over a stenotic lesion that achieves a 2:1 systolic ratio and followed by post-stenotic turbulence indicates a 50% or greater stenosis.

% Stenosis	Peak Velocity	Velocity ratio
Normal	< 150 cm/sec	< 1.5:1
30% - 49%	150 - 200 cm/sec	1.5:1 - 2:1
50% - 75%	200 - 400 cm/sec	2:1 - 4:1
> 75%	> 400 cm/sec	> 4:1
Occlusion	No color saturation	

From Cossman DV, Ellison JE, et al.[4]

TOTAL OCCLUSION

• Positive predictive value is improved for total occlusion if no flow is detected in the segment by color and spectral Doppler, collateral outflow is identified proximal to the occlusion, and reconstituting inflow is identified distal to the occlusion.[2] Pay close attention to flow direction in connecting arteries; flow entering an artery is usually reconstituted flow and is indicative of more proximal disease.

Helpful hints:

⇒ The major arteries lie right beside the major deep veins, so use the veins as landmarks in the event the arteries are occluded.

⇒ Long-standing occluded vessels are often contracted and difficult to identify. To be certain an artery is occluded you have to identify it.

⇒ Use the length of the transducer face as a ruler to measure occlusion distances that are longer than the image field of view.

⇒ Position the patient so that the leg that you're studying is closest to you. This is critical for evaluating calf arteries and useful in other artery segments as well. It's inconsequential if the patient's feet are toward the ultrasound instrument and contrary to the traditional ultrasound patient position; your arms and back will thank you !

⇒   Be aware that blood can flow in either direction in an artery, as there are no valves. It is not uncommon to find total retrograde flow in the profunda femoris artery to supply the SFA in the event of a CFA occlusion, or similarly, reversed flow in the internal iliac artery to feed the external iliac artery. So pay attention to flow direction.

TIBIAL ARTERY SEGMENT

The posterior tibial, peroneal and anterior tibial arteries are difficult and time consuming to study in patients with atherosclerotic occlusive disease. These arteries are small and blood volume and velocity may be low. Their evaluation may be beyond the scope of the routine vascular exam.

They can be studied selectively in patients that will undergo distal bypass procedures. In this case, it is important to identify distal patency, particularly in the posterior and anterior tibial arteries.

Procedure

♦   Begin the longitudinal color Doppler scan of the posterior tibial artery just posterior to the medial malleolus and follow the artery proximally along the course of the tibia.

♦   Identify stenotic regions and confirm with spectral Doppler.

♦   Occluded segments should be noted and confirmed by the presence of collateral outflow and inflow.

♦   If the artery is diseased, use a low color PRF to detect low velocity flow and a narrow color box to maintain suitable frame rate.

♦   Repeat the above procedure for the anterior tibial artery starting at the dorsum of the foot and following its course along the interosseous membrane lateral to the tibia.

Interpretation

Use the same criteria for the femoro-popliteal segment. The more important determination, however, is whether the arteries are patent throughout the calf.

ANEURYSMS

Can occur in:

⇒   Aorta.

⇒   Iliacs and CFA.

⇒   Popliteal artery.

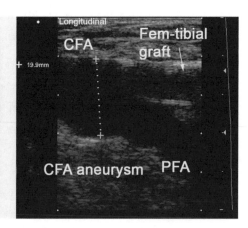

Risks include:

⇒   Thrombosis.

⇒   Embolization.

⇒   Rupture.

⇒   Nerve compression.

Popliteal artery aneurysms

⇒   If thrombosed, 40-75% amputation rate.

⇒   Usually bilateral in 50-70% of patients.

⇒   Likelihood of AAA is 43%.

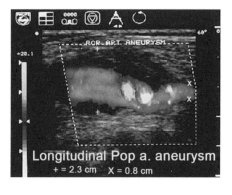

♦   In all aneurysms, measure the anterior-posterior and the lateral dimensions.

♦   Measure the length.

♦   Identify if thrombus is present.

♦   Identify if the artery is occluded or patent.

♦   Measure the diameter of the distal segment to determine if it is normal size (important preoperative information).

PSEUDOANEURYSMS

⇒   High-pressure extravasation of blood into surrounding tissue.

⇒   No arterial wall encapsulating aneurysm.

⇒   "To and fro" flow pattern in aneurysm neck.

Usual causes:

♦   Percutaneous arterial catheterization.

♦   Penetrating trauma.

♦   Graft anastomosis "blowout".

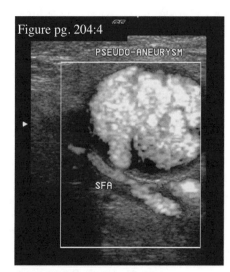

See Color Plate #9: C.

Diagnostic method for pseudoaneurysm caused by interventional arterial vascular procedures.

- Is the pseudoaneurysm directly adjacent to the artery or is there a "neck"?

- Identify the "neck" of the aneurysm.

- Is there "to & fro" flow present? If so, document.

- Is there extrinsic compression of the artery by the pseudo-aneurysm?

- Measure the size of the aneurysm.

- Sample the common femoral vein or external iliac vein to ensure that an arteriovenous fistula has not been created by an inadvertent puncture of the vein during the catheterization procedure.

Pseudoaneurysm flow pattern

Blood flows into the pseudoaneurysm during systole when the pressure in the artery is higher than the pressure with in the pseudo-aneurysm. In diastole, the pressure in the pseudoaneurysm is higher than in the artery, so blood flows back into the artery This fluctuation of pressure results in the "to and fro" pattern in the neck.

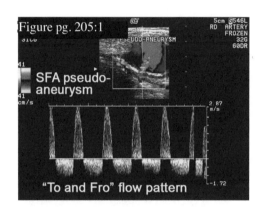

See Color Plate #9: D.

AORTO-ILIAC SEGMENT

- Ideally, the aorta and iliac arteries should be evaluated on all patients with atherosclerotic disease in the lower extremities. However, the lower abdomen and pelvic regions are difficult to interrogate due to the depth and tortuousity of vessels, and to overlying bowel gas.

- If the patient has a 2+ femoral pulse, a normal thigh PVR or normal thigh pressure, and a normal triphasic Doppler spectral waveform in the distal external iliac artery, it is unlikely that a significant (>75%) iliac obstruction exists.

- These indirect methods may not rule out 50% aortoiliac disease[3], so if there is a pressure drop in a symptomatic patient following exercise and the occlusive disease could not be found in the femoro-popliteal segment, then the aorta and iliac arteries must be scanned.

Patient Preparation

- If possible, patients should be NPO for 8 hours prior to the exam to reduce bowel gas.

- It's preferable to perform the exam in the morning after the fast.

- Patients may take clear liquids and any prescription medications.

- Diabetics may take appropriate nourishment.

- The exam is performed with the patient in a supine position.

Scan Technique

- Select an appropriate transducer based on the patient's body habitus, a 2.5-3.5 MHz transducer; in thin patients a 5 MHz transducer.

- Scan the distal abdominal aorta from below the renal arteries to the aortic bifurcation. In transverse plane, look for abdominal aortic aneurysm, and if present, measure outer dimensions and inner residual lumen. SEE CHAPTER ON ABDOMINAL IMAGING FOR MORE INFORMATION.

- Evaluate the aorta with color and spectral Doppler and record a Doppler waveform. Identify the origin of each common iliac artery (CIA) and follow its course with color, or if excessive color flash is present, with just spectral Doppler.

- At the bifurcation of the CIA, identify the internal iliac, or hypogastric artery (IIA), and the external iliac artery (EIA).

- Follow the course of the EIA to the groin crease where it becomes the common femoral artery (CFA).

- The proximal iliacs are best imaged with the transducer placed between the umbilicus and the iliac crest and angled medially.

- Considerable transducer pressure on the abdomen can help to displace bowel gas. If bowel gas still intervenes, place the patient in a lateral decubitus position and try again.

- The diagram below shows three scanning "zones" along the length of the iliac arteries as seen on the ultrasound image. The first zone is usually seen on most patients, as is the third zone. It's the second zone that's the most difficult to interrogate. In difficult patients, scan as distal as you can in zone #1, and as proximal as possible in zone #3. If Doppler waveforms are similar from these two sites, it's unlikely that there is significant disease in zone #2.

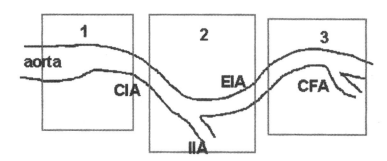

INTERPRETATION

- Because the iliac arteries lie deep and oblique to the face of the transducer, the B-mode image of the lumen is often insufficient to visualize atheromatous plaque. The presence and severity of disease is usually determined by Doppler spectral analysis guided by color Doppler imaging.

- The normal spectral waveform in the distal aorta and iliacs is triphasic and similar to that found in the femoral artery.

> NOTE: In general, if the iliac color image is good, use it to identify regions of stenosis, then confirm and quantify lesions with pulsed Doppler. If the color image is not good, "spot check" with spectral Doppler along the course of the iliacs for the presence of stenosis or occlusion.

- A 2:1 systolic velocity ratio with focal velocity acceleration and followed by post stenotic turbulence[4] is the most reliable indicator for the presence of a 60% or greater stenosis. Beware: high velocity in collateral arteries can be misinterpreted as stenosis.

> NOTE: Although there have been reports in the literature on the ability of spectral Doppler to discriminate lesser degrees of stenosis based on levels of spectral broadening[5], this is impractical and unrealistic in the aortoiliac segments, as spectral broadening occurs in almost all waveforms due to vessel motion, high Doppler angles, and spectral broadening inherent in transducer design.

- The absence of flow in an imaged artery, with markedly decreased velocities proximal and distal to the segment, indicates total occlusion.

- Iliac scanning requires a high degree of technical skill and the "patience of Job". The procedure can be very time-consuming. There is a variable technical failure rate due to obesity, bowel gas, and vessel tortuosity.

REFERENCES

1. Burham S., Jacques P, Burnham C. Noninvasive detection of iliac artery stenosis in the presence of superficial femoral artery obstruction. J Vasc Surg 1992;16:445-52

2. Schroedter WD, Holec SW: The diagnosis of lower extremity arterial occlusion by color flow Doppler. J Vasc Technol 15(5): 245-249. 1991

3. Lewis WA, Bray AE, Harrison CL, Maullin A, Martin RL. A comparison of CFA analysis with Aorto-Iliac Duplex Scanning in Assessment of Aorto-Iliac Disease, J Vasc Technol 18(6): 337-344, 1994

4. Cossman DV, Ellison JE, et al. Comparison of contrast arteriography to arterial mapping with color-flow duplex imaging in the lower extremities. J Vasc Surg 1989;10:522-92.

5. Kohler TR, Nance DR, Cramer MM, Vandenberge NV, Strandness DE Jr.,: Duplex scanning for the diagnosis of aortoiliac and femoro-popliteal disease. A prospective study. Circulation 76(5):1074 -80, 1987

ARTERIAL DUPLEX WORKSHEET

MIC
Medical Imaging
of Colorado
Affiliated with **RIA**

ARTERIAL NIVA:
LOWER EXTREMITIES WORKSHEET

Name: _____ Sex: _____ Age: _____ Date: _____ Page #: _____

Room #: _____ SMC ☐ Craig ☐ Outpatient ☐ Physician: _____

X-ray #: _____ Hospital #: _____ Examiner: _____

History: _____

MI:☐   Hypertension:☐   DM:☐   Smoking:☐ _____

Vascular Operations: _____

Physical Exam: _____

PULSES	CFA	POP	DP	PT
RIGHT				
LEFT				

Color Duplex Imaging: Aorta-iliac ☐, Femoral-popliteal ☐, Tibials ☐.

RT   LT
            AORTA
CIA   CIA
EIA   IIA   EIA

RT   LT
CFA   CFA
PFA   PFA
SFA   SFA
POP   POP
ATA   ATA
PER   PER
PTA   PTA

COMMENTS: _____
_____

A diagram similar to the one above is useful to note what sections were imaged and to draw in regions of stenosis or occlusion.

CHAPTER 12: ARTERIAL BYPASS GRAFTS & STENTS

PREOPERATIVE ASSESSMENT

SAPHENOUS VEIN MAPPING

⇒ Saphenous veins are used as arterial conduit for coronary artery bypass grafts (CABG) or to revascularize the leg with a femoro-popliteal or femoro-tibial bypass graft.

⇒ The great saphenous veins (GSV) and small saphenous veins (SSV) are assessed with duplex ultrasound preoperatively to determine suitability for the above procedures.

⇒ The superficial cephalic and basilic veins in the arm may be used for bypass material, but they are considerably shorter than the GSV. However, these veins are evaluated as part of a pre-op workup for hemodialysis access placement.

⇒ The radial or ulnar artery can be harvested and used for CABG material. Preoperative assessment decreases limb morbidity and increases CABG patency rates.

Saphenous vein mapping for bypass consists of three basic procedures:
1. Procedure #1 determines vein suitability. The goals of this procedure:
    * Is the saphenous vein present and patent?
    * Is it continuous?
    * Does it consist of a double or duplicated system?
    * Does it harbor regions of residual thrombus?
    * Is it of appropriate size?

2. Procedure #2 includes procedure #1 (vein suitability) but also involves mapping and marking the course of the saphenous or the superficial arm vein(s).

3. Procedure #3 determines the suitability of the radial artery for CABG.

ANATOMY

* The *great saphenous vein* (GSV), or long saphenous, courses superficially in an anterio-medial aspect of the leg from its distal end, just anterior to the media malleolus, to the common femoral vein in the groin. This confluence is known as the sapheno-femoral junction (SFJ). The external pudendal, superficial circumflex iliac and the inferior epigastric veins drain into the GSV adjacent to the SFJ.

* A posterior medial branch of the GSV becomes the Giacomini vein in the posterior thigh. This communicates with the small saphenous vein (formerly the lesser saphenous vein) above the sapheno-popliteal junction (SPJ).

- An anterior or accessory saphenous vein is often present and communicates proximally with the GSV. This vein courses anterior-laterally and lies outside of the fascial envelope that contains the GSV.

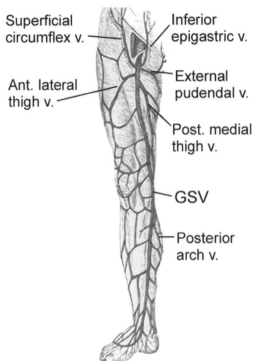

Great saphenous vein

- In the calf a major tributary lying posterio-medial is the *posterior arch vein.* Approximately 65% of individuals have a single GSV in the thigh with 35% having variants, including double systems.

- The *GSV* contains approximately 10-13 semilunar valves with the most proximal valve, called the terminal valve, at the sapheno-femoral junction.

- *Perforating veins* communicate between the deep system and the GSV or SSV. There are numerous perforators in each leg, but most are too small to be visualized with ultrasound unless they're incompetent. They are commonly located in the thigh (Dodd's perforators), near the adductor canal (Hunterian), at the knee (Boyd's perforators), and above the medial malleolus (Cockett's or ankle perforators). Perforating veins may also connect the GSV or SSV with veins of the calf muscles.

- The *small saphenous vein* (SSV) courses along the posterior aspect of the calf and commonly (about 70%) drains into the popliteal vein. It also may enter the distal femoral vein, the GSV or the Giacomini vein. The small and great saphenous veins may communicate via tributaries.

PROCEDURE #1. DETERMINE SUITABILITY OF THE GREAT SAPHENOUS VEIN

Rule out chronic DVT

⇒ With the patient in a reverse Trendelenburg position or with upper body and head elevated (semi-Fowler's position), scan the femoro-popliteal deep veins to ensure they are patent. (Harvesting the GSV when it's functioning as a major outflow channel in chronic deep vein obstruction can have serious sequelae, therefore, check deep vein patency).

Determining Vein Size (diameter)

Technique:

- Using a 7.5-14 MHz transducer, identify the GSV at the sapheno-femoral junction.

- In transverse view, scan the entire length of the GSV and determine the following:

  ⇒ Is it continuous or dichotomous?

  ⇒ Is there a duplicated saphenous system?

  ⇒ Does the vein harbor regions of residual thrombus or wall irregularities?

- To determine if a system is bifid, (vein divides into two segments then rejoins into one) follow any tributaries (branches) to see if they "rejoin" the main GSV. If so, the vein is considered bifid.

- If the vein does not reconnect with the GSV it's one of many saphenous tributaries.

- Measure the diameter of the GSV using system integrated calipers at these locations:

  ⇒ Upper thigh

  ⇒ Mid thigh

  ⇒ Lower thigh

  ⇒ Upper calf

  ⇒ Mid calf

  ⇒ Lower calf

> NOTE: Be careful not to compress the vein with the transducer while obtaining diameter measurements.

- Measure the diameter of both vein segments in a bifid systems.

> NOTE: Vein diameter will expand by about 80-100% when arterialized. Vein diameters of 2.5 mm or greater have higher patency rates for femoro-distal bypass grafts. The graft failure rate is high if preoperative vein diameter is less than 2.5 mm.

- Image the GSV bilaterally. The surgeon may need to use the contralateral vein.

- If the ipsilateral GSV is too small (< 2.0 mm) or unsuitable, evaluate the contralateral GSV as above. The surgeon may need to use the contralateral vein. (Some surgeons may request bilateral GSV assessment routinely).

- If requested, evaluate and measure the diameter of the small saphenous vein at proximal, mid, and distal locations. Identify whether it communicates with the popliteal vein, or above. SSV measurements should be performed with the leg dependent for maximum vein dilatation.

PROCEDURE #2. MAPPING THE VEINS

Limited Mapping for Vein Harvest

The method below is used when complete exposure of the vein will be performed at the time of surgery. The perforators and communicators will not be marked in this technique as they will be identified and ligated during surgery. However, it may be helpful to mark large branches.

Preparation and Method.

- Apply a strip of clear tape on the side of the transducer. Place a small indelible mark on the tape adjacent to the middle of the length of the transducer face. Alternatively, place a thin piece of colored tape in the same location directly on the transducer casing; avoid marking the transducer itself (they're expensive!). This will serve as a reference mark for the center of the ultrasound image.

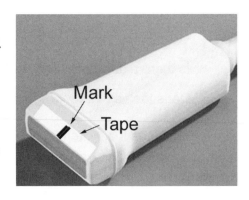

- Various marking devices are available commercially and facilitate this otherwise "messy" job. **

> NOTE: When a patient is referred for a "vein mapping", it is important to find out whether the surgery is planned and scheduled, or whether the surgeon is just interested in "suitability". If surgery is planned, mark the leg, as above. If only suitability is the goal, there is no need to mark the leg during that exam.

- Place patient in reverse Trendelenburg, or semi-Fowler's position.

- Clean the leg along the approximate course of the GSV with 70% alcohol.

- Place a thin layer of WARM acoustic gel along the course of the GSV.

- Identify the proximal *GSV* at the SFJ; position the vein in the center of the ultrasound field of view. This should correspond to the mark on the outside of the transducer casing tape. Use a plastic drinking straw (or commercially available device**) to create an indentation on the skin over the vein (adjacent to the mark on the casing). A ballpoint pen, point retracted, may also be used. Gently press the straw or pen for a few seconds to create the indentation. Move the transducer distally a few centimeters and repeat. Mark the confluences of large tributaries as well.

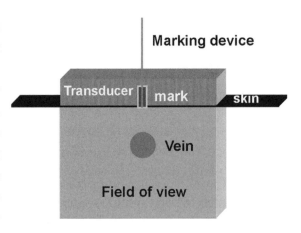

- After the GSV in the thigh has been indented, wipe off the gel and place an indelible (Sanford Marker Deluxe works well) mark over the skin indentations.

- Connect the dots with the marker to map the course of the GSV and major confluences.

** SonoMark. www.sonomarking.com. MPM, Inc. 1775 Gunnison, Delta, CO 81416, 866-477-760

** AIM Medical Technologies. www.vascularmapping.com 866-511-5487

- Regions of the GSV that are less than 2.5 mm can be marked with a dotted line.

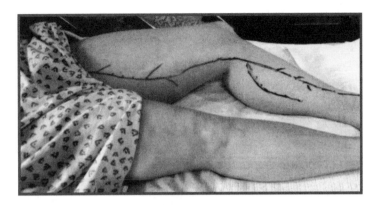

PREOPERATIVE ASSESSMENT OF RADIAL ARTERY

The use of the radial artery for coronary artery bypass conduit was first reported by Carpentier et al., in 1973. Initial results were disappointing due to arterial spasm, and the technique was abandoned for several years. Improvements in radial artery harvest techniques and the realized potential for long-term patency brought about renewed interest in the method.

The radial artery has advantages over the saphenous vein, including:

- Appropriate caliber.

- Thicker wall, less intimal hyperplasia.

- Better availability.

Contraindications for the radial artery harvest include:

- Ischemic digits.

- Raynaud's syndrome.

- Ipsilateral athero-occlusive disease in arm.

- Sclerotic, atretic or occluded radial artery.

- Incomplete palmar arch in hand.

⇒ Raynaud's syndrome can be ruled out by patient history.

⇒ Bilateral brachial pressures, described in the Chapter 13 on upper arterial evaluation, can rule out subclavian artery stenosis. Duplex imaging is required to determine size of radial artery, etc. Physiologic testing can provide a quick, objective means of determining palmar arch patency.

⇒ Generally, the radial artery will be harvested from the non-dominant arm.

Protocol: Radial Artery Duplex Imaging.

- Scan the radial artery in transverse plane, starting from the wrist and continue to the brachial artery. Look for the following and record if found:

  ⇒ Arterial stenosis.

  ⇒ Artery occlusion.

  ⇒ Vessel atresia.

  ⇒ Regions of wall calcification.

- Measure the inside diameter at the distal, mid and proximal segments.

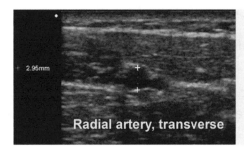
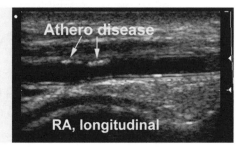

- The average inside diameter of the distal radial artery is 2.8 mm for men, and 2.4 mm for women.

- Surgeons prefer that the diameter of the distal radial artery be at least 2.0 mm for CABG, but 2.5 mm or greater is preferred.

- Note the position of the brachial artery bifurcation into the radial and ulnar arteries. Is it in the antecubital fossa or higher? If it's in the upper arm, as shown in the right image below, inform the surgeon in your report.

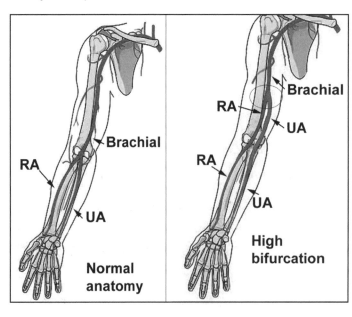

Palmar Arch Test

There are two palmar arches in the hand from which the digital arteries arise; a superficial and a deep. The palmar arch provides a collateral pathway so that the entire hand and all digits can be perfused by the ulnar artery when the radial artery is harvested.

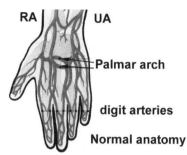

Some individuals have an incomplete palmar arch, or an anomalous anatomy in which the radial artery is dominant and perfuses the entire hand. If the radial artery is removed in these patients, their fingers would most likely become ischemic and fall off!

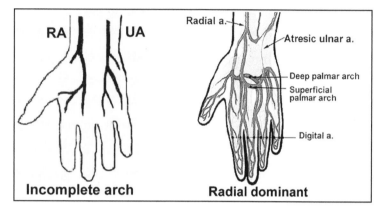

PPG testing for Palmar Arch Patency

The test for Palmar arch patency can be performed with an Allen Test. This test is best performed with physiologic testing devices.

- Photoplethysmography (PPG) sensors are placed on the thumb or index finger and the 5th digit (if a 2 channel system is available).

- The PPG scale or gain controls are adjusted to establish similar amplitudes.

- Use a slow sweep speed and if possible, monitor both digits simultaneously.

- Compress and hold both the radial artery (RA) and ulnar arteries with your thumbs simultaneously, and observe changes in the PPG trace of the two digits. The tracings should be "flat line". This ensures that you're compressions are adequate.

- Compress/hold the RA and observe/ record the PPG waveforms of both digits. There should be no, or little, drop in the PPG amplitudes.

-

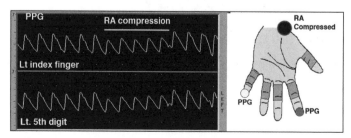

No change with radial artery compression = normal

- If the PPG waveforms drop to flat-line or nearly flat-line, the palmar arch is not intact.

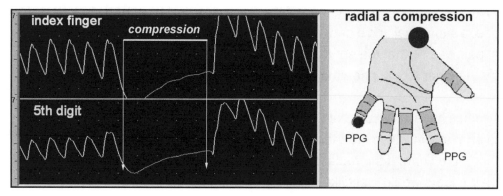

In the figure above, the left radial artery compression significantly decreases flow to both digits. Left radial artery harvest in this patient would be contraindicated.

- Repeat the test, compressing the ulnar artery (UA) this time, and record the waveforms. A normal response is indicated by little or no decrease in PPG waveform amplitude.

- A third test may be performed in which both the radial and ulnar arteries are compressed simultaneously. Flow should stop in both test digits. This 3rd test ensures that the arteries are being adequately compressed.

- Digital pressures are useful when there is a partial decrease in perfusion during radial artery compression with PPG monitoring. This provides a quantitative measure of digit perfusion. It is not necessary (or possible) to attempt to obtain a digit pressure on a finger with a flatline PPG tracing!

Digit pressures with RA compression

- Obtain thumb or index digit pressures at rest.
- While compressing the radial artery, re-obtain digit pressure and compare to resting value.

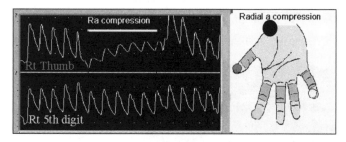

Resting Rt. Thumb P = 147 mmHg. With RA compress, P = 79 mmHg. Patient has decreased PPG amplitude with RA compression indicating a partially intact palmar arch.

POSTOPERATIVE ASSESSMENT- BYPASS GRAFTS AND STENTS

Bypass graft evaluation begins with a patient history and/or surgical record of the type of graft employed. There are basically three types of grafts used for supra-inguinal (above the groin crease) bypass.

Above Inguinal Ligament Grafts

1) Aorto-bifemoral graft ("aortoiliac", if the distal end of the graft is anastomosed above the inguinal ligament).

   • Used to bypass a diseased distal aorta and/or iliac arteries.

   • Patient will have a scar near the umbilicus, and one in each groin region.

2) Femoral to femoral "jump" graft.

   • Scar at each groin, although this can result from endovascular aneurysm stent repair (EVAR) of aortic aneurysm.

   • Used to bypass a single iliac artery.

   • Intended flow direction should be from asymptomatic leg to preoperative symptomatic leg.

3) Axillo-femoral, fem-fem bypass.

   • Used to bypass the abdominal aorta.

   • Proximal anastomosis is at the axillary artery.

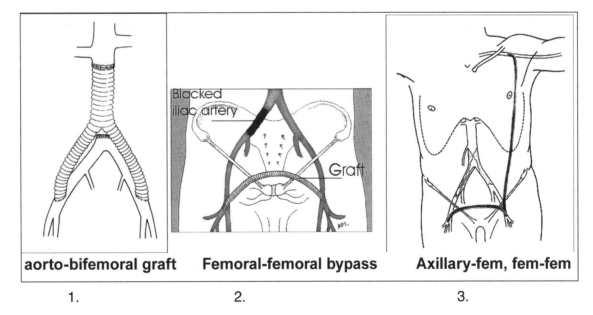

aorto-bifemoral graft	Femoral-femoral bypass	Axillary-fem, fem-fem
1.	2.	3.

The entire graft, as well as the graft inflow and outflow, should be evaluated for stenosis Careful attention should be given to the anastomotic sites as technical problems, graft failure and infection are more likely to occur in these regions.

Below Inguinal Ligament Grafts

1) Synthetic polytetrafluoroethylene (PTFE) graft.

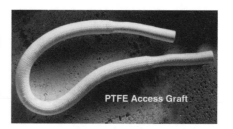

- Common femoral artery (CFA) to distal superficial femoral artery (SFA) or proximal popliteal A.

- Newer flexible fabrication may allow placement to extend below knee. The patency rates of PTFE grafts, when coursing past the knee joint, are limited. Graft kinking is a complication of this type of graft.

2) Synthetic Dacron.

- Often used for fem-fem, and iliac grafts.

- Newer Dacron material is used for femoral-distal bypass grafts.

3) In situ fem-pop or (fem-tibial) vein graft.

- This "autogenous" vein graft is used to bypass femoro-popliteal occlusion.

- The procedure uses the great saphenous vein (GSV) for arterial conduit. The vein is left in place or "in situ".

- The valves are excised with a valvulatome or similar device, and perforating veins and communicating veins are ligated and cut.

- The graft lies superficial in the proximal section, but courses deep towards the SFA, popliteal or tibial anastomosis.

- The proximal anastomosis is usually at the CFA, but the graft may originate at the profunda femoris artery (PFA) or the proximal SFA.

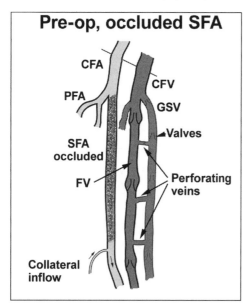

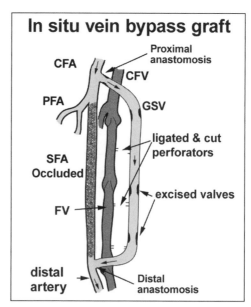

These diagrams demonstrate the pre-operative arterial and venous anatomy, and the post-op in situ vein (GSV) bypass graft.

- Partially excised valve leaflets are not uncommon. These leaflets act as a stenosis within the graft and may reduce blood flow distally.

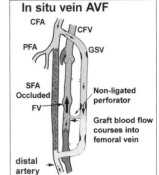

- A potential complication of in situ grafts is a fistula created by a non-ligated perforating vein. Arterial flow courses down the vein graft and crosses into the femoral vein. Small perforating vein fistulas are not a problem, as the volume of the "steal" is low, but in large fistulas blood flow to the distal extremity is reduced and the efficacy of the graft diminished.

4) Reversed vein graft.

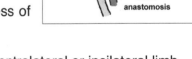

- In this procedure the GSV is removed, turned upside down, and sewn back in.

- The valves are not removed or excised as in the in situ method.

- All perforating veins/ communicators are ligated and cut.

- This graft is smaller proximally, larger distally due to the diameter of the reversed vein.

- Some surgeons prefer this bypass method, as distal anastomotic stenosis (by neointimal hyperplasia) has less of an effect due to the wide bore of the vein.

- The vein for this procedure may be harvested from the contralateral or ipsilateral limb.

5) Other grafts.

- Veins and arteries harvested from cadavers are also used.

- The small saphenous vein (SSV) is used for small segments or for graft revisions.

- The cephalic or basilic veins in the arm may be used for small graft extensions or revisions.

Follow-up Surveillance of Bypass Grafts-Rationale

- Allows the surgeon to detect early graft stenosis prior to thrombosis and occlusion.

- Thrombosed grafts are prone to early failure following thrombectomy.

- Graft defects and stenosis may be followed for progression or resolution.

- Intervention can be initiated with onset of symptoms and confirmation of progressive occlusive disease.

Scan Method

If possible, obtain information from the surgeon's office or medical record regarding the type and the anatomical placement of the graft.

Obtain ABIs and ankle PVRs or Doppler waveforms and compare to previous exams; no need to exercise patient. A drop of 0.15 in the ABI from the previous exam suggests progressive graft stenosis.

> NOTE: Post operatively, do not obtain an ankle pressure in a femoral - distal tibial graft if the graft lies under the cuff, without permission of the surgeon.

Use image, color and spectral Doppler to evaluate:

1. Graft inflow.

2. The entire graft lumen for:

   - Stenosis.

   - Wall irregularity.

   - Aneurysms.

   - Pseudoaneurysm (graft blow-out).

   - A-V fistulas from non-ligated perforators.

   - Partially excised valve leaflets.

3. The anastomoses for stenosis or defects. The proximal vein graft often develops neo-intimal hyperplasia due to the shear stress of arterial flow on a thin vein wall. Intimal hyperplasia is a rapid proliferation of intimal cells causing wall thickening and lumen encroachment.

4. Assess the profunda femoris artery origin.

Obtain and record peak systolic velocities from the following locations:

⇒ Proximal to, at and distal to a stenotic segment.

⇒ The artery segment proximal to the graft.

⇒ Within the graft:

   - Proximal graft

   - Mid graft

   - Distal graft segments

⇒ The artery segment distal to the graft.

TIP: If a specific stenosis is being serially evaluated, place a tape measure on the thigh/calf along the course of the graft and identify its location relative to a major branch vessel. New stenoses can be differentiated from a known stenosis in this fashion.

- Velocity ratios may be unreliable in regions of anastomoses as the vein and the runoff vessel diameters are often of different size. Look for velocity changes over time in these specific areas during serial follow-up exams.

- Doppler waveforms of blood flow in "mature" bypass grafts resemble that of native vessels, i.e., high resistance flow presented as a triphasic waveform. Proximal, distal, or intragraft disease may affect the morphology of the waveform and indicate the presence of disease.

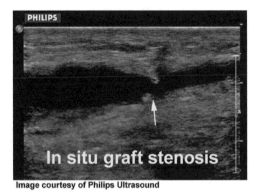

Image courtesy of Philips Ultrasound

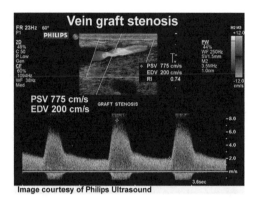

Image courtesy of Philips Ultrasound

- In the early post-operative period (less than 45 days), the Doppler flow pattern may <u>not</u> be triphasic and may exhibit antegrade flow throughout the cardiac cycle. Chronic vasodilation that occurred before the graft or PTA will persist for some weeks and cause the hyperemic flow. After the hyperemic response subsides, the graft waveforms should be triphasic and consistent with normal outflow resistance.

Post-op bypass graft waveform.

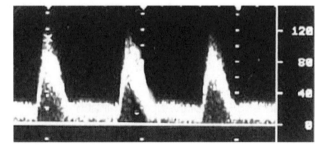

Interpretation

- Graft velocities will vary with vessel diameter, but should be above 40 cm/sec. Velocities in normal reversed vein grafts will decrease distally as the diameter becomes larger.

- For infrainguinal vein grafts focal velocity acceleration followed by post stenotic turbulence, peak velocities of ≥150 cm/sec and velocity ratio of ≥ 2.0 are consistent with a 50% or greater stenosis.[1]

- Absence of color filling, absence of spectral Doppler signal, and visualization of thrombus indicates the graft is occluded.

- If velocity ratios are > 3.5 and peak systolic velocities exceed 300 cm/sec, the stenosis is unlikely to regress and intervention is recommended to prolong graft patency.[2]

Stents

Vascular stenting, used in combination with percutaneous angioplasty, has been successful in the treatment of coronary artery stenosis. The success of this procedure has encouraged its use in the peripheral arterial system.

The diseased segment of the artery is initially dilated with the angioplasty balloon. The stent is then introduced within a catheter sleeve, the sleeve is removed, and the stent is expanded with the underlying balloon catheter. The stent mechanically holds the artery open and improves patency rates compared to angioplasty alone.

Angioplasty with stent deployment

NIH   http://www.nhlbi.nih.gov/health/dci/Diseases/stents/stents_placed.html

Lower extremities

The patency rate of iliac artery stents appears much better compared to that for femoro-popliteal stents.[3] Mechanical factors are more likely to distort the stent and contribute to its failure. Stents appear to have better patency if the stenotic lesion is short. Long lesions may require serial stents and the technique becomes costly compared to a vein bypass graft.

- Stents for peripheral arterial disease are either balloon-deployed or self expanding.

- Stents are made of titanium, nitinol or similar material and can be either open or covered.

- At the time of this writing, there are no established velocity criteria for peripheral arterial stent stenosis. As with carotid stents, it is recommended that post stent velocities be recorded and used as a reference for follow-up examinations.

Aorta

Endovascular treatment of abdominal aortic aneurysm (EVAR) involves the percutaneous placement of a thin Teflon covered stent graft within the aortic aneurysm. The graft is anchored at each end by stents against the normal vessel wall. The risk of aneurysm rupture, thrombosis, and embolization appears to be significantly reduced. It is a relatively minor procedure, requiring much less recovery time, and a shorter hospital stay compared to AAA resection.

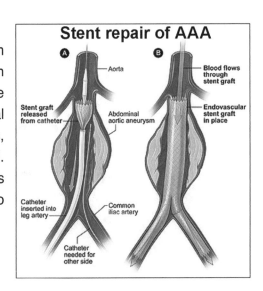

Stent repair of AAA

Complications include:

- Endoleak - an inadequate seal of the proximal or distal wall that allows blood flow into the perigraft region.

- Graft infection.

- Vessel rupture during deployment.

- Embolization.

Pre-stent evaluation [4]

1. Obtain pressure measurements and calculate an ankle to brachial index (ABI).

2. Carefully assess the aorta from the diaphragm to the bifurcation of iliac arteries, and to the CFA bilaterally.

3. Measure aneurysm outside diameter, its length, and residual lumen. Does the aneurysm extend above the renal arteries (RA)?

4. Measure the diameter of the aorta proximal to the aneurysm, and if possible, the distance between the left RA and the aneurysm. To allow for proper stent anchoring, there should be at least 1 cm of normal aorta between the left RA and the aneurysm.

5. Measure the diameter of the iliac arteries. Measurements of the proximal and distal anchoring sites will enable the correct size selection of stent.

Post stent evaluation [4]

1. ABIs.
2. Monitor stent for patency.
3. Is the graft in the same position or has it moved proximally or distally?
4. Look carefully for low velocity endoleaks into the aneurysm sac.
5. Look for retroperitoneal fluid that may represent a leak outside of the aorta.
6. Measure diameter of aorta.
7. DO NOT OBTAIN A SEGMENTAL PRESSURE WITH THE CUFF OVER A FEMORAL, POPLITEAL OR TIBIAL STENT.

Carotid

Investigative trials are now underway to determine the efficacy, safety, and long term outcome of carotid stent placement. Currently, carotid stenting is performed when the patient is a poor operative candidate for endarterectomy. Stenting of the ICA may reduce stroke and mortality rates associated with endarterectomy.[5] Complications of stent movement, intimal hyperplasia, and embolization have been reported, and the peri-procedure stroke rate has yet to be established. As with other stents, the long-term effect of carotid stents is not known.

See carotid chapters for more information.

Color Duplex assessment

Most stents are made of metal mesh that ultrasound will penetrate. Although some shadowing will occur, color and spectral Doppler may be used to evaluate stents for stenosis, occlusion and position shift. In carotid stenting the proximal ECA may occlude if the stent blocks its origin, so careful evaluation of this area is appropriate. Increased velocity has been reported through normal carotid stents, perhaps due to a decrease in wall elasticity.

REFERENCES

1. Mattos MA, van Bemmelen PS, et al. Does correction of stenoses identified with color duplex scanning improve infrainguinal graft patency? J Vasc Surg 1993; 17:54-66

2. Gahtan V, Payne LP, Roper LA, et al. Duplex criteria for predicting progression of vein graft lesions: Which stenoses can be followed? J Vasc Technol 19(4): 211-215. 1995

3. Henry M, et al. Occlusive and aneurysmal peripheral disease: assessment of a stent- graft system. Radiology. 210(3):717-24, 1996 Dec.

4. Johnson BL, Harris EJ, Fogarty TJ, Olcott C IV, Zarins CK. Color duplex evaluation of endoluminal aortic stent grafts J Vasc Technol 22(2):97-104, 1998

5. Wholey MH, et al. Endovascular stents for carotid artery occlusive disease. J. Endovascular surgery. 4(4):326-38,1997 Nov.

6. Criado FJ. Stents in Endovascular Surgery. Union Memorial Hospital, Baltimore MD, 1995

CHAPTER 13: ARTERIAL EVALUATION OF THE UPPER EXTREMITIES

ARTERIAL, UPPER ANATOMY

1. Brachiocephalic a. (innominate) - right side only.

2. Subclavian a.
   - Left: originates at the aortic arch.
   - Right: originates at the brachio-cephalic artery.

3. Axillary a.- from the first rib to the axilla.

4. Brachial a. - from the axilla to the antecubital fossa.

5. Radial a. - from the distal brachial artery to the wrist.

6. Ulnar a. - from the distal brachial artery to the wrist.

7. Palmar arches in hand: deep and superficial.

8. Digital arteries (2 per digit) arise from the palmar arch.

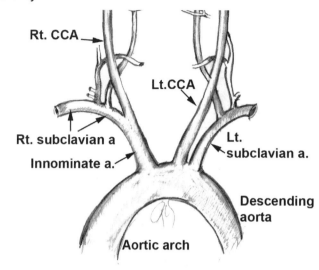

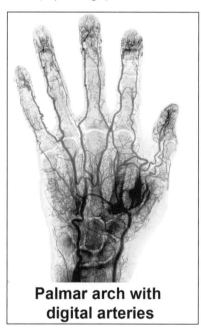

Palmar arch with digital arteries

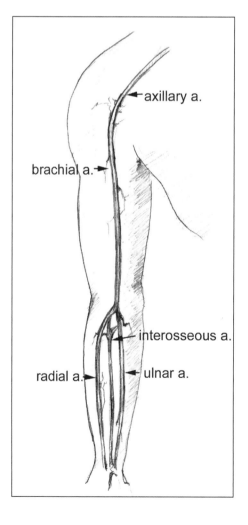

INDICATIONS

- Arterial insufficiency.

- Weakness in the arm.

- Thoracic Outlet Syndrome (TOS).

- Vasospastic disorder -digit cold sensitivity.

- Digital ischemia.

- Abnormal vertebral artery waveform.

- Pre-operative assessment:
  ⇒ Hemodialysis access.
  ⇒ Radial artery harvest for coronary artery bypass graft (CABG).

Contraindications

- No arm pressure measurements should be obtained on an arm with a hemodialysis access. However, PVRs, with reduced inflation pressure, or Doppler waveforms are OK.

DISEASE PROCESSES

Large vessel occlusive disease

- Atherosclerotic obstruction occurs predominately in the subclavian & innominate arteries. The axillary, brachial, radial, & ulnar arteries usually spared.

- Takayasu's and giant cell arteritis are autoimmune disorders that may affect the subclavian arteries.

- Subclavian stenosis/occlusion is diagnosed with comparisons of bilateral brachial systolic pressures: a >20 mmHg gradient suggests subclavian artery disease on the side with the lower pressure. Also, direct interrogation of the subclavian artery with color duplex is more sensitive than a pressure differential in detecting subclavian artery stenosis.

- Thromboembolism: acute obstruction of the distal arteries caused by emboli from subclavian artery disease, proximal aneurysm, or the heart. The site of obstruction depends on the size of the embolus relative to the size of the artery.

Small vessel occlusive disease- fixed

- Buerger's disease (thromboangiitis obliterans): inflammatory condition of the palmar arch and/or digital arteries leading to small vessel obstruction. Found most often in male smokers.

- Thromboemboli: small emboli that occlude the vessels of the hand and digits.

See Color Plate #9: E&F.

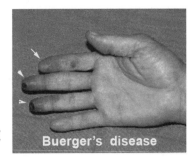
Buerger's disease

Small vessel occlusive disease- vasospastic disorder

- Raynaud's Syndrome: episodic, prolonged digital vasospasm brought about by cold exposure, chemicals (nicotine), emotion, or occupational trauma (vibration injury) to the hands.

  ⇒ Primary Raynaud's Syndrome: a vasospastic disorder without underlying disease. The digital and palmar arteries are without obstruction and perfusion to the digits at rest is normal.

  ⇒ Secondary Raynaud's syndrome: vasospasm associated with an underlying autoimmune disease or connective tissue disease, e.g., scleroderma. The digital/palmar arteries often have fixed obstruction. Even a normal vasoconstrictive response to cold in these patients can cause severe ischemia.

- These were previously differentiated as Raynaud's disease, and Raynaud's phenomenon, respectively.

- Symptoms of the primary syndrome include pallor of digits during vasospasm, followed by cyanosis and rubor upon release of the spasm. The spasm may take 10-30 minutes to release. Small vessel vasospasm occurs normally in response to cold exposure and is triggered by the sympathetic nervous system. In some individuals, however, a sympathetic over-activity occurs that causes the vasospasm to occur with less provocation. Following the vasospastic response, or the removal of the condition that triggered the effect, the spasm does not quit.

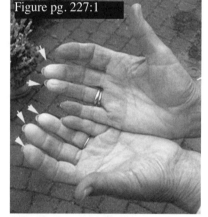

Figure pg. 227:1

See Color Plate #9: F.

- Typically, the affected area turns white, then blue, then often to bright red.

- Symptoms include numbness and pain.

Raynaud's Syndrome:

- 70-90% of cases occur in females.

- 40% related to connective tissue disorders (scleroderma, lupus, rheumatoid arthritis).

- 40% idiopathic.

- 20% other etiology, frostbite, repetitive vibration injury, etc.

Treatment:

- Cessation of smoking.

- Cold/stress avoidance.

- Calcium channel blockers: Procardia, Nicardipine.

- Sympathetic blocking agents.
- Treat associated disease.
- Cervico-thoracic sympathectomy.
- Micro-revascularization.
- Relocation to warm climate.

Thoracic Outlet Syndrome (TOS)

- Intermittent pain, numbness, or weakness of arm(s) related to arm position. Caused by compression of artery or nerve by the anterior scalene muscle, clavicle, rib, or congenital muscular anomalies.
- 95% of TOS is of neurogenic etiology, i.e., compression of the brachial plexus.
- Less than 5% is vascular compression in which the subclavian/axillary artery flow is compromised.
- TOS may cause thrombosis, fibrosis, and aneurysm of the subclavian or axillary arteries.

INDIRECT TEST METHODS

Baseline exam- Rule out arterial occlusive disease

1. Introduce yourself to your patient.

2. Obtain a pertinent history of symptoms, including duration, location, and whether persistent or episodic. Note HX of smoking, diabetes, MI, and vascular bypass operations.

3. With the patient in a sitting position, obtain segmental systolic pressures at the arm and the forearm levels, bilaterally.

4. Obtain pulse volume recordings (PVR) from the same sites, or acquire CW Doppler waveform tracings from the axillary, brachial, radial and ulnar arteries.

5. Obtain a PVR, photoplethysmography (PPG) waveform or pressures from both index fingers.

6. If the patient complains of arm pain/numbness/weakness that is position related, perform Thoracic Outlet Test described below.

Tailor subsequent testing for the patient's symptoms.

⇒ Position-related arm pain, numbness or weakness- perform thoracic outlet test.

⇒ Ischemic digits- perform upper extremity and digit physiologic exam.

⇒ Episodic vasospasm- perform baseline digit exam and cold immersion study.

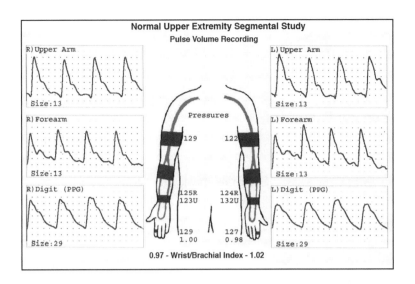

Thoracic Outlet Test Method

- After the baseline study has been performed, obtain a waveform with one following methods to serve as a baseline reference for positional TOS study:

  a) Photoplethysmography (PPG) on the index fingers.

  b) Pulse volume recording (PVRs) of the arms.

  c) CW-Doppler tracings from the radial or ulnar arteries.

- Next, obtain tracings from both arms either bilaterally, if instrumentation allows, or unilaterally in each of the following arm positions:

  1. Abducted 90 degrees to the torso.

  2. Elevated 180 degrees above the head.

  3. Arm abducted 90 degrees, with elbow bend 90 degrees ("pledge" position). Evaluate with the head turned toward, then away from the hand (modified Adson's maneuver).

  4. Elbows at side and pressed backwards, hands up, shoulders pressed downward and back ("stick-up" position).

  5. Symptomatic position.

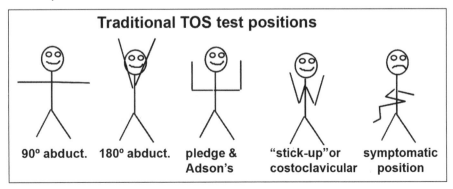

MOST IMPORTANT, evaluate in the symptomatic position.

TOS Interpretation

- The amplitude of waveform tracings should remain similar to or larger than baseline tracings in any of the arm positions.

- A significant and sustained decrease in amplitude suggests vascular compression.

- The definitive positive finding is a loss of pulsatility or "flatline" waveform with the patient in a symptomatic condition.

- Often, in a patient with vascular TOS, small changes in arm position can restore or diminish the waveform tracing. Below is a positive TOS study.

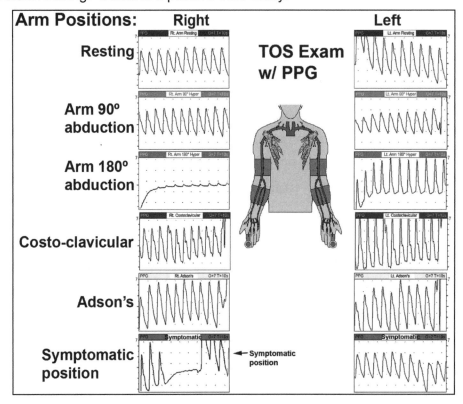

TOS TEST. PPG sensors record perfusion from both index fingers. There is reduced right arm perfusion in the 180° elevated position. This corresponded with the patient's symptomatic position. This is a positive study for right arm vascular TOS.

TOS Pitfalls

In some otherwise normal patients the PPG tracings may go "flatline" when the arm is raised over the head (180°) and if their hand is hyperextended. If this occurs, ask that they relax their fingers then reassess. If the flat line tracings persist, confirm this positive finding with a CW Doppler held over the radial or ulnar artery in the same arm position. Another false positive result can occur if the Doppler probe slips off the radial or ulnar artery in any arm position. This, of course, would result in a reduced or absent Doppler signal and tracing.

Baseline Physiologic Digital Exam

Using the procedures described below, determine whether digital perfusion is normal or abnormal. If abnormal, determine whether the cause is small vessel fixed obstructive disease, e.g., Buerger's disease, or vasospasm disorder.

Digital exams should be performed in a comfortably warm room to avoid vasoconstriction.

- Evaluate all digits with one of the following methods:

    a) PVRs with digital pressure cuffs.

    b) PPGs obtained distally.

    c) Digit pressures using PPG and digital pressure cuffs.

    d) Duplex imaging of the digits (with a high frequency transducers) is an option if there is evidence for fixed obstruction.

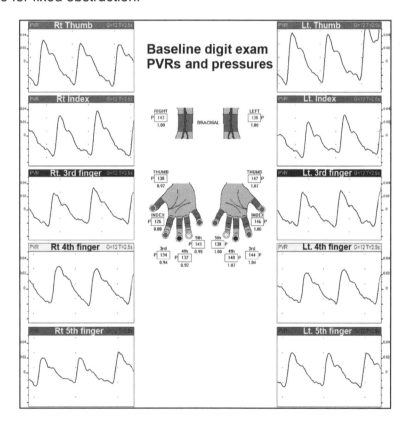

If perfusion is normal or near normal and the patient is symptomatic for Raynaud's Syndrome, perform TEST "A" described below. If digital tracings are abnormal at rest, proceed to TEST "B".

Raynaud's exam

Test "A", Cold Immersion test

⇒   Record pre-submersion PVRs or PPGs on the symptomatic digits.

⇒   Remove the PPG sensors and place the symptomatic hand(s) in a plastic bag. Submerge the hand(s) into a basin of ice water for 1-2 minutes, or less, if the patient is unable to tolerate the discomfort/pain.   This technique keeps the hand dry, and the PVR cuff may be left on. Hands may be immersed without the plastic bag after removing sensors/cuffs, but the hand must be dried and sensors or cuffs reapplied after submersion.

⇒   Obtain post submersion tracings on the symptomatic digits using whatever method was used in pre-submersion test.

⇒   Obtain tracings at 2 or 3 minutes intervals thereafter. If PVR amplitude returns to baseline levels within 5 minutes, you may discontinue testing as this represents a normal exam.

⇒   If waveform amplitude remains low, continue recording at 2 minute intervals until 10 minutes has elapsed since the first post-submersion tracing. A persistent decrease in digital waveform amplitude, as compared to baseline pre-submersion tracings, at 10 minutes or longer confirms a vasospastic disorder, or Raynaud's syndrome.

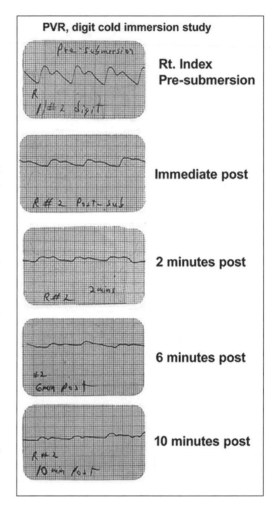

PVR, digit cold immersion study

Rt. Index
Pre-submersion

Immediate post

2 minutes post

6 minutes post

10 minutes post

Abnormal cold immersion test of the right index finger; the PVR waveforms are persistently dampened even 10 minutes after cessation of cold stimulation.

Testing for Raynaud's can also be performed with digit temperature sensors and cold immersion. Infrared temperature sensors or thermistors are used to acquire digital temperatures in a similar sequence to those described above. Failure to return to baseline temperatures within 5 minutes constitutes a positive exam.

Test "B"

If digital PVR or PPG tracings are abnormal at rest, the patient may have occlusive disease, secondary Raynaud's, Buerger's etc., or they may be experiencing vasoconstriction or vasospasm.

⇒   Ensure that the exam room is warm.

⇒   Wrap the affected hand in a heating pad and warm for 5 minutes.

⇒   Repeat digit PVRs or PPGs following re-warming. If waveform amplitudes remain abnormal, small vessel occlusive disease should be suspected. If amplitudes become normal following warming, a vasospasm/vasoconstrictive condition exists.

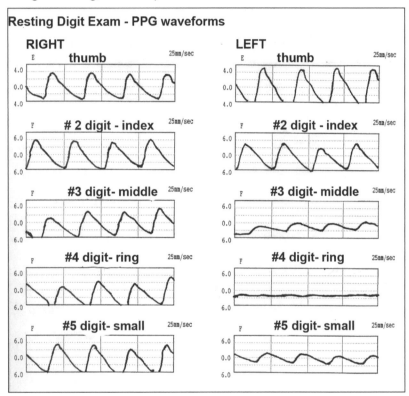

A 62-year-old male presented with numbness and ischemic changed on his left 4th and 5th digits distally. No history of smoking or prior cold sensitivity. The arm physiologic study was normal. PPG waveforms were abnormal in the left 3rd, 4th, and 5th digits indicating reduced perfusion. Both hands were warmed in a heating blanket for 10 minutes and digits were retested.

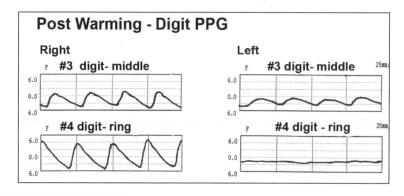

Following rewarming there was no improvement in perfusion to the affected digits on the left hand. This finding suggested fixed occlusive disease, as opposed to vasospasm. The digits were imaged with a high frequency intraoperative ultrasound transducer and digital artery occlusion was found in the involved fingers. Ultrasound scan of the left subclavian artery for aneurysm was negative. Due to a suspicion of thromboemboli as the cause of the occlusions, the patient was scheduled for an echocardiogram. The results were unavailable.

Allen Test for Palmar Arch Patency

This exam is essential prior to radial artery harvest for coronary artery bypass surgery and prior to ipsilateral hemodialysis fistula or graft implantation. If the radial artery is removed in a patient that is "radial dominant", and if the palmar arch is not intact, severe ischemia may result in the fingers and hand. Radial artery "steal" phenomenon is not uncommon in Brescia-Cimino dialysis fistulas. The "steal" condition is usually benign as long as the palmar arch is complete.

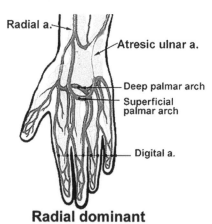

Radial dominant

The Allen test may be performed manually without instrumentation, or with monitoring devices (PPG, PVR or digit pressures) on the thumb or index finger and the little finger. A standard resting digit exam should be performed on all fingers prior to the Allen test.

Manual Exam

1. Occlude the patient's radial and ulnar arteries with your thumbs, and have the patient squeeze their fist 3-4 times to exsanguinate the blood out of the hand.

2. Release only one of the arteries and observe whether the palm becomes pink (perfused) across the entire hand and digits.

3. Repeat arterial compression and hand squeeze, then release the other artery and observe normal or abnormal cutaneous filling.

4. Absence of capillary refilling suggests an occluded palmar arch or radial/ulnar dominance.

Allen Exam with instrumentation: See Chapter 12: Arterial bypass graft chapter, pre-operative mapping.

1. This test is best performed with PPG sensors placed on the thumb or index finger and on the 5th digit. Use scale or gain controls to establish similar waveform amplitudes.

2. Use a slower sweep speed, and if possible, monitor both digits simultaneously.

3. Compress the radial artery (RA) with your thumb and observe/record changes in the PPG trace of the two digits. If the PPG tracing drops to flat-line or nearly flat-line, the palmar arch is not intact.

4. Repeat the test; compress the ulnar artery (UA), and record waveforms.

Preoperative color duplex imaging should also be performed on the radial and ulnar arteries to detect stenosis, occlusion, or atresia.

COLOR DUPLEX IMAGING

Indications:

*   Abnormal vertebral artery spectral waveform.

*   Abnormal right CCA waveform.

*   Subclavian bruit.

*   Decreased arm pressure.

*   Acute ischemia in hand (atheroemboli ?).

*   Additional testing for a positive TOS exam.

*   Suspicion of subclavian aneurysm or mural thrombus.

*   Pre-operative assessment for hemodialysis access or bypass graft.

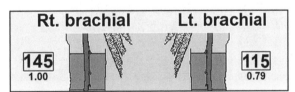

Abnormal pressure gradient indicating left subclavian artery occlusive disease.

This patient (above) had a brachial pressure difference of > 20 mmHg. The patient's subclavian and axillary arteries were imaged, as well as the vertebral artery; the latter had retrograde flow.

Left side evaluation

- Color duplex evaluation of the left subclavian artery is performed by placing a 5.0-9.0 MHz transducer superior to the clavicle and pointed in a caudal direction to identify the subclavian artery as it emerges from the thorax.

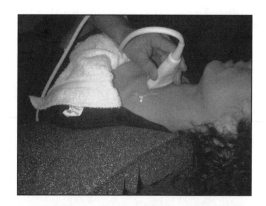

- Place the Doppler sample volume as proximal as possible in the artery (guided by color Doppler) and obtain spectral waveforms.

- In normal subclavian flow, the spectral waveform should be triphasic, or exhibit a high resistance flow pattern.

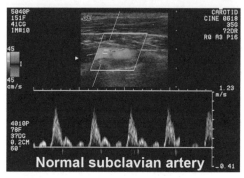

Normal subclavian artery

- Waveforms obtained from within a stenosis will display high velocities and more distally, spectral broadening indicative of post- stenotic turbulence. Depending on the severity of the stenosis, an abnormal waveform may persist in the distal subclavian and beyond.

- With a proximal left subclavian occlusion, spectral waveforms distal to the occlusion may not exhibit spectral broadening, but will be abnormal in contour, and often of the same morphology as the (retrograde) vertebral artery.

- Evaluate flow in the vertebral artery.

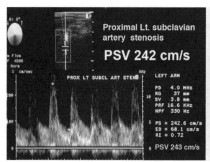
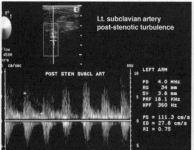
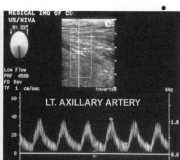

Proximal left subclavian stenosis followed by post-stenotic turbulence and an abnormal axillary artery waveform. Vertebral flow was retrograde- see below.

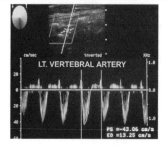

Right side evaluation

The right side exam differs somewhat from the left in than the innominate (brachio-cephalic) artery should be evaluated as well as the subclavian. Remember that the right common carotid artery (CCA) arises from the innominate artery. Just distal to the CCA takeoff, the vessel becomes the subclavian artery. Stenosis or occlusion in the innominate usually affects flow in the CCA as well as the subclavian artery.

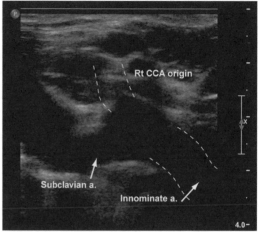

- Locate the innominate in the notch formed by the clavicle and the sternocleidomastoid muscle. Innominate waveforms will exhibit a low resistance pattern until the origin of the subclavian. The subclavian waveforms will appear to be high resistance.

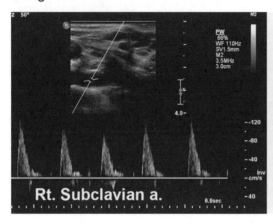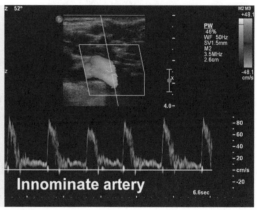

- Evaluate for stenosis and occlusion, and as on the left side, proceed distally along the subclavian artery.

- If innominate artery stenosis or occlusion is detected, evaluate flow in the proximal CCA and obtain Doppler waveforms.

> It's not necessary to routinely scan the innominate artery; only when the CCA, subclavian, or vertebral waveforms are abnormal on the right side.

- Evaluate flow in the vertebral artery and carefully note flow direction. Beware that flow may become retrograde in the proximal subclavian artery in the presence of right subclavian steal. See Chapter 4 on vertebral imaging for additional information.

Radial and Ulnar Arteries

A word of caution about "normal" radial and ulnar waveforms. Hand and digit perfusion is very vasoreactive; Doppler waveform morphology can change rapidly from a high resistance to low resistance, and vice versa, for no particular reason or known provocation. In general, flow into the hand is of high resistance, but the appearance of forward flow throughout the cardiac cycle in a radial or ulnar artery should not be cause for alarm. Images below demonstrate some variations in "normal" radial artery flow.

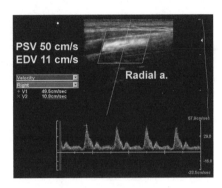
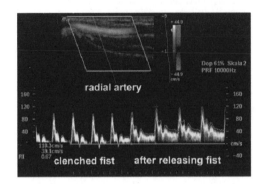

REFERENCES AND ADDITIONAL READING

Taylor DC, Jameson M, Semchuk J. Assessment of Arterial Compression In Patients With Suspected Thoracic Outlet Syndrome, Comparison Of Pressure Indices And Photoplethysmography. J Vasc Technol..13:158-160. July 1989

Harris J, Huang W, Tyrer P, Burnett A, May J. Clinical and Photoplethysmographic Assessment of Thoracic Outlet Arterial Compression. J Vasc Technol 13: 20-23, January 1989

CHAPTER 14: VASCULOGENIC IMPOTENCE

Impotence is a widespread problem that affects as many as one million American men. There are a variety of causes for erectile failure:

1. Hormonal imbalance.

2. Psychogenesis and neurogenic dysfunction.

3. Cavernosal venous leak.

4. Arterial insufficiency.

ANATOMY

Penile blood supply is derived from the:

*   Hypogastric artery.

*   Internal pudendal artery: to the base of the penis.

    Within the penis:
    *   Cavernosal arteries.
    *   Bulbourethral artery.
    *   Dorsal artery.

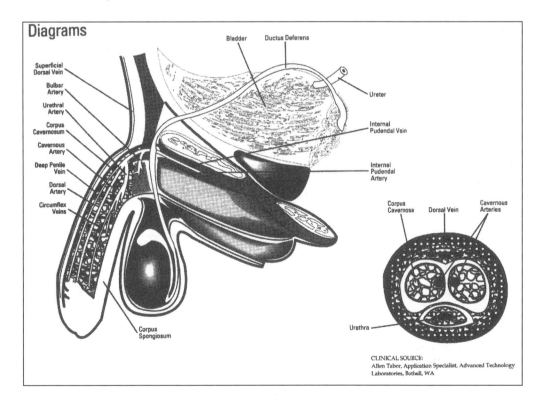

1. The cavernosal arteries supply blood to the main erectile tissue, the corpora cavernosa.

2. The bulbourethral arteries supply the more ventral corpus spongiosum.

3. The dorsal artery courses along the dorsum of the penis and supplies the skin , the glans and other non-erectile tissue.

4. The corpora cavernosa are two bodies consisting of multiple sinusoidal chambers and smooth muscle lying on the dorsal 2/3 of the penis. They are the main erectile tissue for the penis.

5. The sinusoidal chambers are encased in connective tissue called tunic albuginea.

The cavernosa are drained by the:
- Emissary veins.
- Circumflex veins.
- Deep dorsal.
- Internal pudendal vein.
- Hypogastric vein.

A single corpora spongiosum lies on the ventral side of the penis and contains the urethra.

PHYSIOLOGY IN FLACCID STATE

⇒   In a resting, flaccid state there is very little flow into the cavernosa.

⇒   Arterioles in the corpora cavernosa are constricted.

⇒   Contraction of smooth muscle cells in the walls of the sinusoids creates high resistance to inflow.

⇒   Blood courses through pre-cavernosal arterio -venous shunts.

PHYSIOLOGY OF ERECTION

During psycho-erotic stimulation:

⇒   Neurochemical stimulation and parasympathetic innervations produce smooth muscle cell relaxation within the sinusoids.

⇒   Relaxation of vasoconstriction within cavernosal arterioles.

⇒   Closing of pre-cavernous a-v shunts.

⇒   Blood flow increases into the corpora as resistance decreases.

⇒   Sinusoidal chambers distend.

⇒ Emissary veins within the cavernosa are compressed against the tunica albuginea.

⇒ Increased inflow and decreased outflow causes penile tumescence and rigidity.

⇒ With erection, flow resistance in the corpora cavernosa dramatically increases.

⇒ Normal erectile function requires, among other factors, sufficient arterial inflow *and* decreased venous outflow during tumescence.

⇒ An insufficient veno-occlusive mechanism resulting in a cavernosal "venous leak" is thought to be a major cause of impotence.

EXAM PROTOCOL

This protocol will describe two methods:

1. Penile pressure and waveform evaluation.
2. Intracavernosal injection of a vasodilatory agent, followed by color duplex imaging.

Patient history

Risk and contributing factors:
Does the patient have:

- Insulin dependent diabetes (DM).

- Hypertension.

- Peripheral arterial disease (PAD).

- Tobacco abuse.

- Arterial bypass surgeries.

- Prostatectomy.

Ask these questions regarding the patient's condition:

- Is the patient able to achieve an erection? Maintain it?

- Is the problem intermittent or persistent?

- Is the patient able to achieve erection during the night (Nocturnal tumescence)?

- How long has he had the symptoms?

This is a good time to explain the techniques that you'll be using.

Penile pressures and waveforms [1]

Physical exam

- Palpate pedal pulses and evaluate for apparent ischemic changes in feet that may signal the presence of peripheral arterial disease.

Rule out Peripheral Arterial Disease

- With the patient in a supine position obtain bilateral brachial and ankle systolic pressures and calculate ankle/brachial indices (ABI).

- An abnormal ABI should be followed with a full segmental exam or duplex scan to determine if aortoiliac artery disease is presence. This condition can reduce blood flow and pressure in the hypogastic arteries.

Penile Systolic Pressure

1. Apply an appropriately sized penile blood pressure cuff to the base of the penis and connect the cuff to a pressure manometer.

2. Apply acoustic gel to the penis just proximal to the glans and locate a dorsal artery with a hand-held CW-Doppler.

3. Inflate the cuff slowly keeping the probe over the artery to obliterate pulse signal.

4. Slowly deflate the cuff until the Doppler signal returns, and note the penile systolic pressure. Repeat the pressure measurement to assure reproducibility.

5. The penile pressure test may also be performed with PPG instead of Doppler.

Penile/Brachial Index (PBI)

Divide the penile pressure by the higher of the two brachial pressures to calculate this index.[1-3]

> 0.7 - 1.0 = normal.
> 0.6 - 0.7 = borderline abnormal.
> < 0.6   = abnormal.

Pulse Volume Recording (PVR)

1. Connect the penile cuff to the PVR instrument and inflate cuff to 60 mmHg.

2. Record several PVR waveforms.

3. A PVR waveform that is low in amplitude and rounded in contour is abnormal.

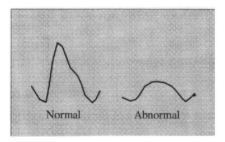

Normal   Abnormal

Photoplethysmography (PPG)

PPG waveforms are obtained with the sensor placed on the glans. Use appropriate gain or size setting and record several waveforms. These are evaluated in a similar fashion to the PVRs.

Reactive Hyperemia (Optional): Record PVR with 60 mmHg pressure in cuff. Inflate cuff to 20 mm Hg above penile systolic pressure for 5 minutes. Release the pressure, reinflate to 60 mmHg and record several PVRs. Amplitude of PVR's should increase by at least 15% over baseline amplitude. Note: this is an older test of dubious value.

EXAM PROTOCOL - DUPLEX IMAGING

Intracavernosal Injection of Papavarine

*   Position flaccid penis in a cephalid direction and place a 7.5 -12 MHz transducer on the ventral side of the penis.

*   Scan the entire penis in transverse and longitudinal views. Identify plaque or echogenic regions within the penis that may be consistent with Peyronne's disease, or other abnormalities.

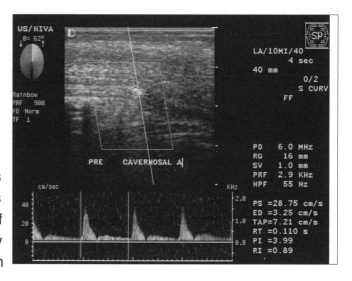

*   Identify both the corpora cavernosa and the cavernosal arteries proximally. The arteries have echogenic walls and are often tortuous. (Some labs attempt to measure the diameter of the cavernosal arteries, but accuracy is limited by the small size, 0.5 mm diameter, of a normal artery).

*   Record a PW Doppler waveform from each cavernosal artery proximally and measure peak systole velocity (PSV) and end diastole velocity (EDV).

Pre-injection Cavernosal Artery

Peak Systolic Velocity = 29 cm/sec

End Diastolic Velocity = 3 cm/sec

An intracavernosal injection of a potent vasodilatory agent (Prostaglandin E-1 or Papavarine (60 mg Papavarine in 2-5 ml) is performed by the patient or by a physician. A rubber band or penile blood pressure cuff is applied to the base of the penis for 2 minutes following injection, then removed.

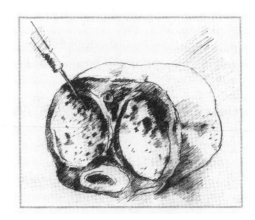

Following injection, cavernosal artery flow will increase temporarily as resistance decreases. There will be a corresponding increase in diastolic flow.

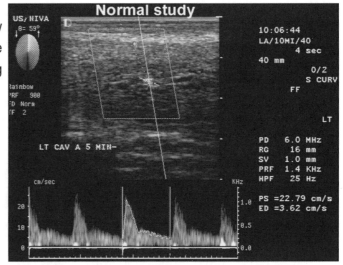

Five minutes post-papavarine injection
PSV = 23 cm/sec
EDV = 4 cm /sec

Obtain Doppler waveforms and measure PSV & EDV from the proximal cavernosal arteries at 5, 10, 15, 20 minutes after the injection.

Normal penile duplex criteria values during erectile state.[2]

• PSV >35 cm/sec.

- EDV < 5 cm/sec.

- 75% or greater increase in diameter.

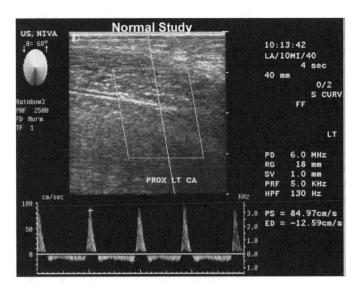

15 minutes post injection
PSV = 85 cm/sec
EDV = -13cm/sec

After full erection is achieved, diastolic velocities should decrease significantly, and flow in diastole often reverses direction due to the high resistance.

Normal erectile response should occur within 10 minutes, and erection should be maintained for 30 minutes.

Abnormal Values

- PSV < 25 cm/sec (insufficient arterial inflow).

- PSV > 35 cm/sec, but EDV is > 6 cm/sec, (venous leak should be suspected).

- Vessel diameter increase less than 75%.

⇒ If diastolic velocities are abnormal in the presence of an unsatisfactory erection, an appropriately-sized rubber band may be placed at the base of the penis, or a penile pressure cuff inflated to restrict venous outflow.

⇒ Remeasure diastolic velocity. If the velocity decreases and erection improves, venous leak is confirmed.

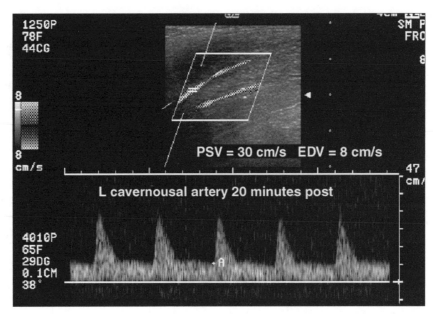

Abnormal, low resistance cavernousal waveform obtained 20 minutes after papavarine injection. Although the arterial inflow is sufficient in this patient, the venous" leak" is occuring, as demonstrated by the high diastolic flow. This prevents sustained erection.

A potential complication of Papavarine injection is priaprism. This is a painful condition is which erection does not subside. If left untreated, it can cause ischemic changes and tissue damage within the penis.

*Penile anatomy diagram courtesy of Allen Tabor

REFERENCES

1. Kempczinski RF, et al. Role of Vascular Diagnostic Laboratory in the evaluation of male impotence. Amer J Surg 138:278 -282, Aug. 1979

2. Bassioumy HS, Levine LA. Penile duplex sonography in the diagnosis of venogenic impotence. J Vasc Surg 1991;13:75-83

3. Stauffer D, DePalma RG. A comparison of penile-brachial index (PBI) and penile pulse volume recording (PVR) for diagnosis of vasculogenic impotence. Bruit 1983;7:29-32

4. DePalma RG, Emseilem HA , et al. A screening sequence for vasculogenic impotence. J Vasc Surgery 1987:5:28-36

CHAPTER 15: HEMODIALYSIS ACCESS FISTULAS & GRAFTS

Hemodialysis access is created to sustain patients with end-stage renal failure.
The purposes of this procedure are:

1. Pre-operative, to assess arterial inflow and to determine the suitability of efferent (outflow) veins for hemodialysis access creation.

2. Post-operatively, to assess fistulas and grafts for defects, stenosis or occlusion.

3. Evaluate the access for aneurysms, pseudoaneurysms and perigraft abscess.

INDICATIONS FOR THE EXAM:

- Pre-op assessment
- Distal limb ischemia
- Absence of fistula palpable "thrill"
- Peri-graft fluids or mass

- Poor dialysis
- Elevated pressures during dialysis
- Access recirculation of 12% or greater
- Unexplained urea reduction ratio < 60%
- Difficult cannulation or thrombus aspiration

TYPES OF ACCESS

Central venous catheter

- IJV or subclavian vein insertion
- Temporary-short term solution, sometimes tunneled

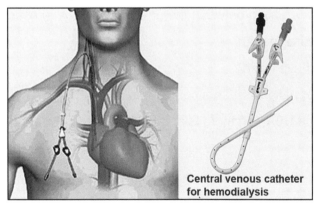

Central venous catheter for hemodialysis

Native Access Fistula

Brescia-Cimino Fistula

- This arterial to venous fistula is usually created in the non-dominant arm.
- Radial artery to cephalic vein fistula is the most common.

- Brachial artery to cephalic or basilic vein fistula is also common.

- Arterial-Venous Fistulas (AVF) are autogenous and known for long term patency, and low complication rate.

- AVF must be allowed to "mature" prior to use, otherwise adequate flow volume may not occur.

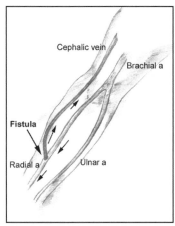

Brescia-Cimino fistula.

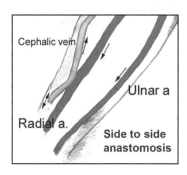

Brescia-Cimino fistula, side to side anastomosis.

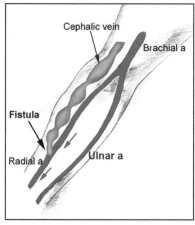

Brescia-Cimino fistula after time due to intraluminal pressure.

- When a fistula is created, the superficial efferent vein, once the fistula has "matured," is used for dialysis puncture. This vein often becomes "lumpy" and sausage shaped due to increased intraluminal pressure.

- Flow volumes are difficult to obtain in the efferent vein due to inconsistent vein diameter.

Access Grafts

- A synthetic tube graft is placed between the artery and vein and used for dialysis puncture.

- Used when veins are inadequate.

- Useful when fistulas have failed.

- Approximately 50% of patients are not candidates for AVF.

- Favored method in the USA, but there is a trend towards fistula creation.

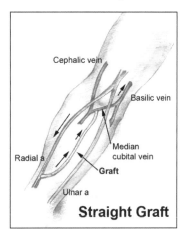

Straight Graft

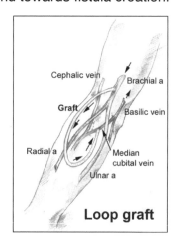

Loop graft

- The graft may be straight or looped, and usually made of Teflon (polytetrafluoroethylene) (PTFE), commercially known as Gore-Tex.

- They may be tapered at the arterial end to reduce flow volume.

- Polyurethane grafts are also used. These can be used soon after implantation as they do not require maturation time. They're also self-sealing.

  ⇒ NOTE: Ultrasound does not penetrate polyurethane grafts (Vectra).

- Grafts tend to have shorter patency rates than fistulas.

- Grafts and fistulas are usually created initially in the forearm. When they fail, the more proximal vasculature is used to create new access.

Other Access Locations

♦ Brachial artery to basilic vein graft.

♦ Subclavian artery to jugular vein graft.

♦ Superficial femoral artery to great saphenous vein loop graft.

PREOPERATIVE PROCEDURE

Arterial Requirements

- Adequate arterial inflow (pressure differential between arms should be less than 20 mmHg).

- Patent palmar arch.

- Arterial lumen diameter >2.0 mm or greater at the point of anastomosis.

Evaluate Arterial Inflow

⇒ Obtain bilateral arm pressures.

⇒ Scan the brachial and radial arteries to look for occlusion, stenoses, and anomalous anatomy.

⇒ Pay careful attention to the brachial bifurcation into the radial and ulnar arteries, and note a common variant: the bifurcation occurring in mid-humeral region rather than in the antecubital fossa.

⇒ In transverse plane measure the inside diameter of the distal radial artery. If < 2.0 mm, scan proximally and locate a segment that is at least 2.0 mm in diameter.

⇒ Identify and note any regions of calcification within the artery.

⇒ Assess the patency of the palmar arch in the hand with the Allen test. (See arterial upper extremity chapter or arterial bypass graft chapter).

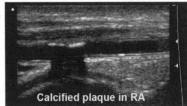

Calcified plaque in RA

Venous Requirements for AVF and Grafts

- For an AVF, vein luminal diameter of ≥ 2.5 mm (with or without tourniquet) at anastomosis point.[1]
- For a dialysis graft, the vein should be ≥4 mm at the anastomotic site.[1]
- Absence of obstruction.
- Straight vein segment for cannulation.
- Vein is within 1 cm of the skin surface.
- Continuity with proximal central veins.
- No central venous outflow obstruction.

Evaluate the Entire Venous Outflow Tract

⇒   Determine presence and patency of the basilic, cephalic, median cubital, axillary, subclavian and innominate veins, or any other veins that may be the recipient of the graft (IJV, GSV, etc.). Note: the brachial veins are rarely used for hemodialysis access.

⇒   Use ultrasound compression methods for the arm veins, and evaluate subclavian vein waveforms with bilateral comparison to rule out subclavian and innominate vein obstruction.

⇒   Are the veins free of defects, residual thrombus or sclerotic?

⇒   Measure the diameter of the cephalic vein and basilic veins in the forearm. If necessary, use a tourniquet (latex glove or Penrose drain) on the upper arm to dilate superficial veins.

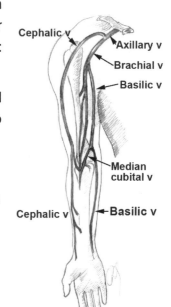

Graft and Fistula Complications

- Thrombosis/occlusion.
- Stenosis:
  - ⇒ Proximal and distal anastomoses.
  - ⇒ Within graft.
  - ⇒ In venous outflow tract, due to intimal hyperplasia or thrombus.
- Arterial steal; may result in digit or hand ischemia.
- Distal venous hypertension.
- Aneurysms and pseudoaneurysms (common).
- Elevated right side heart pressure due to excessive graft flow.
- Infection (mostly with synthetic grafts).

POSTOPERATIVE PROTOCOL- GENERAL CONSIDERATIONS

NOTE: DO NOT TAKE A BLOOD PRESSURE OVER A SYNTHETIC GRAFT

- Determine the location of the fistula, or the type and course of the graft, by patient history or from medical records.

- Determine the indication for the exam. Often the patient will know of problems with dialysis or with their access sites. If not, contact the referring physician or staff.

- Visually examine the graft/fistula location and note puncture sites and lumps.

- Palpate any lumps to determine if they are pulsatile (possible pseudoaneurysms).

COLOR DUPLEX PROTOCOL

Preparation

- Use a transducer with suitable frequency for the depth of the graft/fistula. Some superficial access sites may require a 7.5 - 12 MHz range transducer.

- If access site is bleeding, use plastic wrap, Tegaderm, or a transducer cover and sterile gel.

- Introduce yourself, and explain the exam procedure to the patient.

- Allow plenty of time for the test (60 minutes).

General Ultrasound Survey

1. Perform a general "survey" scan, beginning in transverse orientation, from the upper brachial to the distal radial artery. Identify the origin of the graft or fistula arising from one of these two arteries.

2. Next, perform a survey scan of the graft and outflow vein, or the fistula vein.

3. Repeat the survey in longitudinal plane.

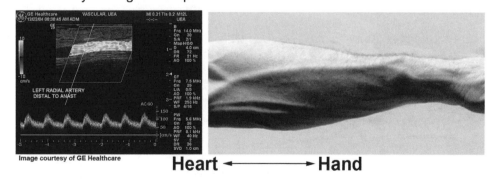

Image courtesy of GE Healthcare

Heart ◄─────► Hand

Helpful Hint: Image orientation: keep the hand (distal) to the <u>right</u> on the ultrasound image. When following a loop graft you'll have to invert the image to maintain this orientation once you've scanned past the distal curve or loop. Without an image "standard", blood flow direction can become very confusing!!

Doppler Exam

4. Evaluate arterial inflow just proximal to the graft or fistula. Doppler waveforms should demonstrate low resistance, i.e., high diastolic flow, as seen in the left image below. High resistance in the brachial or radial artery flow proximal to a graft or AVF is a sign of graft/fistula occlusion or severe stenosis.

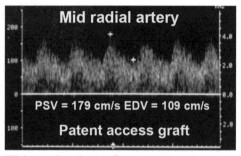

This patient's graft was patent.

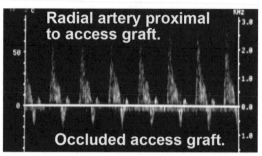

This patient had an occluded graft.

5. Assess arterial flow beyond the distal anastomosis. Flow should be antegrade and demonstrate high resistance.

> NOTE: It is common to find retrograde flow in the radial artery distal to a graft/fistula near the wrist. This "steal" may be asymptomatic if the palmar arch is intact and ulnar artery flow is adequate. Compress the ulnar artery while monitoring the distal radial artery flow; the RA flow will often resort to an antegrade direction.

6. Retrograde flow in the brachial artery distal to the anastomosis will often cause symptoms distally.

7. Carefully assess the proximal anastomosis, the entire graft, and distal anastomosis for stenosis, and of course, occlusion.

8. Record systolic velocities in the proximal, mid and distal graft.

    ⇒ Obtain and record velocity before, at, and after any areas of flow disturbance.

    ⇒ Compare velocities at the distal end of graft to those at the efferent anastomotic site.

    ⇒ Pay close attention to regions within the graft that have been punctured.

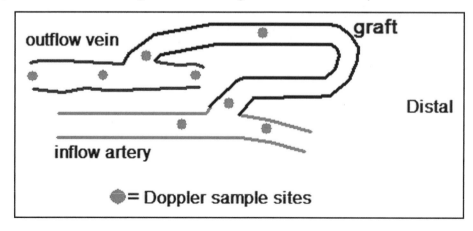

Note. Stenosis in the distal (efferent) anastomosis or AV fistula (Brescia-Cimino) is not uncommon. Ermers et al.,[2] demonstrated >50% stenoses in 72% of new (within one month) fistulas and 80% of new grafts. However, there was no significant relationship between stenotic lesions and graft occlusion. Other investigators have confirmed a high percentage of grafts and fistulas with subclinical 50% stenoses.[1,3]

9. Evaluate the efferent vein for stenosis at these sites:

⇒ Just proximal or cephalad to the anastomosis. This is usually the site of stenosis caused by neo-intimal hyperplasia.

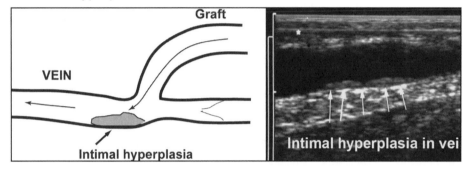

⇒ Vein stenosis is more likely to occur with a graft than a fistula.

⇒ Distal (caudal) to vein anastomosis. Check flow direction, as it's common to have flow reverse back down into the limb under high arterial pressure. This increased venous pressure in itself may cause symptoms, particularly edema in the hand.

⇒ Evaluate the outflow vein to the proximal subclavian artery for stenosis.

10. Obtain a flow volume measurement within graft (optional).

Flow Volume Method-Access Graft

• Select a "clean" intraluminal site with the graft.

• In transverse view, measure the inside diameters of the graft; do this with color Doppler off. The diameter measurement can be converted to area by the US system.

• In longitudinal view, place the sample volume in the region from which the diameter was measured. Expand the sample volume to equal the size of the diameter of the graft.

• Obtain several spectral waveforms, and with system software, obtain a "time average velocity", or TAV, that is, a measurement of the instantaneous AVERAGE, or mean velocity over time. *Some instrumentation will only allow a time average of PEAK velocity. This measurement is acceptable, but flow volume calculations will read a bit high compared to the average of the <u>mean</u> velocities over time.*

• Using system software or manual calculation, determine flow volume.

Patient with recent revision of left radial artery to basilic vein straight PTFE graft.

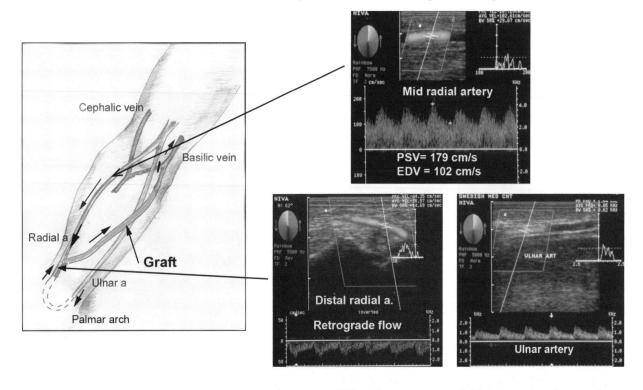

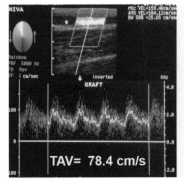

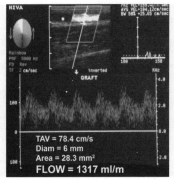

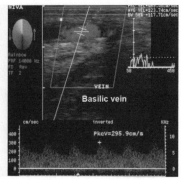

Time average velocity (TAV) within graft.

Based on graft TAV and diameter/area measurement, flow volume is 1317 ml/min.

Normal basilic vein outflow

Normal, functioning dialysis access graft with high flow volume (1317 ml/min). Ulnar artery is perfusing the hand, and retrograde flow exists in the radial artery distal to the graft origin.

Flow Volume (Q) in ml/minute
Q = graft area x TAV x 60 second

11. Obtain 2 or 3 flow volume measurements and compare for consistency.

12. Assess perigraft/fistula tissue for:

⇒ Hematomas (usually old pseudoaneurysms that have thrombosed).

⇒ Pseudoaneurysms (PA) are common and result from dialysis puncture. Measure the PA:

if less than 5 mm they tend to remain stable. If > 5 mm, they should be carefully followed or surgically repaired.

⇒ Aneurysm- more likely to occur in AVF than grafts.

⇒ Seromas- These appear as peri-graft fluid collections and result from serum filtering through the graft wall. Usually a benign condition, as long as there is no extrinsic compression on the graft.

⇒ Infection/ abscess- This perigraft fluid collection can resemble a seroma. Confirmation of infection usually requires analysis of aspirated fluid.

13. Assess for arterial steal.

- High flow into a graft or fistula can cause the distal arterial flow to reverse and "steal" perfusion from the hand and fingers. If the patient has symptoms of **arterial steal**, it will be necessary to assess perfusion distally in the hand or fingers. Use indirect testing methods as an adjunct to color duplex.

  - Obtain pulse volume recording (PVR) or photoplethysmography (PPG) waveforms on all digits and compare to asymptomatic hand.

  - Obtain digital pressures and compare to the asymptomatic hand. Digit pressures lower than 60 mmHg usually result in ischemic symptoms.

  - If possible, temporarily occlude fistula while obtaining PVR / PPG waveforms and see if their amplitudes increase.

- Surgical revision of the graft, fistula or distal artery may be required to alleviate the digit ischemia.

> NOTE: Patients on long term dialysis often have multiple grafts or fistulas configured, as the duration of patency is not long. Surgical solutions can be very creative.

INTERPRETATION

Normal

Grafts and fistulas have very high systolic velocities (100-400 cm/sec), high diastolic velocity (60-200 cm/sec), high flow, and low resistance.

The flow pattern may be disorganized with spectral broadening. Normal high flow volumes may be maintained in the presence of venous stenosis, if there is retrograde flow in vein tributaries distal to the efferent anastomosis.

Occlusion

- No flow detected in graft with color or spectral Doppler.

- No flow in efferent vein distal to fistula.

- High resistance in artery leading into the graft or fistula.

- Low venous outflow.

Note: recently created access grafts may contain air in the wall of the synthetic material for a few days. The Doppler signal may not penetrate the graft wall and this could lead to a false determination of occlusion. In this case, rely on information from the inflow and outflow vessels.

Ultrasound criteria for graft and fistula stenosis include stenosis by B-mode image, peak systolic velocity, velocity ratios and flow volumes. Because the hemodynamic effect of a particular narrowing varies with flow volume, velocity criteria is not precise for estimating a 50% stenosis. Some investigators report a 2:1 ratio for a ≥ 50% stenosis[4,5] whereas others use a 3:1 ratio for a ≥50% stenosis.[3,7] Flow volumes, however, have been correlated a fistula's ability to mature or to fail. Ultrasound-derived flow volume measurements are perhaps more accurate when obtained in a graft than in a fistula, as the area measurement component in a dilated vein tends to be imprecise.

Criteria for > 50% GRAFT stenosis

- Peak systolic velocity > 400 cm/sec [3,6]

- Velocity ratio ≥ 2:1[4]

- Or velocity ratio ≥ 3:1[3]

> The velocity ratio was determined by comparing the velocity at the area of suspected stenosis with the velocity just proximal to the area of suspected stenosis.

Criteria for > 50% FISTULA stenosis

- Peak systolic velocity ≥ 400 cm/sec [3,7]

- Velocity ratio ≥ 2:1[5] or ≥ 3:1.[3,5,7] (Anastomotic stenosis PSV / radial artery PSV). For outflow cephalic vein, ratio of ≥ 3:1.[7]

- Velocity values may be unreliable due to variations in vein diameter.

- A velocity measurement limitation occurs when estimating Doppler angle in a tortuous fistula's anastomosis.[2]

Graft Flow Volumes (milliliters/minute)

Flow volume parameters vary considerably and there is no specific "cutoff point" for normal versus abnormal. However, low volume interferes with dialysis and will result in graft or fistula failure.

Access Grafts

< 350 ml/min = poor dialysis, pending graft failure.[10]

< 500 ml/min = increased risk of graft failure.[8]

> 800 ml/min = normal flow range.[9]

> 1500 ml/min = possible congestive heart failure.

AV Fistula

> 500 ml/ min with 4 mm outflow vein = adequate dialysis.[10]

> 800 ml/ min =normal.[9]

In summation, duplex ultrasound can be a valuable tool in assessing AV fistulas and grafts for stenosis, defects and occlusion. There are a lot of "gaps" in understanding which stenoses are more likely to go on to occlude the graft and which ones will remain stable. Quantitative values have been established for > 50% stenosis in grafts but velocity values are less efficient in quantifying fistula stenoses. Flow volume calculations are performed at some institutions, but are not universally accepted as a method for fistula evaluation.

REFERENCES

1. Silva MB, Hobson RW, Pappas PJ, et al. A strategy for increasing use of autogenous hemodialysis access procedures: impact of preoperative noninvasive evaluation Our results show a high percentage of subclinical access graft stenoses. J Vasc Surg 1998; 27: 302–8

2. Ermers EJM, Langeveld AP, et al. Duplex ultrasound detection in newly created hemodialysis AV fistulas: Its significance in relation to fistula complications. J Vasc Technol 16(6):295-297,19

3. Older RA, Gizienski TA, Wilkowski MJ, Angle JF, Cote DA. Hemodialysis access stenosis : Early detection with Color Doppler US. Radiology 1998;207:161-164

4. Robbins ML, Oser R F, Allon M, Clements M W, Dockery J, Weber T M, Hamrick-Waller K M, Smith J K, Jones B C, Morgan D E, Saddekni S. Hemodialysis access stenosis: US detection. Radiology 1998:208: 655-661

5. Grogan J, Castilla MC, Lozanski L, Griffin A, Loth F, Bassiouny H. Frequency of critical stenosis in primary arteriovenous fistulae before hemodialysis access: Should duplex ultrasound surveillance be the standard of care? J Vasc Surg. 41;6: P 1000-1006 (June 2005)

6   Dumars MC, Thompson WE, Bluth EI, Lindberg JS, Yoselevitz M, Merritt CR. Management of Suspected Hemodialysis Graft Dysfunction: Usefulness of Diagnostic US Radiology 2002;222:103-107.

7. Chao AKH, Daley T , Gruenewald S, et al. Duplex Ultrasound Crteria for Assessment of Stenoses in Radiocephalic Hemodialysis Fistulas. (Sensitivity for 10 lesions at anastomoses, 100%, Specificity 96%, overall Accuracy 97% if both criteria were used). J Vasc Technol 25(4):203-208,2001

8. Bay WH, Henry ML, Lazarus JM, Lew NL, Ling J, Lowrie EG. Predicting Hemodialysis Access Failure with Color Flow Doppler Ultrasound .Am J Nephrol 1998;18:296-304

9. Back MR, Maynard M, Winkler A, Bandyk, DF. Expected Flow Parameters Within Hemodialysis Access and Selection for Remedial Intervention of Nonmaturing Conduits Vascular and Endovascular Surgery, Vol. 42, No. 2, 150-158 (2008)

10. Robbin ML, Chamberlain NE, Lockhart ME, et al. Hemodialysis arteriovenous fistula maturity: US evaluation. Radiology 225:59-64, 2002

Other reading-references

♦ Comeaux ME, Bryant PS, Harkrider WW. Preoperative evaluation of the renal access patients with color Doppler Imaging. J Vasc.Technol 17(5):247-250,1993

♦ Finlay DE, Longley DG, Foshager MC, Letourneau JG. Duplex and color Doppler sonography of hemodialysis A-V fistulas and grafts. Radiographics 1993;13:983-999

♦ Haimov M. Vascular Access: A Practical Guide. Textbook, Mount Kisco, NY, Futura Publishing 1987

♦ Beathard Guide to AVFs : A Practitioner's Resource Guide To Hemodialysis Arteriovenous Fistulas. Fistula First Distributed by: End Stage Renal Disease Network of Texas, Inc. 14114 Dallas Parkway #660, Dallas, Texas 75254 http://www.esrdnetwork.org/

CHAPTER 16: TRANSCRANIAL DOPPLER

Introduction

Transcranial Doppler (TCD) for the noninvasive evaluation of intracranial circulation was first performed by Rune Aaslid and colleagues in 1982.[1] The original clinical utility was found in serial monitoring of MCA flow velocities during cerebral arterial vasospasm.

Traditional TCD is performed with what is referred to as "the free-hand" method. This is a non-imaging method that uses a 2.0 MHz pulsed-wave Doppler with FFT spectral analysis. The operator identifies and differentiates the cerebral vascular anatomy by knowledge of depth, mean velocity and flow direction relative to the Doppler beam. These systems are less expensive and more portable than transcranial color imaging systems described below. This is an advantage in the crowded operating room suite, and for mobile or bedside applications.

Advances in ultrasound imaging technology now allow visualization of the Circle of Willis in many patients with real-time color Doppler. This technique, using 1.8 - 2.5 MHz transducers, enables the user to actually visualize the location and course of the intracranial vessels and allows an accurate placement of the Doppler sample volume for spectral analysis. Transcranial Color Imaging, or TCI, requires somewhat less skill than the traditional non-imaging technique and this is advantageous for those who perform the exam infrequently. TCI transducers, however, have a larger "footprint" than the non imaging, or "free-hand" probes and when they're placed over a small cranial window, the Doppler sensitivity is often reduced. This may result in a higher technical failure rate compared to traditional TCD. Both methods will be discussed in this chapter.

"Free-hand" non-imaging TCD method.

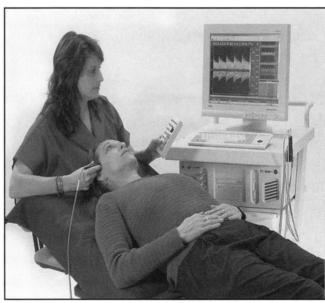

Image courtesy of Cardinal Health

APPLICATIONS OF TCD AND TCI

- Serial monitoring of MCA and other intracranial vessels for vasospasm.

- Evaluation of intracranial aneurysm and arterio-venous malformation.

- Basilar artery occlusion.

- Intracranial ICA stenosis.

- Adjunct to extracranial carotid duplex exam.

- Monitoring vasospastic effect of sickle cell anemia.

- Confirmation of brain death.

EXCLUSIVE APPLICATIONS OF TCD

- Microemboli detection during carotid endarterectomy, coronary bypass surgery, and carotid PTA/stenting.

- Cerebral autoregulation- vasomotor reactivity to CO2 (TCD).

- Detection of patent foramen ovale (PFO).

- Monitoring of real-time blood flow to the brain during a variety of surgical procedures allowing for timely intervention to flow changes.

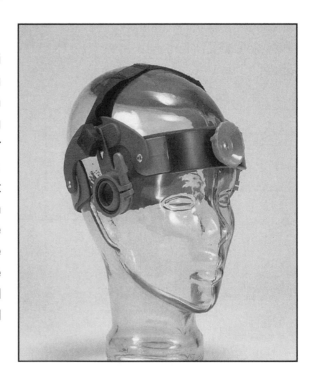

Transcranial surveillance for micro-emboli and CO_2 reactivity typically is performed using bilateral TCD transducers that monitor both hemispheres simultaneously, and record long periods of spectral Doppler information. For emboli monitoring in carotid endarterectomy, one TCD transducer may be used, but it must be held in place with an attachment system similar to that used in bilateral monitoring. These attachment systems are not currently available for transcranial color imaging transducers. The 2 MHz transducers are inserted into the lateral probe holders and adjusted to receive signal from the MCAs.

CEREBROVASCULAR ANATOMY

The internal carotid artery (ICA) is divided into segments:

♦ Cervical ICA

⇒ Extends from the carotid bifurcation to the carotid canal of the petrous portion of the temporal bone.

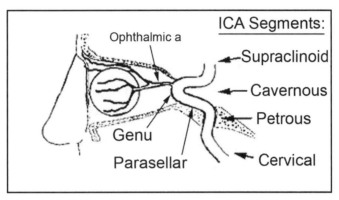

♦ Petrous ICA

⇒ Courses through the petrous portion of the temporal bone and is inaccessible to ultrasound.

♦ Cavernous ICA, also known as the carotid siphon, consists of:

⇒ Parasellar portion.

⇒ Genu portion (the bend).

⇒ Supraclinoid portion (distal segment).

♦ The first major branch of the ICA is the ophthalmic artery (OA): it arises from the cavernous portion of the ICA.

♦ The middle cerebral artery (MCA) and anterior cerebral artery (ACA) bifurcate from the terminus of the ICA.

Middle cerebral arteries (MCA)

♦ Course laterally towards the temporal bone with a number of branches.

♦ Carry 75-80% of ICA flow.

♦ Larger than the ACAs.

♦ M1 segment- from the MCA origin to the first branch.

♦ M2 segment, MCA distal to the first branch.

Anterior cerebral arteries (ACA)

♦ Course medially towards the midbrain (A1 segment).

♦ Give rise to the anterior communicating artery (AcoA). This vessel courses between the two ACAs.

♦ A2 segment then courses anteriorly to supply the anterior segments of the brain.

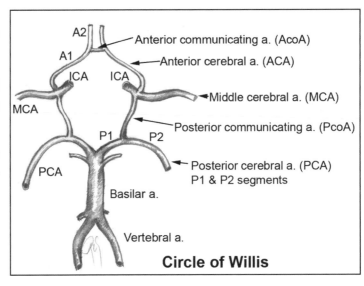

Circle of Willis

Vertebral-Basilar system- Vertebral arteries

♦ Arise from the subclavian arteries.

♦ Course between the transverse processes of the spine.

♦ Enter the skull at the foramen magnum.

♦ Intracranial branches include:

⇒ Anterior spinal artery.

⇒ Posterior inferior cerebellar artery (PICA).

Posterior and anterior communicating arteries provide collateral pathways within the circle of Willis. In the presence of an ICA occlusion, flow from the contralateral ACA can "cross-fill" via the anterior communicating artery, and course retrograde in the ipsilateral ACA to supply the MCA and the lateral hemisphere.

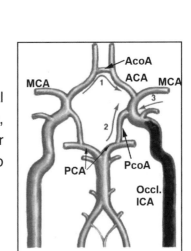

Other collateral pathways that may develop with ICA occlusion include retrograde flow in the supraorbital and supratrochlear arteries, branches of the ophthalmic artery. This pathway reconstitutes the supraclinoid segment of the ICA with blood flow being supplied by communicating ECA branches.

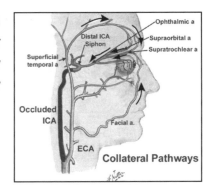

Collateral Pathways

Basilar artery

♦ Formed by the confluence of the 2 intracranial vertebral arteries.

♦ Approximately 3 cm long.

♦ Bifurcates into two posterior cerebral arteries (PCA).

Posterior cerebral arteries (PCA)

♦ Perfuse the posterior hemispheres.

♦ Wrap around the cerebral peduncle.

♦ P1 segment – origin to the posterior communicating arteries (PCoA). The PCoA connects to the anterior circulation.

♦ P2 segment -distal to the PCoA.

⇒ Anatomical variation of the circle of Willis is common. It has been estimated that only 50 percent of people have an intact and functioning circle of Willis, and only 25% have this classic configuration shown above.

⇒ In up to 25% of the population the PCA arises from the ICA.

⇒ In up to 25% the A1 segment of the ACA is atretic or hypoplastic.

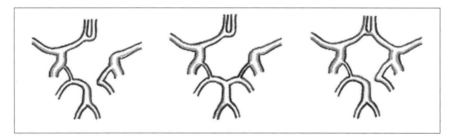

Typical anatomic variations in the Circle of Willis.

⇒ The anterior communicating and posterior communicating arteries can allow cross filling and collateralization in the presence of ICA obstruction.

⇒ Those patients without a functioning circle of Willis may suffer more profound neurologic ischemia in the presence of ICA obstruction.

TCD ACCESS WINDOWS

Transtemporal window

• Over the temporal bone superior to the zygomatic arch.

- Only 35% or less of transmitted ultrasound energy passes through this window.

- In 10% of the population there is no ultrasound penetration due a thickened bone segment (hyperostosis).

Vessels identified from this window:

- Middle cerebral artery (MCA).

- Anterior cerebral artery (ACA).

- Posterior cerebral artery (PCA).

- Terminal internal carotid artery (TICA).

- PCoA and ACoA may be identified if functioning as collateral pathways.

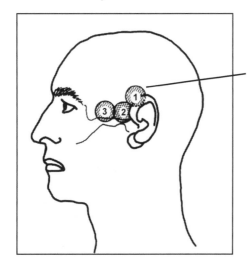

Transtemporal windows, potential locations:

1. posterior
2. middle
3. anterior

Transorbital - through the eye

- ICA siphon

- Ophthalmic artery (OA)

Suboccipital - Foramen Magnum

- Vertebral arteries (VA)

- Basilar artery (BA)

BASIC TCD TECHNIQUE

MCA

- Patient in supine position, operator at head of the bed if possible.

- Apply gel to the temporal region and place transducer against the skull in the posterior transtemporal position shown above.

- Set sample volume (SV) depth to 50 mm.

> NOTE: The TCD sample gate is typically quite large, 5-15 mm in length. Consequently, there is no spectral "window" or "envelope" similar to that found in waveforms in extracranial carotid duplex imaging. Additionally, with the large sample volume, flow from more than one artery is often seen in the spectral display, e.g., the MCA-ACA bifurcation.

- Use a "flashlight" technique, keeping the face of the transducer stationary while the back end of the probe is moved back and forth in small increments to locate the MCA, (flow towards transducer, mean velocity about 60 cm/s).

- Once a Doppler signal has been established, try to optimize the signal while staying on the artery.

- Try the anterior and middle temporal acoustic windows to either gain or improve the MCA signal; always observe for the highest velocity window.

- Once the optimum signal is established interrogate the course of the MCA by "stepping" the Doppler sample gate to a shallow depth, then increase SV depth to the MCA-ACA bifurcation (at approximately 5.5 - 6.5 cm depth in normal adults).

- MCA flow direction should be towards the transducer and displayed above spectral baseline.

- Record representative spectra and measure peak systolic velocity, mean velocity and any other desired parameters.

- In normal subjects the MCA flow velocity will be higher than the ACA and the ACA higher than the PCA.

Typical MCA velocity and depth are listed below-next page.

> NOTE: <u>Mean</u> velocity values are used in both TCD and TCI. The "mean" velocity is a mean of the peak velocities over time, sometimes referred to as TAMX, (Time Average Max). Although TCI allows for Doppler angle correction, most of the mean velocity criteria in use have been derived with the assumption that the Doppler angle was zero. So if you use that criteria, adjust the Doppler angle cursor to zero and leave it there.

MCA-ACA Bifurcation

- Identify the MCA-ACA bifurcation at a SV depth of approximately 5.5- 6.5 mm.

- Flow should be bi-directional.

- This signal serves as an excellent "landmark" for the remaining exam.

ACA

- From the bifurcation increase the SV depth and optimize the signal at each step to follow the course of the ACA.

- Flow should away be from the transducer and below baseline. (Don't invert the spectrum unless it is necessitated by your instrumentation for flow velocity measurements).

- Velocities will ordinarily be less than the MCA.

- Record representative spectra and measure waveform parameters as above.

- Follow the ACA to midline depths of 7.5 - 8.0 cm.

Step the sample volume back to the location of the MCA-ACA bifurcation.
Next, locate the terminal ICA.

TICA

- Direct the transducer slightly inferior keeping the SV at the same depth for the bifurcation.

- The TICA flow should be towards the transducer and it will be low in frequency due to poor angle of insonation.

PCA

- Start at the bifurcation and aim the transducer posteriorly (first) then inferiorly. Keep the SV at same depth initially. Once a signal is identified increase the SV depth to approximately 75 mm.

- Flow in this P1 segment should be towards the transducer.

- The P2 segment is not typically part of the "normal" exam. It is identified with a more posterior aim: flow will be initially bidirectional, then, with increased SV depth, away from the transducer.

Typical Depths and Flow direction from Transtemporal Window			
Artery	Depth of SV	Flow direction	Mean velocity
MCA	3.0 - 6.0 cm	towards	55 ± 12 cm/s
MCA/ACA	5.5 - 6.5 cm	bidirectional	
ACA (A1)	6.0 - 8.0 cm	away	50 ± 11 cm /s
PCA (P1)	6.0 - 7.0 cm	towards	39 ± 10 cm/s
TICA	5.5 - 6.5 cm	towards	39 ± 9 cm/s

Transient oscillation of the ipsilateral and contralateral common carotid arteries while performing TCD may be useful in identifying intracranial anatomy and disease states. *The extracranial carotid should be first interrogated with duplex ultrasound prior to CCA oscillation to identify any potential risks.*

CCA oscillations are usually sufficient. However, in some instances the CCA can be compressed low in the neck for a few cardiac cycles. Compressions may be useful in scenarios in which the contralateral ACA is cross-filling to the ipsilateral MCA. Also, pre-operative determinations of adequate MCA collateral flow with ipsilateral CCA compression may aid in determining whether carotid shunting is required in carotid TEA. However, this method is rarely used today.

Suboccipital Window
Vertebral – basilar arteries (BA)

- Optimal patient position is with the patient lying on his/her side with a pillow under the head and the chin tucked slightly to the chest.

- Place the transducer to one side of midline and about 1 inch below the base of the skull.

- Start with a SV depth of 60 mm and aim at the bridge of the nose.

- Flow should be away from the transducer. If a signal is not detected move the transducer more laterally.

- Follow the course of the VA to the basilar artery at a depth of approximately 80-90 mm.

- Record and measure velocity from both the BA and the VA as above, and follow the BA to its maximum depth of 120 mm.

- Repeat with process on the contralateral VA.

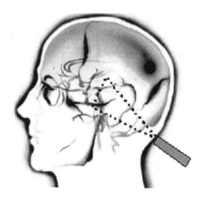

suboccipital window

Typical Depths & Flow Direction - Suboccipital Window			
Artery	Depth of SV	Flow direction	Mean Velocity
Vertebral	6.0 - 9.0 cm	away	38 ± 10 cm/s
Basilar	8.0 - 12 cm	away	41 ± 10 cm/s

Ophthalmic artery (OA), ICA – Siphon - Transorbital Window

NOTE: The system transmit power should be reduced for this approach to prevent damage to the eye.

*   Place the transducer over closed eyelid and aim in a slight posterior direction and slightly towards midline.

*   Set the SV to 50 mm for the OA. The OA supplies a high resistant vascular bed and will have a higher pulsatility than the ICA with mean velocity of about 21 cm/s. Flow should be towards the transducer.

*   Step the SV along the length of the OA to the ICA at approximately 55-70 mm depth. There is wide variation in the depth of the ICA and the examiner should carefully observe a decrease in pulsatility as the ICA is encountered, (i.e., increase in diastolic flow velocity).

Typical Depths & Flow Direction - Transorbital Window			
Artery	Depth of SV	Flow Direction	Mean Velocity
OA	4.0 - 6.0 cm	towards	21 ± 5 cm/s
Carotid Siphon	5.5 - 8.0 cm		
supraclinoid		away	41 ± 11 cm/s
genu		bidirectional	
parasellar		towards	47 ± 14 cm/s

*   ICA flow at the "S" shaped siphon may be towards, bidirectional or away depending on whether the SV is in the parasellar, genu or supraclinoid segments respectively.

*   Record and measure waveforms as above.

TRANSCRANIAL COLOR IMAGING

TCI and TCD methods use the same access windows. TCI allows the operator to identify anatomic landmarks on the 2-D image and then adjust color parameters to optimize frame rate, sensitivity, PRF and depth penetration. The sample volume of the spectral Doppler can be selectively placed to record mean velocities from the intracranial vasculature. Although it is possible to adjust the angle cursor to obtain an angle corrected velocity at any location, it's probably best to set the cursor to zero degrees. Angle correction in the MCA or basilar artery would not dramatically alter the velocity values, as these vessels are within 10-20 degrees of the Doppler beam, but this is not the case with the ACA, or PCA.

TCI ANATOMY

From the transtemporal window:

- Arrange transducer in the longitudinal plane with the anterior (front of head) to the left on the ultrasound image.

- Optimize the gray scale image parameters. Field of view should be set to 12-14 cm.

- Identify the temporal lobe, and the bony intracranial structures demonstrated below.

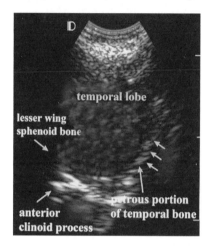 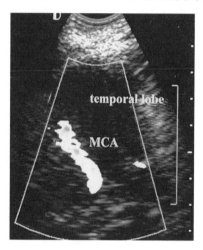

- The MCA will course along the anterior side of the temporal lobe.

- Adjust color Doppler or power Doppler parameters to "illuminate" MCA and other vessels.

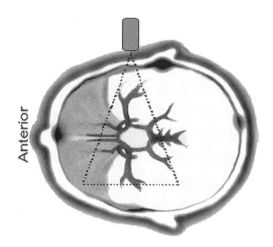 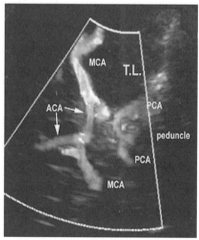

Diagram of TCI anatomy from transtemporal window.

- Place the Doppler sample volume in the ipsilateral MCA and interrogate the entire length.

- Increase the sample volume depth to evaluate the MCA - ACA bifurcation and the ACA. As in TCD, do not use the spectral invert control unless it's warranted for Doppler measurements. Some systems will only perform Doppler calculations on waveforms above baseline.

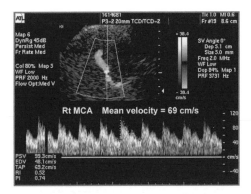 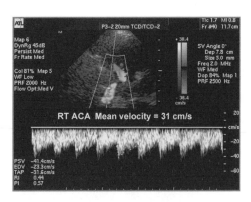

Normal RT MCA and ACA from right transtemporal window

- Identify the mesencephalic brain stem or "peduncle" that lies slightly posterior and deep to the temporal lobe. The PCAs wrap around the peduncle.

- Obtain Doppler samples from the ipsilateral and if possible, the contralateral PCA.

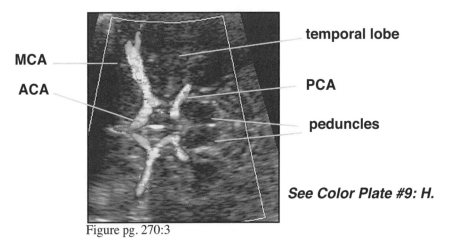

See Color Plate #9: H.

Figure pg. 270:3

Intracranial anatomy from the transtemporal window.

Image courtesy of Philips Ultrasound.

<u>Vertebral -basilar arteries through the suboccipital window.</u>

- Position the patient lying on his/her side with a pillow under the head and the chin tucked slightly to the chest similar to the TCD technique.

- Place the transducer just to one side of midline and about 1 inch below the skull.

- Start with a SV depth of 60 mm and aim at the nose.

- Optimize B-mode image, then turn on color Doppler.

- The dark anechoic area is the foramen magnum. The adjacent bright echoes are the occipital bone.

- The vertebral is located at a depth of 6-9 cm. Flow should be away from the transducer. Both vertebrals may be seen in the same plane on some patients.

- Step the sample volume in deeper along the course of the vertebral artery. The basilar artery will be found at approximately 8 cm. A velocity increase or the demonstration of the vertebral confluence is useful in identifying the basilar artery.

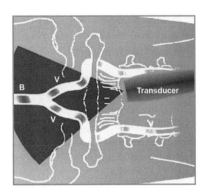 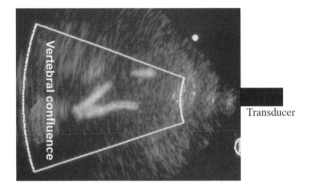

Actual onscreen orientation. Both vertebral arteries are seen as legs of the "Y". The right vertebral artery is on the left of the image. The junction of the two vessels is the basilar artery. Flow direction is from the top of the screen to the bottom.

- If the vertebral is not identified, move the transducer laterally, or move inferior and angle superior.

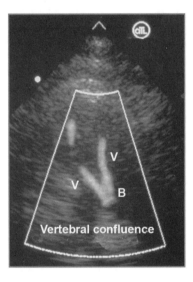

TCD compared to TCI.

Fujioka and associates compared the success rates for TCD and TCI and reported that middle cerebral arteries (MCA's) were identified in 82% of the study population with TCD and only 53% with the color duplex TCI.[2] They advocate the combined use of TCD and TCI to improve diagnostic success.

Cerebral Vasospasm

- Cerebrovascular aneurysm rupture occurs in approximately 28,000 individuals in North America annually with the mortality rate exceeding 50%.[3]

- Those that survive the initial subarachnoid hemorrhage (SAH) and surgical clipping of the aneurysm face the risk of vasospasm in the major intracranial vessels. Mild vasospasm can be asymptomatic, but severe spasm reduces cerebral perfusion and symptomatic ischemic deficit can result. Symptoms include confusion, decreased levels of consciousness, and stroke.

- The mechanism that brings about vasospasm following SAH is not well known. Vasospasm can occur ipsilateral or contralateral to the side of the aneurysm or occur bilaterally, and may involve any of the major intracranial arteries.

- It is common that the spasm is delayed in onset, commencing several days after the aneurysm rupture.

- Serial transcranial Doppler monitoring for the presence of vasospasm not only alerts the physician to the occurrence but also allows the neurosurgeon and neuroradiologist to plan an appropriate course of patient management, particularly in those with decreased neurologic function as a result of the spasm.

- The administration of potent vasodilators, such as Papavarine, selectively applied by catheter directly into the vessel just proximal to the spasm can reduce vasospasm and improve hemispheric perfusion.

- TCD performed before and after percutaneous angioplasty of the MCA can provide valuable information as to the efficacy of the treatment. PTA and Papavarine are often used as a combined therapy.

- TCD and TCI are both effective methods for monitoring the results of this therapy.

Serial monitoring for vasospasm

Patient preparation

- If necessary, have the patient sedated.
- Move or remove temporal bandages to allow access to each transtemporal window.
- Be careful not to disturb the intracranial drain or pressure line.
- Use sterile acoustic gel on the side of the incision.
- A sterile probe sheath should be used as necessary.

TCD and TCI

- Use the transtemporal window.
- Identify the MCA and with the spectral Doppler and interrogate the MCA from its origin to the distal segment.
- Look for regions of focal velocity increase and record the highest mean velocity obtained.
- Measure the mean velocity of the Doppler waveform.

- Note the sample volume depth of the recorded Doppler sample. This will be important for serial follow-up. Often there is more than one area of narrowing.

- If possible, record flow direction and velocity from the ACA and PCA.

- For follow-up exams, try to obtain Doppler samples at the same or nearly the same depth as previous studies. Vessel spasm may occur in a long segment or be focal in nature.

- Optional: compare extracranial ICA velocities and resistive index to MCA flow velocities to determine the effect of changing cardiac output, mean arterial pressure and hydration. This ratio helps to differentiate systemic hyperemic flow from vasospasm

- Repeat the procedure on the contralateral side.

> **NOTE:** Intracranial vessels on the side contralateral to the transducer can often be seen and evaluated with TCI and TCD. This is particularly useful when there is only one good acoustic window.

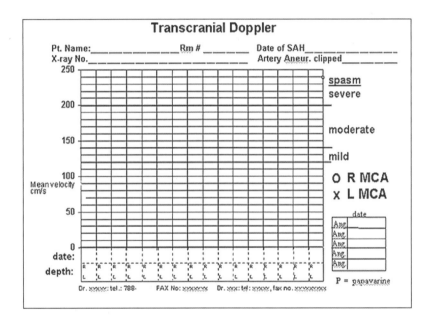

A surveillance chart or graph similar to the one above is indispensable for trending MCA velocities during post operative surveillance for vasospasm. It can be kept on the patient's chart, and also faxed to the neurosurgeon's office after each exam.

Vasospasm Mean Velocity Criteria for MCA (angle corrected to 0 degrees)		
Degree of Vasospasm[4]	Mean Velocity	MCA/ICA mean velocity ratio
Normal	30 -80 cm/s	
Hyperemia	120 - 140 cm/s	< 3.0
Moderate	140 - 200 cm/s	3 - 6
Severe	> 200 cm/s	> 6

The following case study illustrates the utility of transcranial monitoring for intracranial vasospasm.

Patient SG. A 46-year-old female incurred a SAH from a left MCA aneurysm on 6/28/—. The aneurysm was clipped on the same day. On the 7th post-operative day mild to moderate spasm of the left MCA was found during the TCI exam. The increased velocities subsided within a few days. On or about the 14th post-operative day the patient sustained vasospasm in the right MCA that progressed to the severe range. This was accompanied by a decline in her neurological condition.

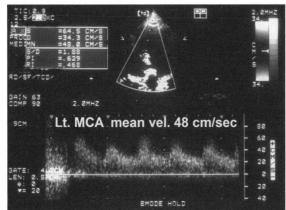
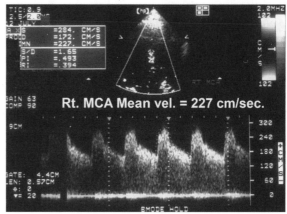

Patient with severe spasm of Rt. MCA following SAH and clipping of Lt MCA aneurysm. Mean MCA velocity on left 48 cm/s, and 227 cm/s on right.

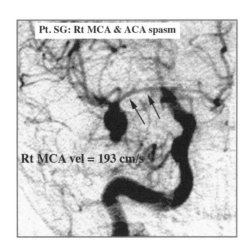
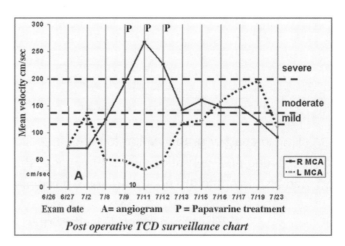

Angio of vasospasm right MCA & ACA. Note aneurysm in MCA distal to spasm.

Useful chart for vasospasm surveillance.

She underwent 3 local Papavarine treatments to the right MCA that resulted in a decline in mean velocities as the spasm subsided. There was a progressive, but transient vasospasm in the left MCA during the 3rd post-op week, but there were no symptoms associated with this episode. The patient went on to a full recovery. The chart below demonstrates the velocities of the MCAs during this post-operative surveillance.

> **NOTE:** Surgical clips can occasionally obscure the MCAs, depending on the location of the clips. Be aware that brain tissue swelling may cause the MCA origin depth to vary from the values listed in this chapter.

• Both TCI and TCD can be effective in monitoring patients with cerebral vasospasm related to subarachnoid hemorrhage.

INTRAOPERATIVE MONITORING

Carotid Artery Endarterectomy (CEA)

During carotid endarterectomy the surgeon may cross-clamp the CCA proximally and the ICA distally. TCD monitoring of the ipsilateral mean MCA flow velocity is useful in determining the potential of ischemia that may result from this procedure.

If collateral pathways in the circle of Willis are insufficient, the surgeon will typically install a temporary intraluminal shunt around the surgical site.

An MCA velocity of 30-40% of the pre-clamp velocity appears to represent adequate collateralization. If MCA mean velocity drops by 60% or greater, a shunt is warranted.[5]

Haley et al., demonstrated that selective shunting based on TCD in ischemic patients may reduce perioperative stroke rate. However, in patients that were not ischemic, there was an increase in perioperative stroke when shunts were used.[6]

CEREBRAL EMBOLI DETECTION

• TCD has shown that air and particulate emboli to the cerebral vasculature can occur during and following a variety of vascular operative procedures.

TCD monitoring of MCA with microembolic signal

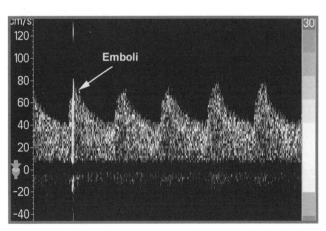

- High Intensity Transient Signals (HITS), sometimes referred to as microembolic signals (MES), are seen and heard with TCD.

- Air emboli, sometimes described as having a "chirp" sound, are of longer duration than particulate matter. They usually have a higher intensity reflection signal on the spectral display than particle emboli.

- Particulate emboli may consist of platelet aggregates, atheromatous material or both.

- Air emboli appear to have less fewer neurologic consequences than particulate emboli. But as of this writing, efforts to differentiate air and particle emboli based on signal patterns have not been satisfactory. Additionally, during many embolic events there is a mixture of both types of emboli.

Instrumentation

- TCD instrumentation is fashioned by its purpose, whether diagnostic or monitoring, but all use low frequency transducers required to penetrate the skull.

- TCI is used for diagnostic purposes, but not for monitoring.

- TCD monitoring for emboli is performed either in a unilateral fashion for ipsilateral carotid TEA, or bilaterally for cardiac or other procedures.

- Monitoring requires an adjustable headset that holds the TCD transducers to the patient's transtemporal window.

- Monitoring is usually performed for at least 20 minutes. An automatic emboli counter is very useful.

- High–end TCD instruments use multiple sample gates simultaneously recording from multiple depths along the course of the MCA, as well as other vessels. Multi-gated units may better differentiate true emboli from artifact, as the recorded signals of an emboli will occur at slightly different times as it passes through the various sample volumes. An artifact appears in all channels simultaneously.

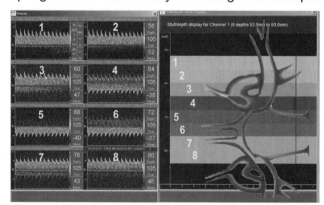

Figure pg. 276:1

Multi-gate PW Doppler with color M-mode.
Diagram of the circle of Willis is superimposed.

See Color Plate #9: I.

- Another method used to differentiate emboli from artifact is to record and display the audio spectrum of the event. Emboli and artifact usually have quite different audio signatures.

- The display on the right shows a distinct microemboli within the Doppler spectral display (top) and as well as in the audio spectrum on the bottom.

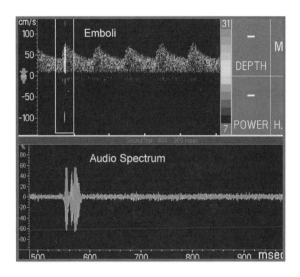

- The Doppler screen on the right demonstrates an artifact in the spectral display and a diffuse audio spectrum that is uncharacteristic for MES

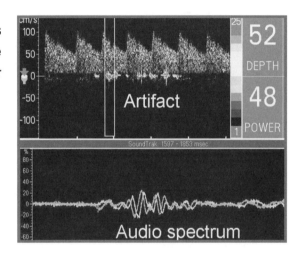

- Occasionally a burst or shower of microembolus occurs in the MCA. The image on the right demonstrates this event. The Doppler signal processing is overloaded by the intensity of the MES and "spikes" appear throughout the vertical dimension of the spectral display.

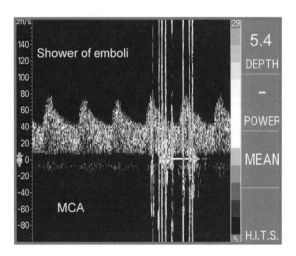

- New TCD technology is employing colored M-mode simultaneously with multi-gated spectral Doppler to distinguish artifact from emboli.

Criteria for identifying a Microembolic signal.

1. Duration is usually less than 300 msec.

2. Amplitude is at least 3 dB higher than that of background blood flow *(see below).

3. A signal is unidirectional within the Doppler velocity spectrum.

4. A signal is accompanied by a snap or chirp on the audible output.[7]

From the consensus committee of the ninth International Cerebral Hemodynamic Symposium.[8]

* This particular criteria was established when TCD units had a relatively narrow dynamic range. Newer Doppler systems have a wider dynamic range and a 3 dB relative difference is not as significant as it once was. Consequently, the 3 dB value is somewhat obsolete.

CLINICAL APPLICATION

Carotid endarterectomy

The stroke rate associated with carotid endarterectomy (CEA) ranges from about 2 - 8%. The majority of perioperative strokes are thought to be caused by emboli that occur with release of the cross-clamped artery, during shunt placement or within the initial 24-hour postoperative period.

HITS occur in almost all patients undergoing CEA. A patient is at increased risk for stroke if the embolic rate is high[9]. Paradoxically, there are some patients with a high emboli rate but no clinically detected neurological deficit. Patients with a high MES rate can be treated with anti-thrombotic agents to reduce the chance of neurological ischemia.

Angioplasty with carotid stenting versus CEA

Cerebral emboli occur during carotid stenting as well as CEA. Investigations are ongoing to determine the peri-procedure stroke rate associated with the placement of carotid stents. Jordan et al., evaluated patients undergoing carotid angioplasty (PTA) with stenting and compared stroke rates and MES count to traditional CEA. The study reported that there were 8 times more emboli (detected with TCD monitoring) with the PTA procedure compared to CEA HIT rate. The stroke rate in the study was 5.6% with PTA and 1.4% with CEA. There was a clear correlation between high MES rate and high neurological complication rate.[9]

TCD monitoring will continue to be a valuable tool in assessing the effectiveness of new techniques and treatments.

Coronary Artery Bypass Grafts (CABG)

Approximately 3-10% of patients undergoing CABG will experience clinically observable neurological deficits. Cerebral emboli are believed to be the most common cause of this complication.[10] The microembolic signals (MES) consist of a mixture of air and particulate emboli. The literature is somewhat varied in what constitutes a dangerous embolic rate: some studies have found neurological ischemia associated with >60 MES where others have reported >100[11]. These findings have led to the ongoing development of intra-arterial filters to prevent cerebral emboli. TCD will be an important tool in monitoring the effectiveness of these devices.

Patent Foramen Ovale

A patent foramen ovale allows an abnormal right to left blood shunt in the heart that bypasses the pulmonary artery and the lungs. Among other effects of this condition is the potential for venous thromboemboli ending up in the peripheral arterial system or in the cerebral vasculature. TCD can be utilized to detect this condition, and has high sensitivity and specificity when compared to TEE, the current gold standard.

Micro air bubbles (agitated saline) are injected into a superficial vein in the arm during bilateral TCD monitoring of the MCA blood flow. The bubbles go to the lungs if the FO is closed. The bubbles will cause HITS in the MCA after a few seconds time delay if the foramen ovale is patent.

There are a number of other unique applications for TCD. A thorough discussion of these methods is beyond the scope of this text.

- Detection of intracranial stenosis.

- Arterio-venous fistula and malformations.

- Sickle cell anemia.

- Vasomotor reactivity and cerebral autoregulation.

References

1. Aslid R, Markwalder TM, Nornes H: Noninvasive transcranial Doppler ultrasound recording of flow velocity in the basal cerebral arteries. J Neurosurg 57: 769-774, 1982.

2. Fujioka KA, Gates DT, Spencer MP. A comparison of transcranial color Doppler imaging and standard static pulsed wave Doppler in the assessment of intracranial hemodynamics. J Vasc Technol 18(1):29-35, 1994

3. Kassell NF, Drake CG: Timing of Aneurysm surgery. Neurosurgery 10:514-519,1982

4. Aaslid R, Huber P, Nornes H. A transcranial Doppler method in the evaluation of cerebrovascular spasm. Neuroradiology 1986, 2 8:11-16

5. Visco E, LAM A. Transcranial Doppler as an intraoperative monitor. J Vasc Technol.24 (1):61-66,2000

6. Haley JHJ. Risks and benefits of shunting in carotid endarterectomy. The International Transcranial Doppler Collaborators. Stroke 23:1583-87, 1992

7. Babikian VL, et al. Detection of Cerebral Embolism with Transcranial Doppler Ultrasound. J Vasc Technol 24(1):35-41, 2000

8. Consensus Committee of the Ninth International Cerebral Hemodynamic Symposium. Basic identification criteria of Doppler microembolic signals. Stroke 26:1123, 1995

9. Jordan WD, Voellinger DC, Doblar DD, Plyushcheva NP, Fisher WS, McDowell HA. Microemboli detected by transcranial monitoring in patients during carotid angioplasty versus carotid endarterectomy. Cardiovascular Surgery

10. Babikian VL, et al. Detection of Cerebral Embolism with Transcranial Doppler Ultrasound. J Vasc. Tecnol 24(1):35-41,2000

11. Hammon J, Stump DA, et al. Risk factors and solutions for the development of neurobehavioral changes after coronary artery bypass grafting. Ann Thorac Surg 63:1613-1618, 1997.

Other reading: A Practical Guide to Transcranial Doppler Examinations. M Katz, A. Alexandrov . Summer Publishing 2003. www.summerpublishing.com

Transcranial Doppler , David Newell, Rune Aaslid, Raven Press 1992

CHAPTER 17: ABDOMINAL DOPPLER FUNDAMENTALS

INTRODUCTION

Color duplex imaging is used to evaluate perfusion in the following organ systems:

- Abdominal Aorta for aneurysm/stenosis.

- Renal artery/vein.

- Mesenteric arteries.

- Portal venous system.

- Hepatic vasculature.

ABDOMINAL AORTA

Aneurysm

- An abdominal aortic aneurysm (AAA) is a permanent pathologic dilation of the aorta with a diameter greater than 1.5 times the expected diameter of that segment, given the patient's gender and body size. In most individuals this is ≥ 3 cm in diameter.[1]

- More than 90% of abdominal aneurysms originate below the renal arteries.[2]

- Annual mortality from ruptured abdominal aneurysms in the United States is about 15,000.[3]

- Only 10-25% of patients survive an aneurysm rupture.

- There is a large risk of rupture once the size has reached 5 cm.

- Aneurysms are thought to be caused by atherosclerotic disease.

Risk factors

⇒ Tobacco abuse.

⇒ Hereditary/family history.

⇒ Advanced age.

⇒ Male gender (men are 5 times more likely to develop AAA than women).

⇒ High cholesterol.

⇒ Obesity.

Symptoms

⇒ Most intact aortic aneurysms do not produce symptoms.

⇒ Palpable pulsatile mass in abdomen on examination.

⇒ Back pain.

⇒ Abdominal pain.

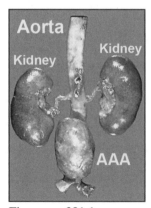

Figure pg. 281:1

See Color Plate #10: A.

IMAGING METHOD

- Place the patient in a supine position.

- Use a 2.5 - 5.0 MHz curved linear array transducer.

- Position the transducer in transverse plane in midline between the xiphoid process and the umbilicus and identify the aorta.

- Scan along the course of the aorta from the renal arteries to the iliac bifurcation and select the area of largest diameter.

- Measure the vessel outside diameter in anterior-posterior (AP) and lateral dimensions using system calipers.

- If an aneurysm is present, measure the dimensions as above; also measure residual lumen if there is thrombus present.

- In longitudinal plane measure the length of the aneurysm.

- Determine if the aneurysm extends distally into the common iliac arteries.

- Also determine if the renal arteries are involved.

- If AAA is within 2 cm of the celiac or SMA, the renal arteries are probably involved.

Aortic Dissection

- The abdominal aorta may also incur dissection.

- Dissection occurs due to a tear in the intima, blood flow then enters the subintimal space.

- The result is a hematoma within the wall of the aorta.

- Dissection can produce vessel stenosis.

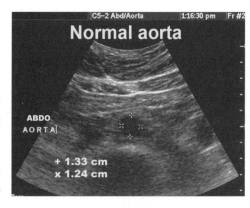

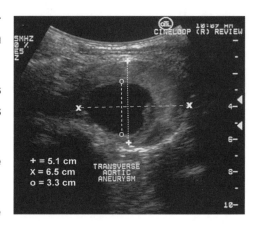

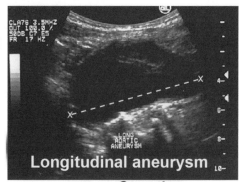

Figure pg. 282:1-3 *See other aneurysms on Color Plate #10: C-E.*

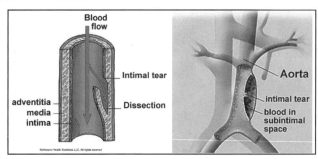

Abdominal aortic flow patterns demonstrate low resistance above the renal arteries, and high resistance distal to the renal arteries.

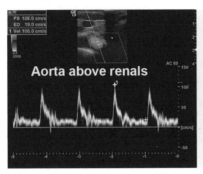 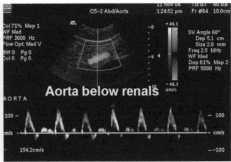

RENAL DOPPLER

- 60 million patients are afflicted by hypertension in the USA.

- ≈10 million with hypertension caused by:

  ⇒ Chronic renal disease.

  ⇒ Renal artery disease (≈ 400,000).

  ⇒ True renovascular hypertension (≈ 260,000), i.e., not everyone with renal artery stenosis has hypertension.

Renovascular Hypertension Etiology

Renovascular hypertension is elevated blood pressure due to stenosis or complete occlusion of one or more renal arteries. There is a resulting decrease in blood pressure and flow within the kidney. The kidney then produces and releases into the blood stream a protein called renin. Renin is converted into an enzyme (angiotensin II) that causes vasoconstriction, and sodium and water retention. The renal artery stenosis must be ≥ 70% before it's likely to cause hypertension.

- Atherosclerosis, usually in the proximal renal artery, is the most common etiology.

- Fibromuscular dysplasia (FMD). This occurs in the mid to distal segments of the renal artery and occurs most frequently in women.

- Dissection and/or extension of an aortic dissection.

Renal Doppler Indications

- Uncontrolled hypertension, especially in younger patients.
- Decreasing renal function.
- Abdominal bruit.

RENAL VASCULAR ANATOMY

- Main renal arteries arise from the aorta just distal to the superior mesenteric artery (SMA).

- The right renal artery courses behind (posterior to) the IVC.

- The right renal artery is longer than the left renal artery.

- The left renal vein lies posterior to SMA and anterior to the aorta.

- The right renal vein is shorter than the left.

- Normal renal veins should demonstrate phasic flow and maybe pulsatile flow transmitted from right atrium.

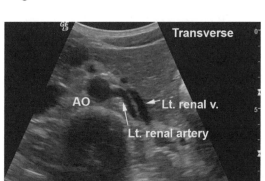

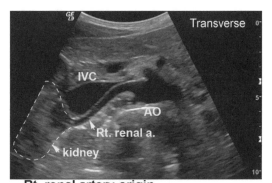

Rt. renal artery origin.
Images courtesy of Cindy Owen and GE Healthcare.

Lt. renal artery origin

- Segmental renal arteries are branches of the main renal artery; they enter through the renal hilum.

- Interlobar arteries arise from the segmentals; they penetrate the renal parenchyma and run between the renal medullary pyramids.

- Arcuate arteries branch from the interlobars and turn at the cortico-medullary junction to course parallel to cortex surface.

- Interlobular arteries (cortical branches) extend into the cortex.

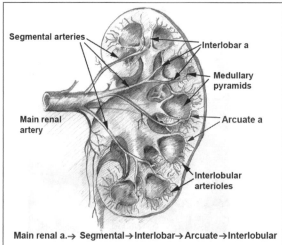

Main renal a.→ Segmental→Interlobar→Arcuate→Interlobular

- Accessory renal arteries (polar arteries) are common. They may arise from the aorta (above or below the main renal arteries), the IMA, SMA or other vessels. On the right side, they may pass anterior to IVC.

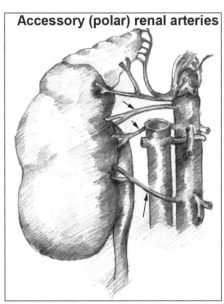

Accessory (polar) renal arteries

Exam Protocol: General Considerations

The Purpose of Renal Doppler:

- Identify a vascular etiology of hypertension.

- Prevent renal failure due to permanent parenchymal changes.

- Evaluate renal transplants for arterial twists, kinks, stenosis, and rejection; also look for renal vein thrombosis.

Indirect Versus Direct Methods

- The direct color duplex method interrogates the both renal arteries from the aorta to the renal parenchyma. Spectral waveforms are obtained from the proximal, mid, and distal renal artery segments, and also from the segmental renal arteries. This method is sometimes limited by obesity, bowel gas, previous abdominal surgery, and prolonged exam time due to inexperience.

- The indirect method interrogates the segmental and/or interlobars arteries of both kidneys. Waveform characteristics within the kidney are analyzed for abnormality associated with main renal artery stenosis or occlusion, as well as for parenchymal disease. The test has a short exam time and high technical success rate. Bilateral comparison of resistance index (RI) aids in detecting parenchymal disease. The indirect method is unlikely to detect main renal artery stenosis unless it's severe, i.e., ≥ 70% stenosis.

METHOD 1 - DIRECT TECHNIQUE

Patient preparation:

⇒ Overnight fast.

⇒ Clear liquids and medications are OK.

⇒ Patients should be well dehydrated: some labs request that patients drink 16 oz. of water 30 minutes before the exam.

⇒ Examination should be performed in the morning.

⇒ No chewing gum or tobacco, and no smoking prior to exam.

Technique for Imaging Kidney

- Use a 2.25 - 3.0 MHz transducer (5.0 MHz on thin patients).

Right Kidney

- Image the right kidney through the liver from right anterior approach.

- Position the transducer obliquely to elongate the kidney.

- Measure each kidney length and compare to the contralateral side. A 2-centimeter difference is significant. Normal adult kidney length is 9-12 cm.

- Look for a mass or cyst within the kidney.

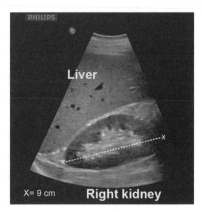

Left Kidney

- With patient in a supine position, scan laterally though intercostal space, or anteriorly (more difficult).

- With the patient in slightly oblique position lying on the right side, scan from lateral or posterior planes.

- Alternatively, with patient in decubitus position, scan through the posterior axillary line.

> NOTE: The spleen may be used as an acoustic window to the left kidney.

- In transverse plane scan the kidney from the superior to the inferior poles; look for masses, cysts, and anomalies.

> TIP: When performing abdominal Doppler exams, do not invert the spectral Doppler waveforms or the color orientation display. Blood flow away from the Doppler beam should be below spectral baseline, and blue should be "away" if using color Doppler.

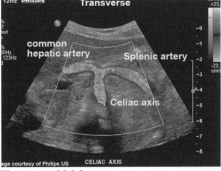

Figure pg. 286:2

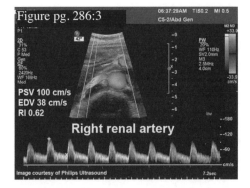

Figure pg. 286:3

See Color Plate #10: F and Plate 11: A.

Scan Technique for Main Renal Arteries [4]

⇒   In transverse plane in midline approach, identify the aorta and locate the celiac artery and the superior mesenteric artery (SMA). Identify the renal artery origins just distal to SMA . In longitudinal plane, 2-3 cm distal to xiphoid process, obtain Doppler waveforms from the aorta and measure/record the aortic peak systolic velocity (PSV).

⇒   With the transducer in transverse plane to the aorta, obtain Doppler waveforms from multiple sites of the renal artery, from the origin to the renal hilum. Also obtain waveforms from the segmental renal arteries within kidney.

⇒   Renal arteries may also be evaluated with patient rolled slightly onto the left side. The aorta and renal arteries lie deep (medial) to the IVC. Scan the aorta from the lateral transducer position. In longitudinal plane, identify the right renal artery coursing towards transducer, and the left renal artery coursing away. Doppler angles are optimal in this position. In transverse plane, the entire course of the right artery is often seen with this approach.

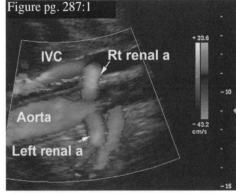

Figure pg. 287:1

See Color Plate #11: B.

To identify stenosis

⇒   Look for regions of velocity increase and post stenotic turbulence. Carefully "map" these regions with spectral Doppler.

⇒   Record the peak systolic velocity from the waveform demonstrating maximum velocity.

⇒   Calculate the Renal/Aortic peak systolic velocity ratio (RAR), which is the highest velocity obtained in the renal artery divided by the peak velocity from the aorta.

⇒   A high velocity alone (without post-stenotic turbulence) at the renal artery origin may be due to a high Doppler angle (>70°), so watch your angle in this inherently difficult region for Doppler.

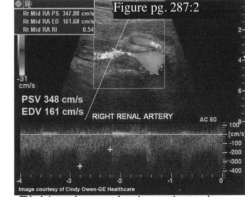

Right main renal artery stenosis
See Color Plate #11: C&D.

NORMAL Characteristics

•   High flow velocity (PSV 100 ± 20 cm/s).

•   Low resistance (RI < 0.75).

•   High diastolic flow (EDV 30 ± 5 cm/s).

Criteria for > 60% stenosis [5,6,7]

- Renal-Aortic Ratio (RAR) (renal PSV divided by aortic PSV) >3.5.

- Peak systolic velocity (PSV) >180 cm/s.

- Post-stenotic turbulence.

- Low flow velocity in distal renal artery.

Renal Artery Occlusion

- No flow detectable in a well-visualized renal artery.

- Low frequency shift in the color and spectral Doppler signal from the parenchyma.

- Small kidney size (< 9 cm).

Renal Parenchymal Disease

Blood flow in the renal artery of a normal kidney is of low resistance. In the presence of renal parenchymal disease velocity is reduced and resistance is high in the main renal artery and in the segmental and interlobar arteries.

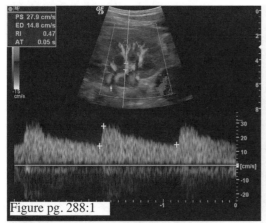

Normal segmental artery flow

See Color Plate #11: E.

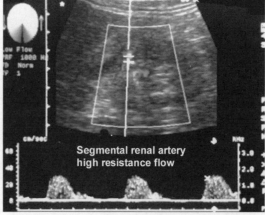

High resistance segmental artery flow due renal parenchymal disease.

Technique Within The Kidney

⇒   Obtain Doppler waveforms from the segmental arteries in the superior pole, mid and inferior pole of the kidney.

⇒   Calculate RIs from segmental arteries.

⇒   Obtain Doppler waveforms and assess waveform morphology from the interlobar and arcuate arteries.

⇒   With color Doppler or Power Doppler, note overall kidney perfusion. Is it reduced unilaterally?

Renal Doppler Physical Limitations

- Excessive depth of the renal arteries.
- Motion of respiration.
- Intra-abdominal gas obscuring the image.
- Obesity.
- Previous abdominal surgery.

Direct Renal Doppler Technical Limitations

- High technical failure rate (12-25% in some reports).

- Accessory renal arteries (polar arteries) occur in >20% of patients and they're difficult, if not impossible, to find with ultrasound. However, it's unlikely that a diseased polar artery, in the absence of main renal artery disease, will cause renovascular hypertension.

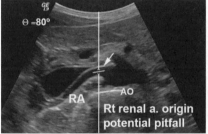

- Poor Doppler angle at the orifice.

- Long exam time (1-2 hours).

- Requires skilled technologist/sonographer.

Beware: high Doppler angle at the renal oriface can cause velocity measurements to be erroneously high.

METHOD 2 - INDIRECT TECHNIQUE

This technique evaluates the segmental and interlobar artery waveforms to indirectly assess for main renal artery stenosis or occlusion and for parenchymal disease. The method requires careful technique and specific setup of Doppler parameters.

Patient Position

Try these different patient positions to optimize access:

⇒ Supine or slightly oblique.

⇒ Right and left lateral decubitus posterolateral approach.

⇒ Use a lateral and /or flank approach.

Doppler Setup

- Doppler frequency should be 3 - 5 MHz.

- Doppler angle in the segmental arteries should be between 0° - 30°.

- Maximize the size of the spectral waveforms by using a low velocity scale, but avoid aliasing.

- Use a large sample volume (4-6 mm).

- Set the Doppler sweep speed time to 2 or 3 seconds (this elongates the waveform along the horizontal axis).

- Use a low wall filter (50-100 Hz).

Indirect Protocol

- Use color Doppler to locate the segmental arteries within the kidney.

- Don't scan through liver as this places the kidney too far from the probe surface. Try to minimize depth.

- Obtain Doppler waveforms from the segmental arteries in the superior pole, mid and inferior pole of the kidney.

- Measure acceleration time (AT), also called rise time (RT), and note the presence (or absence) of the early systolic peak (ESP).

Segmental renal artery waveform

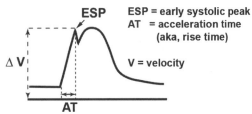

ESP = early systolic peak
AT = acceleration time
(aka, rise time)

V = velocity

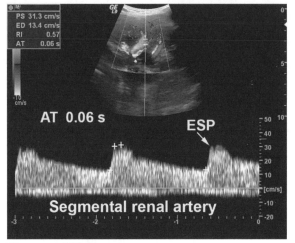

Figure pg. 290:2
See Color Plate #11: E.

Indirect Waveform Parameters- NORMAL

- Presence of an ESP.

- AT less < 0.07 seconds.

- Presence of diastolic flow.

- RI < 0.75

Indirect Criteria for > 60% Stenosis [8,9]

- Acceleration time, AT 0.07 - 0.1 sec. = grey zone.

- Increased (prolonged) acceleration time, > 0.1 sec.

- Tardus - Parvus waveform10 (low amplitude, prolonged rise time, and rounding of the waveforms). Also known as Parvus-Tardus.

- Loss of the early systolic peak (ESP).

- Flattened of the systolic upslope.

- Abnormally lower ipsilateral RI.

- RI > 0.75.

- Reduced color flow in kidney, unilaterally.

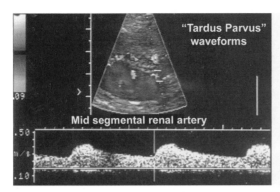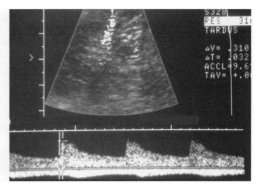

The patient above has a severe stenosis in the main renal artery. Low color flow in the segmental arteries and "tardus parvus" waveforms indicate proximal disease. The image on right was obtained 24 hours after an angioplasty of the main renal artery. Notice the return of normal acceleration times, early systolic peak and increased velocity in the segmental arteries.

Example of a "Tardus-Parvus" waveform in a segmental renal artery. Low amplitude, rounding of the waveform, absence of ESP, and extended acceleration time are all consistent with a severe (>70%) stenosis of the main renal artery.

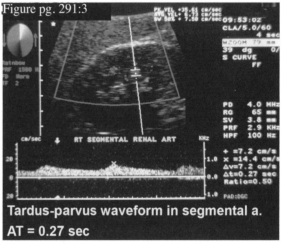

Figure pg. 291:3

See Color Plate # 11: F.

Indirect Method Limitations

- Stenosis in accessory renal arteries may not be detected, as these vessels are difficult to find. Doppler sampling of the segmental arteries in the upper, mid and lower regions of the kidney helps reduce this potential false negative result.

- Although criteria have been developed for stenosis of 60% or greater, this indirect technique is not effective for detecting stenosis of less than 60%. Some authors have shown that the accuracy of the indirect method for main renal artery stenosis is significantly better with ≥70% stenosis.[11]

- A positive study in the segmental arteries cannot differentiate stenosis from occlusion in the main renal artery, nor whether the obstruction is atherosclerosis or fibromuscular dysplasia.

- Parenchymal disease, in the presence of a main renal artery stenosis, may cause the segmental waveform to become "more resistive". This can lead to a false negative result.

- The indirect method should be used in conjunction with the direct method. If the indirect results are positive or equivocal, the renal arteries and the aorta should be scanned.

- When the RI is ≥ 0.8 and indirect results are negative, a careful comparison to the contralateral side is essential.

Despite these limitations, the indirect technique is a relatively quick and effective screening method for patients with suspected renovascular etiology for hypertension. Although a complete exam of the main renal and parenchymal arteries is the optimum procedure, often the main renal arteries are inaccessible and this method will have to suffice.

RENAL FIBROMUSCULAR DYSPLASIA (FMD)

- A non-atherosclerotic, non-inflammatory arterial disease of unknown origin.

- Fibrous thickening of the intima, media, or adventitia.

- Predominance in women (90%).

- Associated with hypertension.

- Usually a bilateral condition.

- Occurs in the mid to distal segments of the renal arteries.

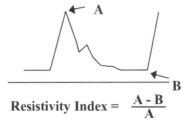

Renal artery FMD

- Also can occur in the carotid arteries.

- If renal artery stenosis is detected distal to the origin in mid segment, FMD should be suspected.

RENAL DOPPLER: TRANSPLANTS

- Transplanted kidneys are evaluated for arterial kinks, stenosis and organ rejection.

- Evaluate the entire renal artery with color and spectral Doppler for flow disturbance associated with kinks or stenosis.

- In kidney transplant rejection, waveforms in the segmental, interlobar and arcuate arteries demonstrate high resistance with absent or minimal diastolic flow. There may be some reversal of flow in diastole.

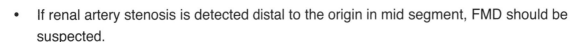

$$\text{Resistivity Index} = \frac{A - B}{A}$$

- Measure RI for rejection:*
    ⇒ Normal value: < 0.73 ± 0.04

⇒ Abnormal: > 0.8 ± 0.07

⇒ * Note: RI is not universally accepted as a solid parameter.

- Acute tubular necrosis within the transplanted kidney and Cyclosporine (an immunosuppressant drug) toxicity can mimic the Doppler findings of rejection. For this reason it is recommended that duplex ultrasound not be the definitive test for kidney rejection.[13]

MESENTERIC DOPPLER

Purpose: To diagnose mesenteric ischemia.

- Mesenteric ischemia is very uncommon due to extensive collateral pathways.

- It is usually caused by athero occlusive disease at vessel origins.

- The celiac, superior mesenteric artery (SMA), and Inferior mesenteric artery (IMA) must be all be involved for bowel ischemia to occur.

- Mesenteric Ischemia.

  ⇒ Can be chronic.

  ⇒ Acute, usually caused by embolization.

  ⇒ Abdominal cramps & pain after eating.

  ⇒ Diarrhea, change in bowel habits.

  ⇒ Weight loss.

  ⇒ AKA: "fear of food" syndrome.

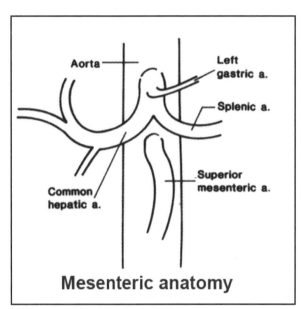

Mesenteric anatomy

MESENTERIC ANATOMY

- <u>Celiac axis.</u> The most cephalad mesenteric vessel; it arises from the anterior surface of the aorta just below the diaphragm and gives rise to:

  ⇒ Lt. gastric artery (a small vessel).

  ⇒ Splenic artery (it can be tortuous). The origin should be viewed in transverse, midline plane. Distally, it may be imaged through the spleen from a lateral scan position.

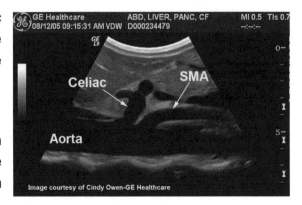

⇒ Common hepatic artery branches into:

- Hepatic artery (at the porta hepatis) divides into right and left hepatic arteries.
- Gastroduodenal artery.
- Pancreaticoduodenal artery.

• Anatomical variants are not uncommon.

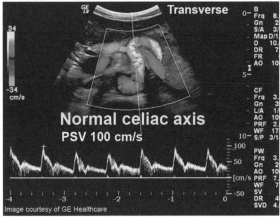

Normal, low resistance celiac axis flow.   Celiac axis stenosis with PSV = 357 cm/s

Figure pg. 294:1 -2 *See Color Plate #12:A-B.*

• Superior mesenteric artery (SMA).

⇒ The next major branch of the aorta caudal to the celiac artery or axis.

⇒ SMA supplies blood to the distal duodenum, small intestine, and the colon.

⇒ In the transverse view, it's surrounded by a triangular region of fat.

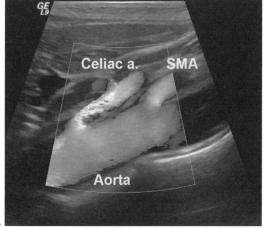

• Inferior mesenteric artery (IMA).

⇒ Arises from the aorta distal to the renal arteries.

⇒ Supplies blood to the transverse, descending, and sigmoid colon.

• Pancreaticoduodenal artery.

⇒ A branch of the gastroduodenal artery.

⇒ Allows communication between the celiac axis and the SMA.

Venous Drainage

• Inferior mesenteric vein joins the splenic vein.

• Superior mesenteric vein joins the splenic vein to form the portal vein.

- Mesenteric flow patterns:

  ⇒ Celiac, hepatic, and splenic arteries- low resistance

  ⇒ SMA & IMA - variable.

  ＊ High resistance when fasting.

  ＊ Low resistance post prandium.

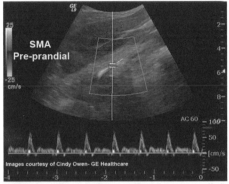

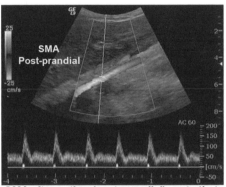

SMA waveform before eating (pre-prandial); note the high resistance waveform.

SMA after eating (post-prandial); note that the flow is now low resistance as more blood flow is needed for digestion.

Mesenteric Doppler Technique

Preparation & Method

- Patients should be in a fasting state for the exam.

- NPO overnight.

- Clear liquids and medications are OK.

- No chewing gum or tobacco, and no smoking prior to exam.

- Patient should be supine, with head elevated 10-30 degrees.

- A 2.5 - 5 MHz transducer is positioned slightly left of midline in longitudinal plane.

- Identify the aorta and obtain Doppler waveforms.

- Obtain spectra from all mesenteric vessels and measure peak systolic and diastolic velocities.

Criteria for >70% stenosis

- Celiac artery: peak systolic velocity > 200 cm/s with post stenotic turbulence.[12]

- SMA: peak systolic velocity > 275 cm/s with post stenotic turbulence.[12]

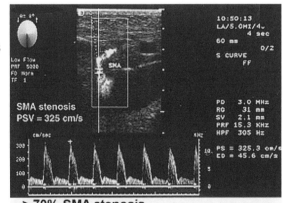

> 70% SMA stenosis
PSV = 325 cm/s

Other Mesenteric Doppler applications

- Median arcuate ligament compression syndrome (MALS). The median arcuate ligament is a ligament of the diaphragm that usually passes superior to the origin of the celiac axis. In some people the ligament inserts low and crosses the proximal segment of the celiac axis, causing compression that often results in abdominal pain. During inspiration the celiac artery becomes trapped by this ligament.

- Median arcuate ligament syndrome can cause a range of symptoms including: nausea, abdominal pain, vomiting, and weight loss.

- SMA compression syndrome. Compression of the third, or transverse, portion of the duodenum against the aorta by the SMA, resulting in chronic, intermittent, or acute complete or partial duodenal obstruction.

PORTAL SYSTEM

The portal venous system drains nutrient-rich blood from the bowel and spleen into liver. It has a capillary bed on each end of system, one in the gut, and the other in the parenchyma of the liver. The portal vein and hepatic artery supply the liver with blood. The hepatic veins drain the liver and enter the inferior vena cava (IVC).

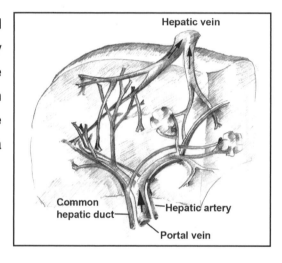

Portal Vein Anatomy

- The portal vein is formed by:
    - ⇒ Superior mesenteric vein (SMV).
    - ⇒ Splenic vein.

- After the porta hepatis, the portal vein divides into:
    - ⇒ Right portal vein: anterior & posterior branches.
    - ⇒ Left portal vein: medial & lateral branches.

- The portal vein courses <u>intra</u>-segmentally in the liver (within the lobes).

- It has very echogenic walls.

- The main portal vein increases in diameter to a maximum of < 13 mm near the porta hepatis. Increased diameter (>13 mm) can be a sign of portal hypertension.

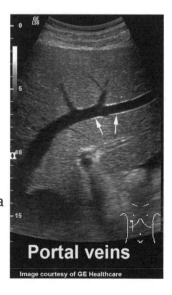

Portal veins

Image courtesy of GE Healthcare

- Portal vein normal flow.

  ⇒ Low velocity (20-40 cm/s), continuous flow, with respiratory phasicity.

  ⇒ No filling defects with color Doppler.

  ⇒ Hepatopetal direction (toward liver). Flow should be in the same direction as the hepatic artery.

  ⇒ Absence of varices.

  ⇒ Normal flow direction in potential collateral vessels.

PORTAL HYPERTENSION

Portal hypertension (PH), or elevated pressure in the portal venous system, is due to increased impedance of flow through the liver. This may be due to:

1. Prehepatic obstruction.

  ⇒ Portal or splenic vein thrombosis.

  ⇒ Extrinsic compression of the portal vein.

2. Intrahepatic.

  ⇒ Cirrhosis (the most common cause; 90% of portal hypertension cases are due to cirrhosis).

  ⇒ Hepatic fibrosis.

  ⇒ Lymphoma.

3. Post hepatic.

  ⇒ IVC obstruction.

  ⇒ Hepatic vein obstruction.

  ⇒ Hepatic artery stenosis.

Portal Hypertension can lead to:
- Ascites.
- Splenomegaly.
- GI - esophageal bleeding.
- Jaundice.
- Signs of hepatic failure.

Proximal IVC thrombosis can cause portal hypertension.
Figure pg. 297:1
See Color Plate #12: C.

Portal Doppler Technique

- Measure portal vein diameter (>13 mm = abnormal).

- For all portal Doppler, use low PRF & wall filter.

- Evaluate PV and branches for patency, flow direction, and measure PSV.

- Measure the spleen length (>13 cm = abnormal).

- Rule out extrinsic compression of the portal vein by a tumor or a mass.

- Evaluate the IVC for obstruction.

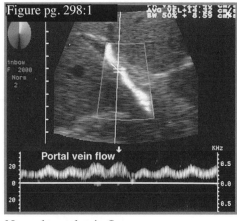

Normal portal vein flow,
See Color Plate #12: D.

Common Porto-systemic shunts (these occur as collateral pathways when flow cannot pass through and out of the liver).

- Left gastric vein, aka, the coronary vein.

  ⇒ Retrograde flow in this vessel occurs in 80-90% of portal hypertension cases.

  ⇒ Increased pressure in this vessel may cause esophageal varices.

- Gastric varices often occur:

  ⇒ Near the stomach (epigastrium).

  ⇒ Under the left lobe of the liver.

  ⇒ Near the spleen.

Other Porto-systemic Shunts

- Recannalized paraumbilical vein with flow is an abnormal finding consistent with portal hypertension.

- Spleno-renal shunt.

  ⇒ Splenic vein to left renal vein.

> Hepatopetal and hepatofugal are terms to describe flow direction in the portal veins and tributaries. An easy way to remember: "petal" is towards, as one would "pedal" a bike forward; fugal is away, as "fugitive" runs away.

Transjugular Intrahepatic Portosystemic Shunts (TIPS)

- Stent placement in the liver parenchyma between the portal vein and hepatic vein.

- The purpose is decompression of the portal venous system.

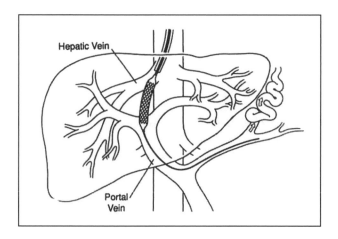

- It does not address the cause of portal hypertension.

HEPATIC VEINS

Hepatic Vein Anatomy

- The hepatic veins drain into the IVC from the liver.

- There are three tributary vessels:

    1. Right hepatic vein drains the right hepatic lobe.

    2. Middle hepatic vein lies between the left and right hepatic lobes.

    3. Left hepatic vein courses between the medial and the lateral segments of the left lobe.

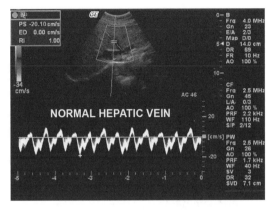

- Left and middle hepatic veins join before the IVC in 96% of individuals.

- Hepatic veins enlarge as they approach the diaphragm.

- These vessels are best imaged in transverse plane, subcostally.

- Normal hepatic vein flow should be:

    ⇒ Hepatofugal.

    ⇒ Pulsatile, due to right atrial pressure changes.

    ⇒ Respiratory variation.

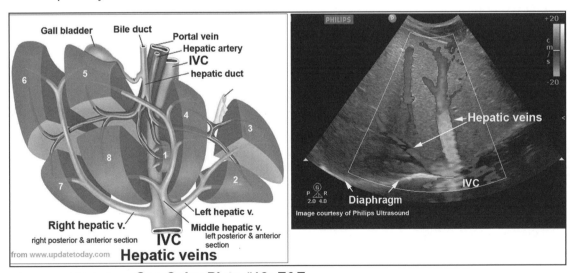

Figure pg. 299:1- 2   *See Color Plate #12: E&F.*

BUDD-CHIARI SYNDROME

- Stenosis or obstruction of the hepatic veins.

- Hepatic outflow obstruction may be caused by:

  ⇒ Hepatomegaly.

  ⇒ Splenomegaly.

  ⇒ Ascites.

  ⇒ Extrinsic compression by a tumor.

  ⇒ Thrombus in the hepatic veins or IVC.

REFERENCES

1. Johnston KW, Rutherford RB, Tilson MD, et al. Suggested standards for reporting on arterial aneurysms. J Vasc Surg. 1991;13:452-458

2. McConathy WJ, Alaupovic P, Woolcock N, et al. Lipids and apolipoprotein profiles in men with aneurysmal and stenosing aorto-iliac atherosclerosis. Eur J Vasc Surg. 1989;3:511-514

3. Emedicine- http://www.emedicinehealth.com

4. Meyers P, Owens C, Renal Doppler: Integrated Ultrasound Reference Guide, SDMS Educational Foundation, Dallas TX 1996

5. Kohler TR, Zeirler RE, Martin RL et al. Nonivasive Diagnosis of Renal Artery Stenosis By Ultrasonic Duplex Scanning. J Vasc Surg 1986;4;450-6.

6. Taylor DC, Kettler MD, Moneta GL, et al. Duplex Ultrasound scaniing in the diagnosis of renal artery stenosis: A prospective evaluation. J Vasc Surg 1988;7:363-9

7. Hansen KJ,Tribble RW, Reavis SW, et al., Renal duplex sonography: Evaluation of clinical utility. J Vasc Surg 1990;12:227-36

8. Martin RL, Nanra RS, Bray AE, et al., Renal Hilar Doppler analysis in the Detection of Renal Artery Stenosis. J Vasc Technol 15(4):173-180 1991

9. Stavros AT, Harchfield D. Renal Doppler, renal artery stenosis, and renovascular hypertension: direct and indirect sonographic abnormalities in patients with renal artery stenosis. Ultrasound Quarterly, Vol.12,No.4, pp. 217-263, 1994 Raven Press Ltd, New York

10. Kotval PS. Doppler Waveform parvus and tardus: a sign of proximal flow obstruction. J Ultrasound Med 1989;8:435-40.

11. Rene CE, Oliva VL, Bui BT et al. Renal Artery Stenosis: Evaluation of Doppler US after Inhibition of Angiotensen - converting enzyme with Captopril. Radiology 1995; 196:675-679.

12. Moneta GL, Lee R, Yeager R, et al. Mesenteric duplex scanning: a blinded prospective study. J Vasc Surg 1993; 17:738

13. Zweibel WJ, Pellerito JS. Introduction to Vascular Ultrasonography. 5th edition, Elsevier 2005 p 268

CHAPTER 18: GLOSSARY

A-MODE - In diagnostic ultrasound, a one-dimensional presentation of a reflected sound wave in which echo amplitude (A) is displayed along the vertical axis and time of rebound (depth) along the horizontal axis; the echo information is presented from interfaces along a single line in the direction of the sound beam.

ABDUCTION - Movement away from the midline of the body.

ABSORPTION - A process of conversion of acoustic energy to heat, resulting in a loss of energy. Absorption is a major player in attenuation.

AC (ALTERNATING CURRENT) COUPLED Output signal to graphic display only responds to changes faster than 0.5 Hz (one complete cycle every two seconds).

ACOUSTIC IMPEDANCE - Property of a medium equal to the product of density and propagation speed.

ACOUSTIC IMPEDANCE MISMATCH - A condition of unequal characteristic acoustic impedances of continuous media, resulting in reflection of acoustic energy at the interface.

ACOUSTIC LENS - A refractive element used to redirect the acoustic beam.

ACOUSTIC PROPAGATION PROPERTIES -Characteristics of a medium that affect the propagation of sound through it.

ACOUSTIC SHADOW -A darkening or loss of image information below an altering structure. "Shadowing" below calcified plaque or bone are examples.

ACROCYANOSIS - Symmetric mottled cyanosis of the hands and feet, associated with coldness and sweating. It is a vasospastic disorder accentuated by cold or emotion and relieved by warmth.

ACUTE - Characterized by a rapid onset, a short course, and pronounced symptoms. Sharp or severe in nature.

ADDUCTION - Movement toward the midline of the body.

ADVENTITIA - The outermost covering of an artery, composed primarily of collagen fibers (tunica adventitia).

AK AMPUTATION - Above knee amputation.

ALGORITHM - An ordered set of discrete steps leading to the solution of a particular problem in such a way as to give a particular result.

ALIASING - An erroneous presentation of the Doppler shift associated with pulsed Doppler systems, due to a low pulse repetition frequency.

ALLEN TEST - A test performed to check the continuity of the palmer arches normally supplied by both the radial and ulnar arteries. The test may be performed using a Doppler, a photoplethysmograph, or a strain gauge plethysmograph.

AMAUROSIS FUGAX - Temporary, partial, or total blindness often resulting from transient occlusion of the retinal arteries. May be a symptom of impending CU.

AMPERE - The unit of electric current used in OHM's law, I = E/R, as I. It measures the rate at which electric current is transferred in Coulomb/sec. See electromotive force, ohm.

AMPLIFICATION - The act of enlarging, increasing, or extending.

AMPUTATION - Traumatic or surgical removal of all or part of a limb.

ANALOGUE - Representing numerical values by physical quantities, so as to allow the manipulation of numerical data over a continuous range of values. A chart recorder is an analogue form of data presentation.

ANASTOMOSIS - A natural or surgical communication between two structures.

ANECHOIC - Describes the property of being echo-free or without echoes. (e.g,. a fluid-filled cyst).

ANEMIA - A condition in which the blood is deficient in oxygen transporting material (red blood cells) in a designated volume of blood.

ANEURYSM - A bulging of the wall of a vein or artery, due to a thinning or weakening by disease or congenital abnormality.

ANGIOPLASTY- Dilatation of an artery or a narrowing within an artery by a balloon-tipped catheter. Procedure is often combined with a stent placement after angioplasty.

ANGLE OF INCIDENCE - Angle at which an ultrasound beam strikes an interface (with respect to the normal or perpendicular angle); in Doppler, angle of the beam with respect to the flow axis.

ANKLE BRACHIAL INDEX (ABI) - A numerical comparison of the systolic blood pressures in the arm and ankle. It is obtained by dividing the ankle pressure by the brachial pressure. Values below 0.9 indicate varying degrees of ischemia.

ANNULAR ARRAY - Array made up of ring-shaped elements arranged concentrically.

ANOXIA - A condition of severe lack of oxygen in the tissues, usually caused by loss of blood supply. Can cause tissue death; synonymous with hypoxia.

ANTEGRADE FLOW - Blood flowing forward, away from the heart.

ANTERIOR - Situated in the frontal plane.

ANTICOAGULANT - A substance which prevents or retards blood clotting, such as Heparin.

APHASIA - Impaired or absent communication by speech or writing centers in the dominant hemisphere due to brain dysfunction.

ARRAY - A spatial arrangement of two or more transducers or transducer elements, arrays may be linear (elements arranged in a line or annular (circular) in configuration.

ARRHYTHMIA - Abnormal rhythm of the heart beat.

ARTERIAL COMPLIANCE - The property of healthy arterial walls to expand and contract with blood flow pulsations.

ARTERIAL INFLOW - Pertaining to blood flow into the lower extremities to the level of the common femoral arteries.

ARTERIAL INSUFFICIENCY - Inadequate blood supply in the arterial system usually caused by stenosis or occlusion proximal to the inadequately supplied area.

ARTERIAL OCCLUSIVE DISEASE - Any disease process which closes (narrows or occludes) the arteries.

ARTERIAL OUTFLOW - Pertaining to blood flow between common femoral artery and trifurcation.

ARTERIAL RUNOFF - Pertaining to blood flow from trifurcation (branching of popliteal artery into anterior tibial, peroneal, and posterior tibial arteries) to the digital arteries of the foot.

ARTERIOGRAPHY - Invasive radiologic procedure involving injection of a radiopaque substance into the arteries. Long recognized as the "gold standard" for arterial evaluation; the procedure carries definite mortality and morbidity risks and gives no functional information, (also termed) the same as angiography.

ARTERIOLES - The smallest arterial vessels (0.2 mm diameter) resulting from repeated branching of the arteries. They are composed of smooth muscle only and conduct blood from the arteries to the capillaries.

ARTERIOSCLEROSIS - Generic term which encompasses a variety of conditions causing the artery walls to thicken, harden, and lose elasticity.

ARTERIOVENOUS FISTULA (AVF)- A direct precapillary communication between an artery and a vein. Can be congenital, traumatic, or surgical, as in dialysis access fistula.

ARTERIOVENOUS MALFORMATION (AVM) -Multiple connection between the arterial and venous systems. Usually congenital in etiology.

ARTERITIS - Inflammation of the arteries.

ARTERY - Blood vessel which carries blood away from the heart, usually contains oxygenated blood for distribution to the tissues. Exceptions are pulmonary arteries that carry deoxygenated blood from heart to lungs.

ARTIFACT - An artificial or extraneous feature introduced into an observation which may simulate a relevant feature of that observation. Limb movement can cause artifact in plethysmography.

ASPHYXIA - Systemic oxygen deficiency and CO_2 accumulation, usually due to impaired respiration.

ATHEROMA - A deposit of fatty (or other) substances in the inner lining of the artery wall. Plural is atheromata.

ATHEROSCLEROSIS - A form of arteriosclerosis by which the inner layer of the artery wall is made thick and irregular by deposits of atheroma. These deposits result in a decrease in vessel diameter.

ATHEROSCLEROTIC ANEURYSM - The most prevalent type of aneurysm occurring in the abdominal aorta and other large medium arteries: due to the weakening of the media by severe atherosclerosis.

ATRIOVENTRICULAR (HEART) BLOCK - A cardiac conduction abnormality in which transmission of the excitatory impulse from the atrium to the ventricle is slowed or stopped.

ATRIUM - One of the two upper chambers of the heart. The right atrium receives deoxygenated venous blood from the inferior and superior vena cava. Blood passes from the right atrium into the right ventricle. The left atrium receives oxygenated blood from the lungs.

ATTENUATION - Decrease in amplitude and/or intensity as a wave travels through a medium.

ATTENUATION COEFFICIENT - Attenuation per unit length of wave travel.

AUGMENTATION - The normal increase in the Doppler sound of venous flow upon compression distal to the Doppler probe or release of compression proximal to the probe. Augmentation resulting from release of distal compression or application of proximal compression indicates valvular incompetence.

AUSCULTATION - The act of listening to sounds within the body, usually with a standard stethoscope.

AUTOCORRELATION- Signal processing used in color Doppler.

AXIAL RESOLUTION -The clarity and shapness of the image in a vertical dimension; the ability to distinguish small structures that are close in the vertical plane is related to axial resolution. Axial resolution is related to transducer frequency (the higher the better) and pulse burst length.

B-MODE - A two-dimensional diagnostic ultrasound presentation of echo-producing interfaces in a single plane; the intensity of the echo is represented by modulation of the brightness (B) of the spot, and the position of the echo is determined from the position of the transducer and the transit time of the acoustical pulse.

BACK PRESSURE - The pressure increase, engorgement and dilatation proximal to a narrowed blood vessel (such as the internal carotid).

BACKSCATTER - Sound scattered back in the direction from which it originally came.

BANDWIDTH -The range of frequencies transmitted by the transducer; like a chord on a piano, multiple notes transmitted instead of one note.

BASILAR ARTERY - An artery formed by the union of the two vertebral arteries, which supply the posterior brain and terminate in the Circle of Willis.

BEAM DIVERGENCE - Spreading of the ultrasound beam from the face of the transducer.

B-FLOW- Imaging method used by GE to see blood flow in grayscale, almost like Color Doppler but in black and white.

BI-DIRECTIONAL DOPPLER - A Doppler instrument capable of determining whether the frequency of the Doppler shift is above or below the transmission frequency, permitting determination of blood flow towards or away from probe.

BIFURCATION - The site of division into two branches, as in an artery. Often the area of atherosclerotic deposits.

BILATERAL - Pertaining to or affecting both sides of the body.

BK AMPUTATION - Below knee amputation.

BLOOD PRESSURE - Pressure of blood against the walls of the blood vessels, usually refers to pressure within the arteries. Arterial blood pressure is indicated by two numbers, systolic over diastolic, -expressed as mm of mercury (mmHg)
1. Systolic Pressure - Pressure in artery when heart muscle is contracted (systole).

2. Diastolic Pressure - Pressure in artery when heart is not contracted, or between beats (diastole).

BRACHIAL ARTERY - Originates as a continuation of the axillary artery and terminally branches into the radial and ulnar arteries. Frequently used artery for arm blood pressure which is then compared with blood pressures in other limbs.

BRADYCARDIA - Abnormally slow heart rate (under 60 beats per minute).

BRUIT - A sound heard on auscultation caused by wall vibration due to blood turbulence.

BUERGER'S DISEASE - Thrombosis with a variable degree of associated inflammation in the arteries and veins of the extremities, complicated by ischemic changes in the parts supplied. Usually a disease of young and middle-aged tobacco-smoking males and synonymous with thromboangiitis obliterans. (From L. Buerger, U.S. Physician, 1879-1943).

BYPASS - A surgically created detour between two points in a physiologic obstruction. Similar to shunt.

BYTE - A set of adjacent binary digits (bits) operated on as a unit by the computer; the most common size byte contains eight bits.

CALCIFICATION - A process in which tissue in the body becomes hardened as the result of deposits of insoluble salts of calcium. In arterial walls calcium absorbs ultrasound energy. Often results in ultrasound acoustic shadowing , or incompressible vessels during pressure assessment.

CANNULATION - The process of inserting an artificial tube into a part of the body, such as an artery.

CAPILLARIES - Extremely narrow vessels forming a network between the arterioles and the veins. The walls are composed of a single layer of cells through which oxygen and nutritive materials pass out to the tissues, and carbon dioxide and waste products are admitted from the tissues into the blood stream (osmosis).

CARDIOVASCULAR - Pertaining to the heart and blood vessels.

CAROTID ARTERIES - Right and left common carotid arteries are the major arteries supplying blood to the head and neck. The common carot1d bifurcates into the external (supplies skin and muscle tissue of the face) and the internal (supplies eye and brain tissue).

CAROTID BODY - A small oval mass of cells and nerve endings about 5 mm long located in the carotid sinus. These cells respond to chemical changes in the blood by altering rate of respiration and other bodily changes.

CAROTID SINUS - A slight dilatation at the point of carotid bifurcation. This sinus contains cells and nerve endings which respond to a change in blood pressure by altering heart rate.

CAT SCAN - (CT) Computerized Axial Tomography. Medical imaging method employing tomography where digital geometry processing is used to generate a three-dimensional image of the internal structure of an object from a large series of two-dimensional X-ray images taken around a single axis of rotation.

CTA- Computerized Axial Tomography Angiography. Medical imaging method employing high speed contrast media injection via a superficial vein, and axial tomography. Used to image arteries and veins.

CATHETER - A thin tube of plastic or other material to which blood will not adhere. This may be inserted into a vein or artery for diagnostic or therapeutic purposes.

CAUDAL - A direction (towards the feet).

CAUTERIZATION - Coagulation of blood by the application of chemicals or heat. Electrocautery is often used in surgery to reduce blood loss.

CAVITATION - A phenomenon produced by sound in liquids or liquid-like media involving the formation of bubbles or cavities containing gas or vapor.

CENTRAL PROCESSING UNIT (CPU) - That part of a computer that includes the arithmetic/logic unit and circuits that control the interpretation and execution of instruction.

CENTRAL VENOUS PRESSURE (CVP) - The pressure representative of the filling pressure of the right ventricle, measured peripherally or centrally, corrected for hydrostatic pressure between the heart and point of measurement. Used to monitor fluid replacement.

CEPHALAD - Toward the head.

CEREBRAL ANGIOGRAPHY - Radiographic visualization of blood vessels supplying the brain after injection of a radiopaque material into an artery.

CEREBRAL VASCULAR ACCIDENT (CVA) -Impeded blood supply to a part of the brain generally caused by one of the following:

1. Blood clot formation in the vessel (thrombosis).

2. Rupture of the vessel wall (hemorrhage) .

3. An obstruction in the form of a clot or other material from another part of the vascular system which flows to the brain (embolism).

4. Pressure on the vessel, as by a tumor.

CEREBROVASCULAR - Pertaining to blood vessels and circulation in the brain.

CHRONIC - Of long duration or frequent recurrence.

CIRCLE OF WILLIS - Arterial circle of the cerebrum composed of left and right internal, anterior, posterior and middle cerebral arteries as well as anterior, and posterior communicating arteries. This important anastomosis connects the bilateral carotid circulation with the vertebral circulation and may be a source of collateralization in internal carotid occlusive disease.

CLAUDICATION - Repetitive pain and dysfunction of the extremity due to arterial insufficiency during exercise and relieved with a brief rest.

COARCTATION - A stricture or narrowing of a vessel, usually congenital in origin.

COLLAGEN DISEASE - Any of various clinical syndromes characterized by widespread alterations of connective tissue including inflammation and degeneration. Included are: poly-arteritis, systemic lupus erythematosis, Marfan's syndrome.

COLLATERAL CIRCULATION - The circulation established through anastomotic communicating channels, when the normal blood supply is compromised or abolished.

COLOR FLOW MAPPING- Color Doppler

COLOR-WRITE PRIORITY– A color Doppler threshold control that sets whether color or gray scale will be assigned to individual pixels on the display screen.

COMMON FEMORAL ARTERY - A major artery of the thigh at the level of the inguinal ligament, arising from the external iliac artery and terminating in the superficial femoral artery.

COMMON FEMORAL VEIN - A major vein adjacent to the femoral artery in the thigh at the level of the inguinal ligament. It arises from the external iliac and continues into the superficial, femoral vein.

COMMON ILIAC ARTERY - Major arterial branch of the distal aorta conducting blood to pelvis and legs.

COMPRESSION - Decreasing differences between small and large amplitudes.

CONGENITAL ANOMALY - An abnormality present at birth.

CONGESTIVE HEART FAILURE (CHF) - A situation in which the heart is unable to adequately pump out all the venous blood returning to it. This results in a pooling of venous blood and accumulation of fluid in various parts of the body (lungs, legs, etc.).

CONTINUOUS WAVE (CW) DOPPLER - A Doppler instrument which emits an ultrasound beam without interruption. It is not range specific and so will detect flow at any depth of penetration governed by the frequency of the probe.

CONTRALATERAL - Pertaining to the opposite side of the body.

CONTRAST RESOLUTION -The ability or lack of, to differentiate subtle differences in tissue echogenicity or gray scale. Good contrast resolution is imperative in tumor identification.

CRESCENDO TIAs - TIAs that are increasing in frequency over a given period of time.

CUFF ARTIFACT - Consistently high segmental blood pressure in the lower extremity resulting from the use of narrow segmental cuffs which may not completely transmit cuff pressure to the vessels in the central part of the limb (i.e. femoral artery). This effect is most pronounced in the upper thigh where true normal blood pressure corresponds closely to brachial pressure. Cuff artifact must be considered to avoid false negative examinations.

CYANOSIS - A bluish-purple discoloration of the membranes and skin, due to the presence of excessive amounts of reduced hemoglobin (deoxygenated) blood in the capillary arteries.

CYCLE - Complete variation of an acoustic variable.

DAMPING - Material placed behind the rear face of a transducer element to reduce pulse duration; also, the process of pulse duration reduction.

DAMPING FACTOR - The ratio of two adjacent pulsatility indices (Gosling, 1971).

DC (DIRECT CURRENT) COUPLE - Output signal to graphic display responds to steady state conditions as slow shifts from baseline. Gives baseline information as well as changes above or below.

DEAD ZONE - Distance closest to the transducer in which imaging cannot be performed.

DECIBEL (dB) - Unit of power or intensity ratio; the number of decibels is 10 times the logarithm (to the base 10) of the power or intensity ratio.

DEEP VEIN THROMBOSIS - The presence of a blood clot in the deep venous system of the lower or upper extremities.

DENSITY - Mass divided by volume.

DEPENDENT RUBOR- Foot or lower leg will turn a light purple or deep red-violet color as it is held in a dependent condition (lower than the heart), and will blanch on elevation. This is a sign of significant leg ischemia.

DEPTH - Distance along the beam path from the point of entry into the patient. Increasing time of return corresponds to increasing depth of penetration in the tissue.

DEPTH OF PENETRATION - Depth in tissue at which intensity is reduced to some fraction of what it was at the transducer surface.

DIABETES MELLITUS - A chronic systemic disease characterized by disorders of the metabolism of insulin, carbohydrate, fat, and protein, impairing function of blood vessels. May be juvenile, onset with insulin dependence, or adult onset usually non-insulin dependent.

DIASTOLE - The period in the cardiac cycle in which a chamber, either the atrium or ventricles, relaxes and fills with blood.

DICOM– DIgital COmmunication in Medicine. A standard for digital transfer of information from medical imaging devices (Ultrasound, cat scanners, MRI etc, to digital storage, display and retrieval systems.

DIGITAL SCAN CONVERTER - A computerized means of displaying, storing, and analyzing information by transforming analog into digital (binary) information.

DISSECTING ANEURYSM - Splitting or dissection of an arterial wall by blood entering through an intimal tear or interwall hemorrhage. Usually in aortic arch and thoracic aorta.

DISTAL - In circulation, farther or farthest from the heart; opposite of proximal.

DOOHICKEY-Something seen on the ultrasound image whose name you've forgotten.

DOPPLER - A diagnostic instrument which emits an ultrasonic beam into the body. This ultrasound is reflected back from moving structures within the body at a frequency higher or lower than this transmitted frequency (Doppler shift). This shift is amplified and presented as a sound or graphic (chart) display.

DOPPLER ANGLE– The angle at which the Doppler beam intersects blood flow

DOPPLER EFFECT - Observed frequency change of reflected sound due to reflector movement relative to the source or the observer.

DOPPLER SHIFT - Reflected frequency minus incident frequency.

DOPPLER STEERING ANGLE– The angle of the Doppler beam off the face of the transducer. Straight down, unsteered, is zero °, steering is usually out to 15 ,20, 25, or 30° depending on the frequency and number of elements of the transducer.

DORSALIS PEDIS ARTERY - The main artery in the dorsum of the foot.

DORSUM - The back or analogous to the back - dorsal.

DUTY FACTOR - Fraction of time that pulsed ultrasound is actually on.

DYNAMIC RANGE -The ratio of the largest and smallest signals that a system can handle simultaneously; expressed in decibels (dB). The contrast of the ultrasound image; a low DR has fewer shades of gray, so it's contrasty. A high DR is a softer image with more levels of gray.

DYSARTHRIA -imperfect articulation, due to disturbances in muscle control

DYSFUNCTION - Impairment of function.

DYSPHASIA - Lack of coordination in speech, failure to arrange words in an understandable way.

ECHO - Reflection of acoustic energy.

ECHO ARTIFACT - An apparent echo for which distance, direction, or amplitude do not correspond to a real target and is generally produced by multiple reflection or scattering pathways.

ECHOCARDIOGRAPHY - Examination of the heart by diagnostic ultrasound.

ECHOGENIC - Relating to the reflectivity of a medium which contains structures capable of producing echoes.

ECHOGENICITY- the ability to create an ultrasound echo

ECHOLUCENT-permitting the passage of ultrasonic waves without echoes, the representative areas appearing black on the sonogram.

EDEMA - Swelling due to increased fluid in the tissues.

EFFECTIVE REFLECTING AREA - The area of a reflector from which sound is received by a transducer.

ELASTICITY - Willingness of a medium to distort from its original size and shape and restore to its original form after the external influence is removed.

ELECTROCARDIOGRAM (EKG or ECG) - A graphic recording of the electrical activity of the heart.

ELEVATION PLANE–The slice thickness of the ultrasound beam.. The "z" axis.

EMBOLECTOMY - Removal of an embolus.

EMBOLUS - An obstruction or occlusion of a vessel by a transported material composed of blood clot, air, fat, tumor, or other foreign material. Plural is emboli.

ENDARTERECTOMY - The surgical removal of endarterium and atheromatous material from an arterial segment which has become stenosed.

ENDOTHELIUM - A layer of flat cells lining blood and lymph vessels.

ENHANCEMENT - (ENHANCED THROUGH-TRANSMISSION) -Increase in reflection amplitude from reflectors that lie behind a weakly attenuating structure.

ENSEMBLE, ENSEMBLE LENGTH– See Packet size

ERGOTISM - Acute or chronic intoxication from use of Ergot-containing drugs. Symptoms include vomiting, colic, convulsions, paresthesias, psychotic behavior, and ischemic gangrene.

ERYTHEMA - Inflammatory redness of the skin.

ERYTHROCYTE - Red blood cell, which contains hemoglobin, an oxygen-carrying protein responsible for the red color of blood.

ETIOLOGY - The study of the cause of disease - pathogenesis.

EXTRACRANIAL - Anatomic structures outside the cranial vault (skull).

FALSE ANEURYSM - High pressure extravasation of blood out of an artery and into surrounding tissue. Can happen at sites of surgical anastomosis, and arterial catheterization.

FALSE NEGATIVE RATE - Statistical research term indicating the rate of negative results on a diagnostic test when disease was actually present.

FALSE POSITIVE RATE - Statistical research term indicating the rate of positive results on a diagnostic test when no disease was actually present.

FAR ZONE (FAR FIELD, FRAUNHOFER ZONE) -The region of a sound beam in which the beam diameter increases as the distance from the transducer increases.

FAST FOURIER TRANSFORM - A mathematical formula used to derive an amplitude frequency profile in Doppler.

FISTULA, ARTERIOVENOUS - An abnormal communication between an artery and a vein, often resulting in cavity or aneurysm formation and abnormal Doppler flow dynamics.

FOCAL LENGTH - Distance from focused transducer to center of focal region or to the location of the spatial peak intensity.

FOCAL REGION - Region of minimum beam diameter and area.

FOCUS - To concentrate the sound beam into a smaller beam area than would exist without focusing.

FRAME - Display image produced by one complete scan of the sound beam. One frame is one completed "picture" produced by multiple, individual scanlines.

FRAME RATE - Number of frames displayed per second. Frame rates slower than 10 FPS looks choppy and noticeable.

FRAUNHOFER ZONE - See FAR ZONE

FREQUENCY - Number of cycles per unit of time (usually seconds), usually expressed in Hertz (Hz), Kilohertz (KHz) and Megahertz (MHz).

FREQUENCY - Number of regular recurrences in a given time, e.g. heartbeats or sound vibrations.

FRESNEL ZONE - See NEAR ZONE.

FRONTAL ARTERY - A terminal branch of the ophthalmic artery often used as the site for indirect internal carotid artery Doppler evaluation.

GAIN - Ratio of output to input electrical power.

GAITER AREA - Region on the lower, medial aspect of the calf; frequent site of venous stasis changes.

GANGRENE - Tissue death due to failure of blood supply, disease, or direct injury.

GATING - Electronically controlled device which controls transmission or reception of signal.

GRAFT - The replacement of a defect in the body with a portion of suitable material, either organic or inorganic. Material used for such replacement.

GRAY-SCALE DISPLAY - A display in which the intensity (amplitude) information is recorded as changes in brightness.

GREAT SAPHENOUS VEIN - One of two major superficial veins of the lower limb. Originating on the dorsum of the foot, it ascends medially along the calf and thigh, draining into the femoral vein. Longest vein in the body, with no direct communication to deep veins in lower leg. See POSTERIOR ARCH VEIN.

HARMONIC IMAGING – A special processing of returning echoes from tissue. The returning frequency is usually the same as transmitted frequency, but in Harmonic imaging, there is a higher returning frequency (from tissue vibration) that is processed. Image resolution is improved.

HEMANGIOMA - A tumor composed of blood vessels.

HEMATOMA - Localized mass of extravasated blood.

HEMIANOPIA - Loss of vision for one half of the visual field of one or both eyes.

HEMIPARESIS - A slight paralysis or incomplete loss of muscular tone on one side of the body.

HEMIPLEGIA - Paralysis of one side of the body. May be temporary (TIA) or permanent (stroke).

HEMISPHERIC - Relating to one side of the brain.

HEMODYNAMICS - The study of the interrelationship of blood pressure, blood flow, vascular volumes, physical properties of the blood, heart rate, and ventricular function.

HEMOGLOBIN - The respiratory protein of erythrocytes, having the reversible property of taking up oxygen (oxyhemoglobin) or of releasing it (reduced hemoglobin), depending primarily on the oxygen tension of the surrounding medium.

HEMORRHAGE - Bleeding, profuse flow of blood.

HEPATOFUGAL-flow away from the liver.

HEPATOPETAL- Flow towards the liver.

HERTZ - Unit of frequency, one cycle per second; unit of pulse repetition frequency, one pulse per second.

HETEROGENEOUS - Composed of structures having dissimilar characteristics or properties.

HOMAN'S' SIGN - Pain in the calf and popliteal area on passive dorsiflexion of the foot (from J. Homan's, U.S. Surgeon, 1872-1954).

HOMOGENEOUS - Of uniform composition.

HYDROSTATIC PRESSURE - A pressure created in a fluid system, such as the circulatory system.

HYPERCHOLESTEROLEMIA - An excess of blood cholesterol.

HYPERECHOIC - Producing echoes of higher amplitude than normal for the surrounding medium.

HYPEREMIA - The presence of an increased amount of blood in a body part. See reactive hyperemia.

HYPERLIPIDEMIA - Presence of increased amounts of lipids in the circulating blood.

HYPERTENSION - Elevated blood pressure.

HYPOECHOIC - Producing echoes of lower amplitude than normal for the surrounding medium.

HYPOTENSION - Diminished blood pressure.

HYPOVOLEMIA - Decreased blood volume usually due to blood or plasma loss in trauma.

HYPOXIA - Any state wherein an inadequate amount of oxygen is available to the tissues, without respect to cause or degree.

IMPEDANCE - Alterations of resistance with application of current. OHM'S law applies.

IMPEDANCE PLETHYSMOGRAPH - An instrument employing measurement electrodes which sense changes in a minute electric current sent through a portion of the body by means of separate electrodes proximal and distal to the sensing electrodes. Changes in electrical impedance of a limb are a reflection of the change in blood content and limb volume.

IMPOTENCE - Inability to achieve penile erection, a manifestation usually of a neurological or emotional dysfunction.

INCIDENCE ANGLE - Angle between propagated sound beam direction and line perpendicular to media boundary.

INFARCT - A localized area of ischemic tissue necrosis due to inadequate arterial blood supply. .

INTENSITY - The energy of an acoustic wave, equal to the power in the wave divided by the area over which the power is spread. Intensity = power (watts)/area (CM2).

INTENSITY REFLECTION COEFFICIENT -Reflected intensity divided by incident intensity.

INTENSITY TRANSMISSION COEFFICIENT -Transmitted intensity divided by incident intensity.

INTER- Between or among, eg., interosseous membrane, a membrane between bones.

INTERFACE - The surface forming the boundary between two media having different properties (i.e., acoustic impedances).

INTIMA - The innermost section of the arterial wall. Tunica intima.

INTRA - within, inside.

INTRACRANIAL - Refers to structures located within the cranium (skull).

INVASIVE PROCEDURES - A procedure characterized by instrumental penetration of the tissues; arteriography and venography are invasive procedures.

IPSILATERAL - Pertaining to anatomical structures on the same side of the body.

ISCHEMIA - Local reduction of blood supply, due to obstruction of inflow of arterial blood, or to vasoconstriction. Symptoms may include pallor, coldness, impairment of function, pain, and gangrene.

ISOECHOIC-Areas which have similar echogenicity are said to be isoechoic to each other. Makes it more difficult to "see" the desired tissue structure

JUGULAR VEIN - Major neck vein subdivided into anterior, external and internal jugular veins, bilaterally.

KILOHERTZ (KHz) - One thousand cycles per second.

LAMINAR FLOW - Fluid moving in concentric rings parallel to the axis of a tube. The center steam of fluid has the greatest velocity, with diminished velocities in successive rings from the axis, and slowest at the tube wall for fully developed steady flow.

LATERAL - Perpendicular to the direction of sound; or referring to a point away from the midline.

LATERAL RESOLUTION - Minimum reflector separation perpendicular to the sound path required for separate reflections to be produced. LR is improved with beam focusing.

LESSER SAPHENOUS VEIN - One of two major superficial veins of the lower limb. Originating on the lateral side of the foot, it extends along the posterior aspect of the calf and drains into the popliteal vein. See Small Saphenous Vein- (new nomenclature)

LINEAR ARRAY - Array made up of rectangular elements in a line.

LIPID - Anyone of a group of fats which are insoluble in water and may be deposited on arterial intima, contributing to arteriosclerosis.

LOGARITHM (BASE 10) - The logarithm of a number is equal to 1 plus the number of times 10 must be multiplied by itself to result in that number.

LONGITUDINAL - Parallel to the beam path (as in resolution) or parallel to the long axis of the vessel (as in scanning).

LONGITUDINAL RESOLUTION - Minimum reflector separation along the sound path required for separate reflections to be produced.

LONGITUDINAL WAVE - Wave in which the particle motion is parallel to the direction of wave travel.

LUMEN - The internal space of a blood vessel or duct.

LYMPHANGITIS - Inflammation of the lymphatic vessels.

LYMPHEDEMA - Swelling resulting from obstruction of lymphatic vessels or lymph nodes with accumulation of lymph in the affected area.

M -MODE (MOTION MODE) - Mode of operation in which the display records a spot brightening for each pulse delivered from the receiver, producing a one-dimensional time display of reflector position (motion).

MATCHING LAYER - Material placed in front of the front face of a transducer element to reduce the reflection at the transducer surface.

MATRIX ARRAY TRANSDUCER– A flat, linear array transducer with elements diced into a grid. Allows electronic focusing in the elevation plane, results in a uniformly narrow slice thickness.

MEAN FREQUENCY - The average frequency in one line of the Doppler spectrum. May be computed with several different algorithms.

MEDIA - Middle layer of an artery, mostly made up of smooth muscle cells, tunica media.

MEDIAL - Nearer to the middle or center.

MEDIUM - Material through which a wave travels.

MEGAHERTZ (MHz) - One million cycles per second. Doppler transducer crystals usually operate at 2-10 megahertz.

MEMORY - -Forgot!

MODE FREQUENCY - The strongest (brightest) frequency in one line of the Doppler spectrum.

MONCKEBERG'S SCLEROSIS - Medial arteriosclerosis - calcification of the middle coat of the small and medium sized muscular arteries (from J. G. Monckeberg, German Pathologist, 1877-1925).

MORBIDITY - The ratio of unhealthy individuals to the total population of a given group.

MORTALITY - The ratio of total number of deaths to the total number of population.

MULTIPLE REFLECTION - Several reflections produced by a pulse encountering a pair of reflectors.

MURAL - Pertaining to the wall of a vessel or cavity.

MYOCARDIAL INFARCTION (M.I.) - Damage or death to an area of heart muscle resulting from reduction of blood supply - heart attack.

NASAL ARTERY - A small artery arising from the ophthalmic artery and running across the dorsum of the nose. May be a source of collateral circulation in internal carotid occlusive disease.

NEAR ZONE (NEAR FIELD, FRESNEL ZONE) -The region of a sound beam in which the beam diameter decreases as the distance from the transducer increases.

NECROSIS - The pathologic death of a cell or group of cells in contact with living cells.

NEGATIVE PREDICTIVE VALUE - Ability of a diagnostic test to predict normal findings. NPV = true negative/all negative tests (true negative + false negative) X I00.

NEOPLASM - New growth. May be benign as in benign growth, or malignant as in cancer.

NEUROGENIC - Caused or affected by a dysfunction of the nervous system i.e. neurogenic impotence.

NEUROPATHY- a disease of the peripheral nerve or nerves.

NOISE - Any signal which interferes with the information being presented from a system; the interference may be electrical in nature or result from reverberation artifact.

NON-SPECULAR REFLECTION (Rayleigh scattering) - Reflection which occurs when boundary dimensions are comparable to or small compared with the wavelength, or if the boundary is irregular; the sound is redirected in many directions.

NORMAL INCIDENCE - Sound direction is perpendicular to media boundary.

NORMOTENSIVE - Characterized by normal blood pressure.

NYQUIST LIMIT– The point at which aliasing occurs. When Doppler frequency shift reaches 1/2 of the PRF.

OBLIQUE INCIDENCE - Sound direction is not perpendicular to media boundary.

OCCLUSIVE - The state of being closed or shut, as a venous or arterial occlusion.

OCULAR - Pertaining to the eye.

OHM - The ohm is the unit used to measure electrical resistance. One ohm is the resistance which will permit one ampere of current to flow under an electromotive force of one volt.

OHM'S LAW - I = E/R where I = current in amperes, E = electromotive force or potential difference in volts and R = resistance.

OPHTHALMIC ARTERY - The major artery of the eye, arising as the first branch of the internal carotid artery and terminating in frontal, supraorbital, and nasal arteries.

OVERALL ACCURACY - Sum of true positive tests and true negative tests divided by the total number of tests performed.

PACKET SIZE– The number of pulses per scan line in color Doppler. Several lines make up one frame of color. There must be at least 3 pulses per line (small packet size); the more pulses per line, the more robust the color.

PACS– Picture Archiving, Communication and Storage system

PALMAR ARCHES - The arterial anastomoses formed by the ulnar artery in the palm with a branch from the radial artery. Includes the deep and superficial palmar arches.

PALPATION - Examination by touch for diagnostic purposes. Arteries are often palpated.

PALPITATION - A throbbing of the heart, often associated with a rapid heart rate or irregular rhythm.

PANSYSTOLIC BRUIT - A bruit that extends throughout systole from the first to second heart sounds. Usually highly significant for arteriosclerotic disease. May be tapering or crescendo.

PARAPLEGIA - Paralysis of both lower extremities and occasionally the lower trunk.

PARESIS - Partial or slight paralysis.

PATENCY - The condition of blood flow through an open vessel. Opposite of occluded.

PATHOGENESIS - The origin and course of disease development, etiology.

PEAK FREQUENCY - The highest visible frequency in a Doppler spectrum.

PEDAL PULSE - Pulses of the foot.

PENILE-BRACHIAL INDEX - An index obtained by dividing the penile systolic pressure by the brachial systolic pressure. Low values may suggest vasculogenic etiology for impotence.

PERCUTANEOUS TRANSLUMINAL ANGIO-PLASTY (PTA) - A procedure involving the peripheral introduction of a balloon-tip catheter and dilating a stenotic region with inflation of the catheter tip.

PERFORATING VEINS (Perforators) - Venous channels that link the superficial and deep venous systems. Found predominantly below the knee, containing valves enabling unidirectional flow from superficial to deep veins, they vary in number from 90-200 over the entire course of the leg.

PERIORBITAL - Enclosing or affecting the tissues around the orbit (eye).

PERIPHERAL RESISTANCE - Impedance to blood flow in the systemic vascular bed.

PERIPHERAL SYMPATHETIC TONE - A state of normal tension in the peripheral vasculature caused by the sympathetic nervous system. Under certain conditions· this-tone may be altered by sympathectomy.

PETECHIA - Pinhead, minute hemorrhages in the skin.

PHANTOM - A device which simulates some parameters of the human body, and allows meaningful measurements of ultrasound system parameters. (Example. - longitudinal and axial resolution measurements).

PHASED ARRAY - A transducer configuration which consists of multiple elements which can be excited independently and allows for beam steering and focusing.

PHLEBITIS - Inflammation of a vein, with or without infection and thrombus formation.

PHLEBOGRAPHY - (VENOGRAPHY) Radio-graphic imaging of a vein or veins following intravenous injection of a radiopaque substance. An invasive procedure with known morbidity. .

PHOTOPLETHYSMOGRAPH (PPG) - An instrument which uses light to assess changes in skin blood perfusion; related to blood flow and limb volume change.

PIEZOELECTRIC CRYSTAL - A crystal that is used to transmit and receive ultrasound information. When excited by electrical charge the crystal vibrates and sends ultrasound waves. When excited by reflected ultrasound waves the piezoelectric crystal emits an electric signal which in turn is processed to indicate frequency of ultrasound energy received.

PIEZOELECTRICITY - Conversion of pressure to electrical voltage.

PIXEL - Picture elements (dots) on the video display of an imager or spectrum analyzer.

PLAQUE - In vascular disease usually refers to vessel disturbances of the intima. Consists of a collection of platelets, fibrin, lipids, and smooth muscle within the intima and media of the artery

PLASMA - The fluid portion of blood, composed of a mixture of many proteins in a crystalloid (crystal-like) solution.

PLETHYSMOGRAPH - Any instrument which measures volume change through a change in quantity of blood therein. Types: air, water, impedance, strain gauge, and photo.

PLUG FLOW - Fluid motion is entirely axial and at the same velocity at every point in the vessel. This type of flow is found in early systole when blood flow is accelerating.

POISEIULLE'S LAW - A formula which corresponds changes in flow in relation to changes in pressure, radius, length of segment, and fluid viscosity.

POPLITEAL ARTERY - A major leg artery, located behind the knee, arising from the superficial femoral arteries and terminating in the anterior tibial and posterior tibial, and peroneal artery.

POPLITEAL VEIN - A major leg vein behind the knee, medial to the popliteal artery. It arises from the superficial femoral vein and continues into the anterior tibial, posterior tibial, and peroneal veins.

POSITIVE PREDICTIVE VALUE - Ability of a diagnostic test result to predict abnormal findings. PPV = true positives/all positive tests (true positive + false positive) x l00.

POSTERIOR - Referring to the back surface of the body, or towards the back surface of the body.

POSTERIOR ARCH VEIN - The major tributary of the great saphenous vein in the lower leg. The vessel arises as a result of the confluence of a series of branches posterior to the medial malleolus, and ascends the posteromedial aspect of the leg terminating distal to the knee by entering the great saphenous veins. This vein communicates directly with the deep veins via medial leg perforators.

POSTPHLEBETIC SYNDROME - Chronic venous insufficiency resulting from deep venous thrombosis of the lower extremity. Symptoms may include edema, pain, varicose veins, and leg ulceration.

POWER - Rate at which work is done; rate at which energy is transferred.

POWER DOPPLER– (aka Color Angio, Convergence Color Doppler, Color Power Doppler) A color flow display based on signal amplitude. Advantages include color fill at 90° angles, and high sensitivity to low flow states. Some systems can color code for flow direction.

PRF-See Pulse Repetition Frequency

PROPAGATION SPEED - Speed with which a wave moves through a medium.

PROPHYLAXIS - A measure preventing the development or spread of disease.

PROXIMAL - Nearest the point of origin (usually heart) along the course of any asymmetrical structure; nearer to the attached end.

PSEUDOCLAUDICATION - Pain on walking, usually in the thigh and buttocks, which may or may not be relieved by rest. It can be distinguished from intermittent claudication usually by determining walk-pain-rest cycle and by location of the pain.

PSYCHOGENIC - The causation of a symptom or illness by psychic (mental) rather than organic factors.

PULMONARY EMBOLISM (PE) - Any obstruction to circulation lodged in the lung vasculature. Such obstruction often results from deep vein thrombosis of the lower extremity.

PULSATILITY INDEX - A Doppler wave form index defined by Gosling as: PI = peak to peak frequency mean frequency. The PI is a direct measure of severity of waveform dampening which is independent of probe angle.

PULSE DURATION - Time from start to finish of a pulse.

PULSE REPETITION FREQUENCY - Number of pulses transmitted per second. Sometimes called pulse repetition rate.

PULSE REPETITION PERIOD - Time from the beginning of one pulse to the beginning of the next.

PULSED WAVE - Short bursts of sound produced by electrical impulses applied to the transducer.

PULSED WAVE DOPPLER - Single transducer system in which bursts of ultrasound are transmitted; reception of returning signals determined by gate which allows flow to be assessed at specific sites and depths.

QUADRIPLEGIA - Paralysis of all four limbs.

QUALITY FACTOR - Operating frequency divided by bandwidth.

RADIAL ARTERY - A major artery of the forearm, arising from the brachial artery descending laterally and terminating in the palmar arch.

RANGE EQUATION - Relationship between round-trip pulse travel time and distance to a reflector.

RAYLEIGH SCATTERING - See Non-specular reflection.

RAYNAUD'S SYNDROME -PRIMARY -Intermittent pallor, cyanosis, or rubor of the digits usually induced by cold or emotion, with normal arterial flow and the absence of other primary causal disease, (from M. Raynaud, French Physician, 1834-1881).

RAYNAUD'S SYNDROME -SECONDARY) - Intermittent pallor, cyanosis, or rubor of the digits usually induced by cold or emotion, often secondary to chronic arterial occlusive disease.

REACTIVE HYPEREMIA - Increased blood flow to a body part in response to temporary occlusion..

RECANALIZATION - Restoration of a lumen in a blood vessel following thrombotic occlusion, by organization of the thrombus with formation of new channels.

REFLECTION - Acoustic energy reflected from a structure; intensity of reflection dependent upon acoustic impedance ratios at the interface.

REFLECTION ANGLE - Angle between reflected sound direction and line perpendicular to media boundary.

REFLECTOR - Media boundary that produces a reflection; reflecting surface.

REFRACTION - Change of sound direction on passing from one medium to another.

REGISTRATION - Positioning of reflectors in the display.

REJECTION - Eliminating smaller-amplitude voltage pulses.

RESISTANCE - Opposition to flow of current in electricity and blood in the vascular system.

REST PAIN - Pain in an extremity at rest, due to chronic ischemia of arterial occlusive disease. Such patients typically have an ankle/arm index of 0.5 or less.

RETROGRADE FLOW - Blood flowing in the opposite direction than is normal.

REVERBERATION - Multiple reflections within a confined space; a source of false information.

REYNOLD'S NUMBER - Abstract dimensionless number used to describe the flow of a fluid in a tube or past obstruction.

RIND - Reversible ischemic neurologic deficit.

RUBOR - Redness. See Dependent Rubor

SAGITTAL PLANE - Any set of anterior-posterior planes parallel to the long axis of the body.

SAMPLE VOLUME - Site of flow detection; size of sample volume determined by beam diameter and length of ultrasound burst.

SCAN CONVERTER - Device that stores a gray-scale image and allows it to be displayed on a television monitor.

SCATTERING - Diffusion or redirection of sound in several directions on encountering a particle suspension or a rough surface.

SCLEROSIS - A hardening or thickening of the arteries, produced by proliferation of fibrous connective tissue and deposit of lipids and calcium salts.

SECTOR SCAN - A system of scanning in which the transducer or transmitted beam is rotated through an angle, the center of rotation being near or behind the surface of the transducer.

SENSITIVITY - Statistical research term indicating the ability of a diagnostic test to detect disease when disease is actually present. Poor sensitivity is a high false negative rate.

SENSITIVITY - The minimum signal that can be satisfactorily detected and is generally limited by the input noise level of &he system.

SHADOWING - Reduction in reflection amplitude from reflectors that lie behind a strongly reflecting or attenuating structure.

SIDE LOBES - Minor beams of sound traveling out in directions not included in the primary beam.

SIGNAL-TO-NOISE RATIO - The ratio of peak amplitude of the signal to the standard deviation of the noise in the signal; the ratio is poor (low) when the Doppler signals have low amplitude relative to background noise.

SNELL'S LAW - Relates incidence and transmission angles of refraction.

SONOLUCENT-Allowing passage of ultrasonic waves without production of echoes that are due to reflection of some of the waves,

SOUND - Propagating, vibrational energy within a medium; gases, liquids and solids support these longitudinal or compression waves.

SPATIAL PULSE LENGTH - Length of space over which a burst occurs.

SPECIFICITY - Statistical research term relating the ability of a diagnostic test to indicate normalcy when no disease is actually present. Poor specificity is a high false positive rate.

SPECTRUM - The complete range of Doppler shift frequencies and amplitudes.

SPECTRUM ANALYZER - A spectrum analyzer employs microprocessing to display and analyze the complete frequency range of the Doppler shift for more complete diagnostic information.

SPECULAR REFLECTION - A highly directional reflection which occurs when the wavelength is small compared with the boundary dimensions and with boundary roughness.

SPHYGMOMANOMETER - An instrument for measuring the arterial blood pressure.

STASIS - A stagnation of blood flow or other fluids. In the lower extremity venous system stasis may contribute to deep vein thrombosis.

STENOSIS - Constriction or narrowing of vessel lumen.

STIFFNESS - Resistance of a medium to distort from original size and shape, and in ability to restore to original form after external influence is removed.

STOKES-ADAM'S SYNDROME - Syncope of cardiac origin occurring most often in patients with a pulse rate of less than 40 beats per minute and complete atrioventricular block. (From W. Stokes, Irish physician, 1804-1878 and R. Adams.)

STRAIN GAUGE PLETHYSMOGRAPH (SPG) - An instrument which assesses blood flow through detection of limb volume changes as reflected by impedance changes in an elastic tube filled with an electro-conductive metal, placed around the limb being examined.

STROKE - Informal term for cerebrovascular accident (CVA).

STROKE VOLUME - The volume of blood ejected by the left ventrical during a single systole.

SUPINE POSITION - Lying on the back, face upward.

SUPRAORBITAL ARTERY - The first terminal branch of the ophthalmic artery. The supraorbital artery is often the site of an indirect Doppler internal carotid evaluation.

SUPRASYSTOLIC PRESSURE - Cuff pressure above arterial systolic pressure producing total arterial occlusion.

SYMPATHECTOMY - Excision (removal) of a portion of the sympathetic (autonomic) nervous system. May be used as surgical therapy for chronic arterial vasoconstriction.

SYNCOPE - Episodic fainting, of brief duration, with complete recovery.

SYNDROME - A group of signs and symptoms, which, when considered together, are presumed to characterize a disease.

SYSTOLE - The contraction phase of the cardiac cycle.

TACHYCARDIA - Abnormally fast heart rate (over 100 beats per minute).

THORACIC OUTLET SYNDROME (TOS) - A condition in which nerves and arteries serving the upper extremity may be compressed at the outlet from the thoracic cavity. Primarily a mechanical neurological dysfunction.

THROMBECTOMY - Surgical removal of a thrombus.

THROMBOPHLEBITIS - Inflammation of a vein associated with thrombosis.

THROMBOSIS - The formation of a thrombus.

THROMBUS - A blood clot formed within the heart or blood vessels.

TIME GAIN COMPENSATION - Selective gain amplification with time to compensate for loss in echo intensity due to attenuation; permits echoes from greater depths to have same intensity as those from shallow sites.

TRANSCUTANEOUS (PERCUTANEOUS) -Performed through the skin.

TRANSIENT ISCHEMIC ATTACK (TIA) - An episode of transient cerebral symptoms including visual disturbances, memory loss, hemiparesis, numbness, dizziness, and speech difficulties which are of brief duration and resolved with no residual dysfunction. Usually related to atherosclerotic thrombotic disease and often a prelude to CVA.

TRANSMETATARSAL AMPUTATION - Amputation of toes across the metatarsals.

TRAPEZOID IMAGING– Combination of straight linear array and phased array on the same transducer. It extends the width of the field of view (FOV) along the sides of the image.

TRIPLEX MODE– Simultaneous operation of the image, color Doppler, and pulsed Doppler. Usually one modality is compromised.

TURBULENCE - The occurrence of eddies and vortices in blood flow, usually caused by a stenotic process which reduces vessel lumen diameter.

ULCERATION - The formation of a lesion on the surface of the skin or mucous tissue caused by arterial, venous, or neurogenic factors.

ULNAR ARTERY - A major artery of the forearm arising from the brachial artery, descending medially and terminating in the palmar arch.

ULTRASOUND - Sound of frequency greater than 20 KHz.

UNI-DIRECTIONAL - A Doppler instrument which assesses flow via frequency shift, in one direction only and gives no information as to which direction in relation to the probe.

VALSALVA MANEUVER - Forcible exhalation against the closed glottis (vocal folds) which increases intrathoracic pressure and impedes venous return. (From A. M. Valsalva, Italian anatomist, 1666-1723.)

VALVULAR INCOMPETENCE (INSUFFICIENCY) -A condition in which a vascular valve does not completely close, causing blood to leak in an abnormal direction (backflow, reflux).

VARICOCELE - A mass of tortuous and dilated scrotal veins most commonly found on the left resulting from valvular insufficiency in the internal spermatic vein. This condition may result in infertility and can be corrected surgically. Doppler ultrasound has been found useful in the diagnosis of clinical and subclinical varicoceles.

VASCULOGENIC - Originating from, or relating to, the vascular system.

VASOCONSTRICTION - Narrowing of the vessel lumen caused by contraction of the muscular vessel walls.

VASODILATION - Enlargement of vessel lumen due to relaxing of the muscular vessel walls.

VASOSPASTIC - A localized, intermittent contraction of a blood vessel.

VENOGRAPHY - Radiographic examination of veins following injection of a contrast medium. This is an invasive procedure with associated morbidity.

VENOUS INCOMPETENCE (INSUFFICIENCY, REFLUX) - Malfunction of the venous valves which allows blood to flow in a retrograde direction. See postphlebitic syndrome.

VENULE - A small vein.

VOLUME PULSE RECORDER (VPR) - Segmental air plethysmograph which employs changes in cuff pressure to indicate changes in limb volume due to blood flow. Same as PVR.

WALL FILTER–A filter in the Doppler system to eliminate high intensity, low frequency "noise" in the spectral display. Filtering occurs along the spectral baseline.

WAVELENGTH - Length of space over which a cycle occurs.

WHICHAMACALLIT- an object seen in the ultrasound image for which there is no name, or that you forgot the name. See Doohickey

ZERO CROSSING DETECTOR - An electrical circuit for Doppler signals. Also known as analog Doppler, it produces a single trace representing average frequency shift.

CME POST-TEST APPLICATION INFORMATION

Introduction

- Due to changing requirements for continuing medical education (CME) credits by issuing organizations, we have elected to offer the CME application and post-test online. This will allow us to stay current and meet any new requirements in the CME process.

- Upon successful completion of the textbook and CME self-test, participants can earn 15 Society of Vascular Ultrasound (SVU) CME credits.

- SVU CME credits may be applied towards the CME requirements of the ARDMS, the ARRT, CCI, and CARDUP, as well as ICAVL and ACR accreditation organizations.

- CME credits have been authorized by the SVU until April 1, 2014. CME credits may or may not be authorized after that date. Please check our website (www.summerpublishing.com) for updates on CME credits.

- ***The CME post-test application and test can be found on our website: www. Summerpublishing.com.***

- Select the CME Information page, and download the PDF document. You must have Adobe Reader software to read the PDF document. A free download of the Reader software is available at www.adobe.com.

- Complete the CME self-test; send the answer sheet, the information section, and the evaluation form to the address below. Please note that the number of multiple choice questions has increased due to the requirements of SVU.

- In the future we may provide the opportunity to take the CME post-test directly online. Information will be provided on the website in CME Information section.

- Additional and up-to-date instructions will be found in the CME section of our website.

- Enter the book code found below on the CME Post-test Application.

Book Code: 102011

Mail the application, completed test answer sheet, and evaluation form, along with check or credit card number to:

Summer Publishing
CME administrator
4572 Christensen Circle
Littleton, CO 80123

The CME self-test answer sheet, the information section, and the evaluation form may also be faxed (credit card number required) to **1-866-519-0674.**

CME Self-test Course Objectives: Upon completion of reading and studying " Techniques in Noninvasive Vascular Diagnosis", the participant should be able to:

1. Describe basic Doppler and color Doppler fundamentals as they apply to vascular diagnosis.

2. Describe cerebrovascular, upper and lower venous and arterial anatomy .

3. List and apply diagnostic criteria for carotid, venous, and arterial disease determination.

4. Describe normal venous and arterial hemodynamics and how flow patterns are altered by disease.

5. Describe abdominal vascular anatomy.

6. List diagnostic criteria for abdominal vascular duplex ultrasound exams.

7. Describe bypass and hemodialysis grafts/fistulas, and list normal and abnormal flow velocity parameters.

8. Describe methods of physiologic, indirect testing for upper and lower arterial disease.

9. Describe potential collateral pathways, and Doppler waveforms in the presence of subclavian or innominate artery obstruction.

10. Change and adjust appropriate imaging, Doppler and Color Doppler controls to optimize exam quality.

11. Recognize Doppler and imaging artifacts and describe how they occur.

12. Recite methods to evaluate vasculogenic impotence.

13. Describe methods for evaluating superficial and deep venous insufficiency.

14. Describe various disease processes that affect upper and lower extremity arteries and veins.

15. Describe intracranial vascular anatomy and transcranial Doppler (TCD) methods.

Index

A

B

C

T

U

V

W

Z

LAB AND PERSONAL RESOURCES

The Society of Vascular Ultrasound: The Voice for the Vascular Profession.
SVU represents vascular technologists, sonographers, vascular physicians, vascular lab managers, nurses, and other allied medical ultrasound professionals. SVU, 4601 Presidents Drive, Suite 260, Lanham, MD 20706-4831, tel: 301-459-7550. web site: www.SVUNET.ORG

The Society of Diagnostic Medical Sonography (SDMS) was founded in 1970 to promote, advance, and educate its members and the medical community in the science of Diagnostic Medical Sonography. Society of Diagnostic Medical Sonography, 2745 Dallas Pkwy. STE 350, Plano, TX 75093-873, tel: (800) 229-9506. web site www.SDMS.org.

Intersocietal Accreditation Commission. The IAC is dedicated to promoting quality health care by providing a peer review process of accreditation for Vascular Laboratories (ICAVL), Echocardiography Laboratories (ICAEL), Magnetic Resonance Laboratories (ICAMRL), and Computed Tomography Laboratories (ICACTL). Intersocietal Accreditation Commission , 8830 Stanford Boulevard, Suite 306 Columbia, MD 21045, tel: 800.838.2110. web site www.intersocietal.org web

---

KRP Accreditation Specialists, Inc. provides expert consultation in working with echo and vascular laboratories in the accreditation process. We essentially become your project coordinator and can lead you through the entire accreditation process. Acquiring accreditation requires not only a thorough, detailed investigation of the laboratory operation, but also a dedicated commitment from the laboratory staff.

Our goal is to ensure integrity and enhance efficiency within your laboratory. KRP Accreditation Specialists, Inc. can help by:

- Assisting with writing policies and procedures.

- Creating quality assurance and peer review programs.

- Review case studies to ensure technical compliance and improve overall imaging quality.

- Preparing the application for submission to the accreditation commission; providing copies of both the application and the data.

For further information, check our web site at www.krpaccreditation.com. E-mail to kpalmieri@ krpaccreditation.com. tel: (315) 685-0631.

Shugart Consulting provides practical tips, tools, resources, and approaches designed to improve vascular lab efficiency, quality, and patient experience while minimizing unnecessary expenses, <u>maximizing legitimate reimbursements,</u> and redirecting inappropriate costs.

On-site evaluation of personnel, operations, and systems results in a written report, containing analysis, recommendations, time lines, sample forms, etc, customized for your lab, to work within your existing systems. Limited services and telephone consultations are also available.
Rita Shugart, RN, RVT, FSVU, President, Shugart Consulting, worked as a vascular lab and surgical practice manager for 27 years.

Rita has also participated in numerous professional activities, serving as President of the North Carolina Vascular Technologists, North Carolina Vascular Nurses, the Society for Vascular Ultrasound, the Intersocietal Commission for the Accreditation of Vascular Laboratories, and the Intersocietal Accreditation Commission.   Shugart Consulting   rshugart@triad.rr.com   tel: 336-339-4323

CHAPTER-BASED EDUCATIONAL EXERCISES

The following self-quiz is designed to test your knowledge based on the book material. There are no continuing medical education (CME) credits offered for this section. The answer sheet can be down-loaded from www.summerpublishing.com. The exercises do not cover all chapters in the book.

CHAPTER 1: DOPPLER FUNDAMENTALS

I-1. What would happen to the frequency component of this waveform if the transmitted Doppler frequency (Ft) was 2.5 MHz?

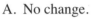

A. No change.
B. Increase by a factor of 2.
C. Increase by a factor of 4.
D. Decrease by a factor of 2.

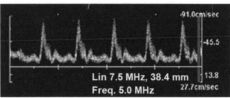

I-2. In the Doppler equation for velocity, what is Cos Θ (theta) ?

A. The Doppler beam angle of incidence to flow.
B. The Doppler steering angle.
C. The propagation speed.
D. The sample volume depth.

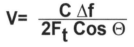

$$V= \frac{C \, \Delta f}{2F_t \, Cos \, \Theta}$$

I-3. In linear array transducers, Doppler steering is accomplished by which of the following methods?

A. An optical lens.
B. A mirror.
C. Mechanical adjustment of piezo elements.
D. Phasing.

I-4. What's causing this peripheral arterial waveform to look "goofy"?

A. Low wall filter.
B. No diastolic flow.
C. Wrong PRF.
D. High wall filter.

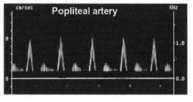

I-5. A Color Doppler image on most ultrasound systems is generated by which process?

A. Quadrature detection.
B. Autocorrelation.
C. Time Domain imaging.
D. Fourier Transformation.

I-6. Which of the following is an advantage of continuous-wave Doppler over pulsed-wave Doppler specifically for <u>segmental pressure</u> determination ?

A. B-mode image is not necessary for vessel location.
B. Higher transmit frequency.
C. Can process venous and arterial signal together.
D. No aliasing.

I-7.   Which of the following is <u>not</u> a product of color autocorrelation?

    A. Variance.
    B. Power.
    C. Peak frequency shift.
    D. Flow direction.

I-8.   Why is the measured velocity in this image inaccurate?

    A. Insufficient Doppler beam steering.
    B. Incorrect placement of measurement caliper.
    C. Angle adjustment cursor not aligned correctly.
    D. Sample volume misplaced.

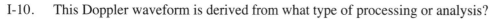

I-9.   Some ultrasound systems can enable a high PRF mode in which the spectral Doppler PRF is doubled. Which of the following is a resulting artifact?

    A. Mirror imaging.
    B. Increased aliasing.
    C. Spectral broadening.
    D. Multiple sample gates.

I-10.   This Doppler waveform is derived from what type of processing or analysis?

    A. Autocorrelation.
    B. Fast Fourier Transform.
    C. Zero crossing detection.
    D. Time interval histogram.

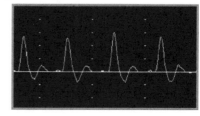

I-11.   Which of the following does not affect color frame rate?

    A. Packet size.
    B. Color gain.
    C. Color scan line density.
    D. Color box width.

I-12.   What pulsed-wave Doppler parameter is decreased when the range gate is reduced in size?

    A. Gain.
    B. PRF.
    C. Lateral resolution.
    D. Spatial pulse length.

I-13.   To improve the AXIAL resolution of an image, you could:

    A. Increase the transmit frequency.
    B. Decrease the transmit frequency.
    C. Add focal zones.
    D. Adjust the elevation plane focus.

I-14.   When obtaining a peak systolic velocity measurement using duplex ultrasound, the Doppler angle cursor should be adjusted to be _____ to the vessel wall.

    A. Perpendicular.

    B. Parallel.

    C. Transverse.

    D. Oblique.

I-15.   Is the flow direction in this vertebral artery normal?

    A. YES

    B. NO

I-16.   Name 3 indicators in the image that are used to determine flow direction.

    1._____

    2._____

    3._____

I-17.   The spectral Doppler display on a duplex ultrasound system is generated by which of the following processes?

    A. Autocorrelation.

    B. Zero-crossing detection.

    C. Analog processing.

    D. Fast Fourier Transform.

CHAPTERS 2 & 3: CAROTID IMAGING AND INTERPRETATION

II-1.   Which normal cerebrovascular vessel demonstrates the highest flow resistance?

    A. Common carotid artery.

    B. Internal carotid artery.

    C. External carotid artery.

    D. Vertebral artery.

II-2.   Which of the following best describes the position of the ICA in the neck ?

    A. It lies more posterior to the ECA.

    B. It's situated lateral to the ECA.

    C. It lies in the far-field of the ultrasound image.

    D. It appears in the near field of the ultrasound image.

II-3.   A high resistance flow pattern in the distal portion of the ICA suggests which of the following conditions?

    A. Proximal CCA disease.

    B. Proximal ICA disease.

    C. Intracranial AV fistula.

    D. Severe distal ICA stenosis.

II-4.   A stroke symptom when a patient cannot speak or express themselves is called :

   A. Dysarthria.
   B. Syncope.
   C. Amaurosis.
   D. Aphasia.

II-5.   In the following sonographic image, how would you describe the arterial wall?

   A. Normal.
   B. Heterogeneous plaque with irregular surface.
   C. Calcified plaque with ulcerated surface.
   D. Homogeneous plaque with smooth surface
      characteristics.

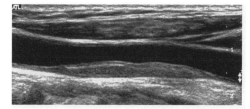

II-6.   What is the first branch of the ECA?

   A. Lingual artery.
   B. Superior thyroid artery.
   C. Facial artery.
   D. Occipital artery.

II-7.   What is the first branch of the ICA?

   A. External carotid artery.
   B. Middle cerebral artery.
   C. Ophthalmic artery.
   D. Retinal artery.

II-8.   The NASCET study clearly demonstrated benefits of carotid endarterectomy over medical
        management in patients who are symptomatic and have stenosis greater than or equal to ____ %.

   A. 80
   B. 70
   C. 65
   D. 40

II-9.   A patient presents with the classic cerebrovascular symptom of left amaurosis fugax. Of the
        choices below, what is the most likely cause?

   A. Atheroemboli from the left ICA.
   B. Atheroemboli from the right ICA.
   C. Occlusion of the left vertebral artery.
   D. Occlusion of the left ICA.

II-10. Which of the following is the most common cause of re-stenosis following carotid
        endarterectomy.

   A. Thrombosis.
   B. Atherosclerosis.
   C. Dissection.
   D. Neointimal hyperplasia.

II-11.   Which of the following is a non-atherosclerotic disease involving the mid segment of the ICA and found predominately in females?

 A. Takayasu's arteritis.
 B. Fibromuscular dysplasia.
 C. Arteriosclerosis.
 D. Scleroderma.

II-12.   Which of the following is the angiographic measurement method recommended by the SRU Consensus Conference of 2003, also known as the "NASCET" method?

 A. The estimated bulb diameter compared to the residual ICA lumen.
 B. The diameter of the CCA compared to the residual ICA lumen.
 C. The distal ICA lumen compared to the residual ICA lumen.
 D. The distal ICA diameter compared to the CCA diameter.

II-13.   A longitudinal image of carotid plaque can sometimes be misleading as to the diameter reduction due to which of the following?

 A. Slice thickness of the beam.
 B. Poor lateral resolution.
 C. Poor Contrast resolution.
 D. Calcium in the far field wall.

II-14.   A patient with a ICA plaque has a 2 mm residual lumen. The distal ICA lumen is 6 mm. What is the percent stenosis (via NASCET method)?

 A. 25%
 B. 33%
 C. 56%
 D. 67%

II-15.   In this example, the ICA velocities may underestimate the category of stenosis. Why?

 A. Doppler gain was too low.
 B. Sample was not obtained at maximum stenosis.
 C. Doppler was steered in the wrong direction.
 D. PRF scale was set incorrectly.

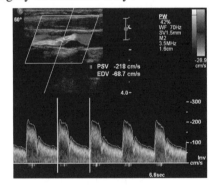

CHAPTER 4: VERTEBRAL-SUBCLAVIAN IMAGING

IV-1.   Which of the following statements regarding subclavian steal is most likely true?

 A. Subclavian steal occurs most frequently on the right side.
 B. Subclavian steal usually results in neurological symptoms.
 C. In left subclavian steal, the right vertebral artery supplies the left arm.
 D. The left common carotid artery flow is reduced.

IV-2.   The appearance of "early systolic deceleration" in the left vertebral artery waveform is usually due to which of the following conditions?

    A. Basilar artery obstruction.
    B. Left distal vertebral.
    C. Proximal left vertebral artery stenosis.
    D. Proximal left subclavian stenosis.

IV-3.   A subclavian artery aneurysm is a possible complication of:

    A. Thoracic outlet compression.
    B. Raynaud's disease.
    C. Fibromuscular dysplasia.
    D. Marfan's syndrome.

IV-4.   In the presence of an innominate artery occlusion, the ipsilateral common carotid artery (CCA) is often supplied by _____ flow in the right _____ artery.

    A. Retrograde, external carotid.
    B. Retrograde, subclavian.
    C. Antegrade, vertebral.
    D. Antegrade, external carotid.

IV-5.   Is the flow direction in this right vertebral artery normal?

    A. YES
    B. NO

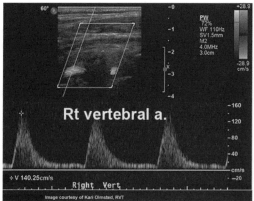

IV-6.   Name 2 indicators in the image that are used to determine flow direction.

    1._____
    2._____

IV-7.   How would you characterize this left subclavian waveform?

    A. Normal.
    B. Abnormal-distal to a stenosis.
    C. Abnormal-proximal to a stenosis.
    D. Hyperemic.

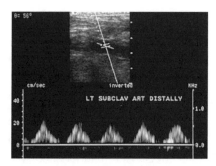

CHAPTER 5: VENOUS ANATOMY AND HEMODYNAMICS

V-1.   The gastrocnemius veins drain into what deep vein?

    A. Soleal vein.
    B. Posterior tibial vein.
    C. Popliteal vein.
    D. Femoral vein.

V-2.   Which of the following does not contribute to chronic venous insufficiency?

    A. Incompetent superficial vein valves.
    B. Chronic venous outflow obstruction.
    C. Dysfunctional veno-motor pump.
    D. Stasis dermatitis.

V-3.   Normal flow direction in perforating veins of the lower extremities is from the deep to superficial veins.

    A. True
    B. False

V-4.   What paired veins lie closest to the fibula?

    A. Posterior tibial.
    B. Peroneal.
    C. Anterior Tibial.
    D. Plantar.

V-5.   What is the name for the perforating veins found in the medial side of the mid to lower calf?

    A. Cockett's.
    B. Dodd's
    C. Hunterian
    D. Sherman's

V-6.   Return blood flow from the legs decreases during inspiration due to which of the following?

    A. An increase in intra-abdominal pressure.
    B. A decrease in intra-abdominal pressure.
    C. An increase in right side heart pressure.
    D. A decrease in intra-thoracic pressure.

V-7.   Pulsatile flow in the popliteal veins, bilateral, may be a sign of which of the following conditions?

    A. Proximal venous thrombosis.
    B. Distal thrombosis.
    C. Incompetent venous valves.
    D. Congestive heart failure.

V-8.   What is the main impediment to blood return from the legs to the heart when sitting?

  A. Small vein diameter
  B. Right-sided heart pressure
  C. Hydrostatic pressure
  D. Extrinsic compression of the popliteal vein

V-9.   In the exercise below, connect a letter that relates to a vein or structure to the description on the left.

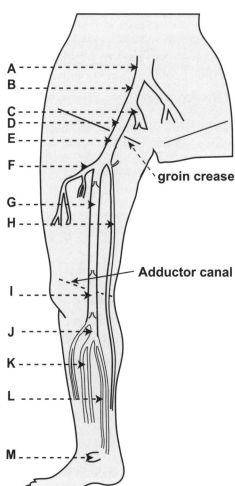

femoral vein.   1)_____
external iliac vein.   2)_____
inferior vena cava.   3)_____
peroneal veins.   4)_____
common iliac vein.   5)_____
internal iliac vein.   6)_____
posterior tibial veins.   7)_____
great saphenous vein.   8)_____
common femoral vein.   9)_____
popliteal vein.   10)_____
deep femoral vein.   11)_____
medial malleolus.   12)_____
tibial-peroneal trunk.   13)_____

V-10.   The calf muscle veins that drain into the posterior tibial or peroneal veins are known as:

  A. Small saphenous veins.
  B. Soleal veins.
  C. Gastrocnemius veins.
  D. Perforator veins.

V-11.   The small saphenous vein usually drains into which of the following veins?

A. Common femoral.
B. Femoral.
C. Gastrocnemius.
D. Popliteal.

V-12.   The vein of Giacomini courses between what two vein segments?

A. Great saphenous to accessory saphenous.
B. Small saphenous to popliteal vein.
C. Small saphenous to great saphenous.
D. Gastrocnemius to soleal.

CHAPTERS 6 & 7: VENOUS IMAGING & INSUFFICIENCY

VI-1.   A venous Doppler exam of the popliteal vein reveals a sustained flow signal upon release of distal compression. This would indicate which of the following:

A. Proximal obstruction.
B. Venous reflux.
C. Normal venous flow.
D. Distal obstruction.

VI-2.   Virchow's triad is best described as the following:

A. Circulatory stasis and hypocoagulability with intimal injury.
B. Circulatory stasis, hypercoagulability and intimal injury.
C. High cardiac output and intimal injury.
D. Intimal injury, hypercoagulability and poor stroke volume.

VI-3.   Continuous, non-phasic venous flow unilaterally in a common femoral vein suggests which of the following conditions.

A. Normal flow.
B. Femoral vein thrombosis.
C. IVC obstruction.
D. Iliac vein obstruction.

VI-4.   What is another name for an abnormal popliteal structure containing synovial fluid?

A. Hematoma.
B. Ganglion cyst.
C. Baker's cyst.
D. Lymph node.

VI-5.   The presence of respiratory variation in the femoral vein rules out DVT in the ipsilateral popliteal vein. True or False?

A. True
B. False

VI-6.   A condition resulting in a grossly swollen and cyanotic leg that is caused by iliofemoral venous thrombosis is known as:

    A. Stasis dermatitis.
    B. Lymph edema.
    C. Homan's sign.
    D. Phlegmasia cerulea dolens.

VI-7.   What is the name of the perforating veins located in the upper thigh?

    A. Cockett's.
    B. Boyd's.
    C. Hunterian.
    D. Dodd's.

VI-8.   Incompetence in this valve often leads to the entire GSV being incompetent. Name this valve?

    A. External iliac valve.
    B. Terminal valve.
    C. Mitral valve.
    D. Sapheno-popliteal valve.

VI-9.   In addition to incompetent valves, which of the following is a cause of venous insufficiency?

    A. Arterial occlusive disease.
    B. IVC filter.
    C. Chronic venous outflow obstruction.
    D. Atresic great saphenous vein.

VI-10. With the patient standing, what time value is the threshold between normal and abnormal reflux in the deep veins?

    A. 0.35 second.
    B. 0.5 second.
    C. 1 second.
    D. 2 seconds.

VI-11. Perforating veins exceeded this diameter have a high predictive value for being incompetent.

    A. > 1 mm
    B. > 1.5 mm
    C. > 2 mm
    D. > 2.5 mm
    E. > 3.5 mm

VI-12. Which of the following describes the anatomical position of the popliteal vein compared to the popliteal artery?

    A. It lies posterior to the artery.
    B. It's lateral to the artery.
    C. It's medial to the artery.
    D. It lies anterior to the artery.

VI-13. Thrombosis of the left common iliac vein by extrinsic compression of the right iliac artery is known as:

    A. Marfan's syndrome.
    B. Nutcracker syndrome.
    C. Arcuate ligament syndrome.
    D. May-Thurner syndrome.

VI-14. Which of the following best describes primary venous insufficiency?

    A. Insufficiency caused by chronic outflow obstruction
    B. Insufficiency caused by congenital absence of valves.
    C. Insufficiency resulting from previous deep vein thrombosis.
    D. Insufficiency resulting from poor arterial inflow.

VI-15. Which of the following veins should not be evaluated with the valsalva maneuver for reflux?

    A. Popliteal.
    B. Great saphenous.
    C. Common femoral.
    D. Proximal femoral.

VI-16. Perforating veins should be evaluated with the patient in which of the following positions?

    A. Supine.
    B. Sitting, leg dependent.
    C. Trendelenburg.
    D. Semi-Fowler's.

VI-17. Why is Doppler angle correction not necessary in venous imaging.?

    A. Velocity is already known.
    B. Velocity calculation is not necessary.
    C. Doppler angle can be at 90 degrees.
    D. Flow direction is not important.

CHAPTER 8: VENOUS UPPER EXTREMITY IMAGING

VIII-1. During inspiration, what condition listed below occurs in the upper extremity veins?

    A. Intra-thoracic pressure is decreased causing an increase in flow.
    B. Intra-thoracic pressure is increased causing an increase in flow.
    C. Intra-thoracic pressure is increased causing a decrease in flow.
    D. Inspiration only affects flow in the leg veins.

VIII-2. The cephalic and the basilic veins are connected distally by which of the following vein?

    A. Median cubital.
    B. Brachial.
    C. Subclavian.
    D. Radial.

VIII-3. The innominate vein is formed by the confluence of what two veins?

    A. Axillary, subclavian.
    B. Internal jugular, subclavian.
    C. External jugular, internal jugular.
    D. Brachiocephalic, subclavian.

VIII-4. Which of the following is a sign of normalcy in a subclavian vein that is usually not present in the lower extremity veins?

    A. Respiratory variation.
    B. Augmentation.
    C. Prominent cardiac pulsatility.
    D. Steady, continuous, non-phasic flow.

VIII-5. What is the best ultrasound method for assessing the central veins?

    A. Compressibility-coaptation.
    B. Spectral Doppler flow pattern assessment.
    C. Color Doppler.
    D. Augmentation from the arm.

CHAPTER 9: ARTERIAL HEMODYNAMICS, ANATOMY, PHYSIOLOGY

IX-1. Which of the following principles, effects or laws apply to decreased pressure with increase flow speed?

    A. Bernoulli's effect.
    B. Poiseuille's law.
    C. Reynolds law.
    D. Murphy's law.

IX-2. Laminar flow is disrupted and turbulence occurs when the Reynold's number meets or exceeds what value?

    A. 100.
    B. 200.
    C. 1000.
    D. 2000.

IX-3. This equation: E (energy) = I (current) x R (resistance) is called _____ and is often used as an analogy to _____.

    A. Ohm's law, Poiseuille's law.
    B. Reynolds law, Bernoulli's principle.
    C. Ohms law, Newton's law.
    D. Continuity rule, Ohm's law.

IX-4.   The highest pressure in the arterial system is found in what region or organ?

    A. Posterior tibial arteries.

    B. Left ventricle of the heart.

    C. Abdominal aorta.

    D. Internal carotid artery.

IX-5.   Which of the following arterial wall structures is in direct contact with blood flow?

    A. Intima.

    B. Media.

    C. Adventitia.

    D. Endothelium.

IX-6.   Perfusion in tissue is controlled by vasoconstriction and vasodilatation in which of the following structures?

    A. Capillaries.

    B. Arterioles.

    C. Large feeding arteries.

    D. Small veins.

IX-7.   Which of the following is not a risk factor for peripheral arterial disease?

    A. Venous reflux/insufficiency.

    B. Diabetes Mellitus.

    C. Hypercholesterolemia.

    D. Tobacco abuse.

IX-8.   What is the most significant factor affecting diastolic blood flow in the lower extremities?

    A. Cardiac output.

    B. Systemic blood pressure.

    C. Vasodilation in the capillary bed.

    D. Vasoconstriction/dilation in the arterioles.

IX-9.   The vaso vasorum supplies blood flow to what structure?

    A. Arterial wall.

    B. Vas deferens.

    C. Capillaries.

    D. Toes.

IX-10. Of the symptoms listed below, which is generally not associated with arterial insufficiency?

    A. "Blue Toe" syndrome.

    B. Dependent rubor.

    C. Limb swelling.

    D. Rest pain in feet and toes.

IX-11. Which of the following is another name for the internal Iliac artery?

  A. Profunda Iliac.
  B. Profunda femoris.
  C. Inferior epigastric.
  D. Hypogastric.

IX-12. What is the first major tibial artery branching off the distal popliteal artery?

  A. Dorsalis pedis artery.
  B. Peroneal artery.
  C. Gastrocnemius artery.
  D. Anterior tibial artery.

IX-13. What is the most common symptom of peripheral arterial disease?

  A. Rest Pain
  B. Claudication
  C. Trophic nails
  D. Reduced pedal pulses

IX-14. Thromboangiitis obliterans is a fixed occlusive disease of the digits. What is another name for this condition?

  A. Marfan's syndrome.
  B. Raynaud's syndrome.
  C. Takayasu's arteritis.
  D. Buerger's disease.

IX-15. The "blue toe" syndrome is a symptoms of what condition?

  A. Vasospasm.
  B. Arteritis.
  C. Atheroemboli.
  D. Popliteal entrapment

IX-16. Which artery supplies the most blood to the gluteus maximus muscle?

  A. External iliac artery
  B. Inferior buttock artery
  C. Inferior epigastric artery
  D. Internal pudendal artery
  E. Hypogastric artery

CHAPTER 10: PHYSIOLOGIC TESTING-LOWER EXTREMITIES.

X-1.   When obtaining ankle blood pressures, what is the primary reason for having the patient in a flat, supine position?

  A. Patient comfort.
  B. Venous pressure reduction.
  C.. Easier Doppler placement.
  D. Reduce/eliminate hydrostatic pressure.

X-2.   Which of the following statements best describes the flow profiles at "X" and "Y" in this spectral Doppler waveform?

   A. X is plug flow, Y is turbulent flow.
   B. X is parabolic flow, Y is turbulent flow.
   C. X is plug flow, Y is parabolic flow.
   D. X is laminar flow, Y is non-laminar flow.

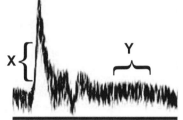

X-3.   Which of the following ankle/brachial indices (ABI) is most consistent with the symptom of ischemic rest pain?

   A. 0.3
   B. 0.5
   C. 0.8
   D. 1.0

X-4.   Which of the following conditions would cause an abnormal pulse volume recording (PVR) at the high-thigh location?

   A. Superficial femoral artery occlusion.
   B. Internal iliac artery stenosis.
   C. Popliteal artery occlusion.
   D. Significant aortoiliac disease.

X-5.   The reported advantage of a four-cuff segmental pressure test over a three-cuff method is differentiating which of these diseased segments?

   A. Aorta disease from iliac disease.
   B. Femoral artery from popliteal artery disease.
   C. Aortoiliac from femoral artery disease.
   D. Common femoral artery from profunda femoris disease.

X-6.   Photoplethysmography uses which of the following modalities for blood flow evaluation.

   A. Pulse volume recording.
   B. Ultrasound.
   C. Ultraviolet.
   D. Infrared.

X-7.   Which of the following lower arterial test modalities provides diagnostic quantitative information?

   A. Segmental pressures.
   B. Continuous-wave Doppler waveforms.
   C. Photoplethysmography.
   D. Pulse volume recording.

X-8.   For accurate blood pressure determination, the cuff bladder should be_____of the limb circumference.

    A. 10%
    B. 20%
    C. 30%
    D. 40%

X-9.   Pulse volume recording is a form of which of the following methods/techniques?

    A. Impedance plethysmography.
    B. Pneumo-plethysmography.
    C. Photoplethysmography.
    D. Segmental pressures.

X-10.   Please review this PVR and segmental pressure study and select an appropriate comment below.

    A. The study is normal.
    B. The study is abnormal on the left.
    C. The left ankle pressures are probably erroneous.
    D. The study is abnormal on the right.
    E. The arteries in the thigh are calcified.

X-11.   In the image about, how is the ankle to brachial index (ABI) calculated?

    A. Left ankle pressure divided by left brachial pressure and right ankle pressure divided by right brachial pressure.
    B. Both right and left ankle pressures divided by the highest brachial pressure.
    C. The right brachial pressure divided by both ankle pressures.
    D. Both right and left ankle pressures divided by the left brachial pressure.

X-12.   While performing segmental pressures on a lower extremity, you note a pressure gradient between two cuffs to equal 15 mmHg. What does this finding indicate?

    A. Normal result, no big deal.
    B. Stenosis in the arterial segment proximal to the lowest cuff.
    C. Total occlusion of the arterial segment.
    D. Stenosis in the arterial segment distal to the lowest cuff.

X-13.   Leg pain with exercise that is not due to arterial occlusive disease is often referred to as:

    A. Buerger's disease.
    B. Pseudo-claudication.
    C. Rest pain.
    D. Arteritis.

X-14. Which of the following is a disadvantage of photoplethysmography compared to CW-Doppler in segmental pressure acquisition?

    A. PPG cannot be heard.
    B. PPG uses analog processing.
    C. PPG has no waveforms.
    D. PPG can only be used for digit pressures.

X-15. The dorsalis pedis artery is a continuation of which vessel?

    A. Peroneal artery.
    B. Gastrocnemius artery.
    C. Posterior tibial artery.
    D. Anterior tibial artery.

CHAPTER 11: COLOR DOPPLER IMAGING: LOWER EXTREMITY.

XI-1. A high-pressure extravasation of blood out of an artery and into the surrounding tissue is called a(n):

    A. Aneurysm.
    B. Arterial-Venous fistula.
    C. Pseudo-aneurysm.
    D. A-V malformation.

XI-2. PW-Doppler spectral waveforms obtained from the common femoral arteries bilaterally are measured for rise time (RT). The right RT is 0.09 seconds, and the left is 0.19 seconds. What is the anatomic level of the occlusive disease?

    A. Aortoiliac disease.
    B. Left iliac disease.
    C. Left superficial femoral artery disease.
    D. Right iliac disease.

XI-3. What is the threshold diameter for the popliteal artery to be considered aneurysmal?

    A. 0.5 cm
    B. 1.0 cm
    C. 2.0 cm
    D. 3.0 cm

XI-4.   In the presence of an SFA occlusion, what vessel usually provides collateral flow?

    A. Popliteal artery.
    B. Common femoral artery.
    C. Great saphenous vein.
    D. Deep femoral artery.

XI-5. The common femoral artery Doppler waveform will always be abnormal in the presence of a >50% common iliac artery stenosis. True or False?

    A. True
    B. False

CHAPTER 12: ARTERIAL BYPASS GRAFTS

XII-1. The most common vein used for "in situ" bypass grafts is:

    A. Small saphenous vein.
    B. Popliteal vein.
    C. Basilic vein.
    D. Great saphenous vein.

XII-2. Which of the following is <u>not</u> a potential complication of a reversed femoro-popliteal vein graft?

    A. Neointimal hyperplasia.
    B. Graft aneurysm.
    C. Fistula via non-ligated perforator vein.
    D. Graft kink.

XII-3. What is the minimum diameter of the great saphenous vein considered to be appropriate for a successful in situ arterial bypass?

    A. 1.0 mm
    B. 1.5 mm
    C. 2.0 mm
    D. 2.5 mm

XII-4. The radial artery terminates in which vessel?

    A. Palmar arch.
    B. Ulnar artery.
    C. Brachial artery.
    D. Interosseous artery.

XII-5. In which bypass graft procedure is a valvulotome used?

    A. In situ vein bypass.
    B. Radial artery harvest.
    C. Reversed vein bypass.
    D. Aorto-bifemoral.

XII-6. During arterial mapping of the radial artery, you should do all of the following except:

    A. Determine if there is a calcified wall.
    B. Measure the peak systolic velocities proximal and distal.
    C. Perform reactive hyperemia on the arm.
    D. Check for stenosis.
    E. Measure the diameter of the vessel.

XII-7. A hyperemic waveform existing in the posterior tibial artery 3 weeks status-post a femoral to distal vein bypass is most likely due to which of these conditions?

    A. Graft occlusion.
    B. Vasoconstriction.
    C. Graft stenosis.
    D. Chronic vasodilation.

XII-8. What is the most common cause of in situ vein bypass graft stenosis?

    A. Atherosclerosis.
    B. Intimal hyperplasia.
    C. Collagen vascular disease.
    D. Arteritis.

XII-9. A photoplethysmography (PPG) tracing on the 5th hand digit (small finger) that goes from normal to "flat-line with radial artery compression indicates which of the following?

    A. Patient has ulnar artery perfusion dominance.
    B. Patient has radial artery dominance.
    C. Patient has a radial artery stenosis.
    D. Patient has disease in the digital arteries.

CHAPTER 13: ARTERIAL UPPER

XIII-1. The left brachial pressure is 20 mmHg lower than the right brachial pressure. What's up?

    A. Stenosis of the brachiocephalic artery.
    B. Stenosis of the subclavian artery.
    C. Stenosis of the brachial artery.
    D. It's a normal pressure gradient.

XIII-2. Buerger's disease is an arterial disorder involving which of the following vessels?

    A. Renal arteries.
    B. Coronary arteries.
    C. Pelvic arteries.
    D. Digital arteries.

XIII-3. What is cold or vibration induced digital vasospasm?

    A. Marfan's syndrome.
    B. Arteritis.
    C. Buerger's disease.
    D. Raynaud's syndrome.

XIII-4. Thoracic outlet syndrome is usually caused by extrinsic compression of the subclavian artery. True or False?

    A. True.
    B. False.

XIII-5. Which of the following is the standard recovery time following a cold immersion test for Raynaud's?

    A. 2 minutes.
    B. 5 Minutes.
    C. 7 minutes.
    D. 10 minutes.

XIII-6. The innominate artery is also called the:

    A. Brachiocephalic.

    B. Subclavian.

    C. Brachiobasilic.

    D. Axillary.

XIII-7. Which of the following is the manual test for palmar arch patency?

    A. Adson test.

    B. TOS test.

    C. Allen's test.

    D. PPG.

CHAPTER 15: HEMODIALYSIS ACCESS GRAFTS AND FISTULAS

XV-1. Which of the following best describes the Brescia-Cimino procedure?

    A. A brachial artery to median cubital vein fistula.

    B. A straight Teflon graft from radial artery to the basilic vein.

    C. A radial artery to cephalic vein fistula.

    D. An indwelling hemodialysis catheter.

XV-2. In a patient with a hemodialysis access forearm loop graft, digital ischemia can result from which of the following conditions?

    A. Thrombosed hemodialysis access graft.

    B. Incomplete palmar arch.

    C. Pseudoaneurysm.

    D. Venous outflow obstruction.

XV-3. Which of the following veins does not have an accompanying artery?

    A. Subclavian.

    B. Axillary.

    C. Brachial.

    D. Basilic.

XV-4. What is considered to be the lowest vein diameter suitable for an arterial to venous hemodialysis fistula?

    A. 1.5 mm

    B. 2.0 mm

    C. 2.5 mm

    D. 2.0 cm

XV-5. Which of the following grafts is impenetrable by ultrasound?

    A. Gore-tex.

    B. Bovine.

    C. Atrium.

    D. Vectra.

XV-6.   Reverse flow detected in the distal radial artery of an ipsilateral radial artery to basilic vein graft indicates which of the following conditions?

    A. Impending graft failure.
    B. Occluded ulnar artery.
    C. Incompetent palmar arch.
    D. Patent palmar arch.

XV-7.   Which of the following vessels is not usually used hemodialysis access grafts of fistulas?

    A. Cephalic vein.
    B. Brachial vein.
    C. Basilic vein.
    D. Median cubital vein.

XV-8.   Antegrade, triphasic flow in a radial artery distal to a brachial artery to basilic vein loop hemodialysis access graft indicates which of the following?

    A .   Normal radial artery flow.
    B. Venous outflow obstruction.
    C. Pseudoaneurysm at anastomosis.
    D. Graft failure.

XV-9.   Which access graft does not require maturation time?

    A. Vectra (polyurethane).
    B. Gore-tex.
    C. Atrium.
    D. Impra PTFE.

XV-10. Antegrade, triphasic flow in a brachial artery proximal to a radial artery to basilic vein hemodialysis access graft indicates which of the following?

    A. Normal radial artery flow.
    B. Venous outflow obstruction.
    C. Pseudoaneurysm at anastomosis.
    D. Graft failure.

CHAPTER 16: TRANSCRANIAL DOPPLER

XVI-1. In transcranial Doppler, the MCA is accessed through _____ "window" and typically demonstrates flow direction _____ the transducer.

    A. Suboccipital, away from.
    B. Transtemporal, away from.
    C. Transorbital, towards.
    D. Transtemporal, towards.

XVI-2. The optimal window for evaluation of the vertebral and basilar arteries with transcranial Doppler is the:

    A. Suboccipital window.
    B. Suborbital window.

C. Transtemporal window.

D. Transorbital window.

XVI-3. The blood flow velocity parameter commonly reported in transcranial Doppler is:

A. Peak systolic velocity.

B. Flow volume.

C. Time-averaged peak velocity.

D. Time-averaged mean velocity.

XVI-4. Intracranial cross-filling often occurs in which of the following vessels in the presence of an occluded ICA?

A. Anterior communicating artery.

B. Vertebral artery

C. Basilar artery

D. Posterior cerebral artery

XVI-5. Which of the following becomes an extracranial to intracranial collateral route in the presence of significant ICA disease?

A. Basilar artery to the two posterior cerebral arteries

B. Supraorbital and ophthalmic arteries via ECA branches

C. Bilateral anterior communicating arteries

D. Posterior communicating artery

XVI-6. Match the letter with the vessel name on the left.

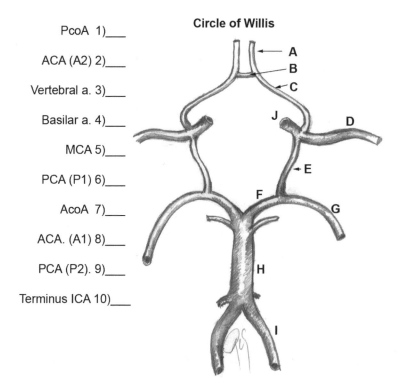

PcoA 1)____

ACA (A2) 2)____

Vertebral a. 3)____

Basilar a. 4)____

MCA 5)____

PCA (P1) 6)____

AcoA 7)____

ACA. (A1) 8)____

PCA (P2). 9)____

Terminus ICA 10)____

Circle of Willis

CHAPTER 17: ABDOMINAL DOPPLER

XVII-1.   The portal vein is formed by the confluence of which two veins?

       A. Splenic, superior mesenteric vein.
       B. Celiac, duodenal.
       C. Hepatic, IVC.
       D. Inferior mesenteric, renal.

XVII-2.   The celiac and hepatic arteries should normally exhibit a _____ waveform pattern.

       A. High resistance.
       B. Low resistance.
       C. Monophasic.
       D. Respiratory.

XVII-3.   What relationship does the right renal artery (RRA) have to the inferior vena cava (IVC)?

       A. RRA passes transverse to the IVC.
       B. RRA passes anterior to the IVC.
       C. RRA passes superior to the IVC.
       D. RRA passes posterior to the IVC.

XVII-4.   Flow direction into the liver is called:

       A. Hepatopetal flow.
       B. Hepatofugal flow.
       C. High resistant flow.
       D. Collateral flow.

XVII-5.   Which of the following is the first branch off the abdominal aorta?

       A. Celiac axis.
       B. Renal artery.
       C. Superior mesenteric artery.
       D. Common iliac artery.

XVII-6.   Which of the following is the threshold for an abnormal renal artery to aortic ratio (RAR)?

       A. 1.5
       B. 2.0
       C. 2.5
       D. 3.5

XVII-7.   What happens to the Doppler waveform in the celiac axis when the patient eats?

       A. Remains the same.
       B. Demonstrates a decrease in systolic velocity.
       C. Demonstrates an increase in systolic velocity.
       D. Demonstrates a decrease in diastolic velocity
       E. Demonstrates an increase in diastolic velocity

XVII-8.   Abdominal pain that develops 15-30 minutes after eating is sometimes called "fear of food" syndrome. Which of the following is a possible cause?

A. Cardiac angina.

B. Nutcracker syndrome.

C. Mesenteric ischemia.

D. Median arcuate ligament compression syndrome.

XVII-9.   A tardus parvus waveform in a segmental renal artery suggests what condition?

A. Renal parenchymal disease.

B. Coarctation of the aorta.

C. Stenosis or occlusion of the main renal artery.

D. Renal vein thrombosis.

XVII-10. Renal fibromuscular dysplasia (FMD) usually occurs in what vessel segment?

A. At the origin of the main renal arteries.

B. In the segmental arteries.

C. In the interlobar arteries.

D. In the mid to distal main renal artery.

XVII-11. Which of the items below describes the course of the left renal vein.

A. Posterior to the celiac axis and anterior to the aorta to enter the IVC.

B. Anterior to the SMA and inferior to the aorta to enter the IVC.

C. Posterior to the SMA and anterior to the aorta to enter the IVC.

D. Lateral to the SMA and medial to the aorta to enter the IVC.

XVII-12. A normal Doppler signal in the SMA postprandial should be:

A. A low resistance waveform.

B. A high resistance waveform with a peak systolic velocity of 220 cm/sec.

C. A low resistance waveform with a peak systolic velocity of 250 cm/sec.

D. A high resistance waveform.

XVII-13. Which of the following is not a cause of portal hypertension?

A. Thrombosis of the portal vein.

B. Hepatic artery stenosis.

C. IVC obstruction.

D. Hepatic fibrosis.

XVII-14. What is the criteria threshold for an SMA >70% stenosis?

A. PSV of 180 cm/sec.

B. EDV of 50 cm/sec.

C. PSV of 220 cm/sec.

D. PSV of 275 cm/sec.

XVII-15. At what dimension point does the portal vein size become abnormal?

A. 5 cm.

B. 8 cm.

C. 13 cm.

D. 16 cm.

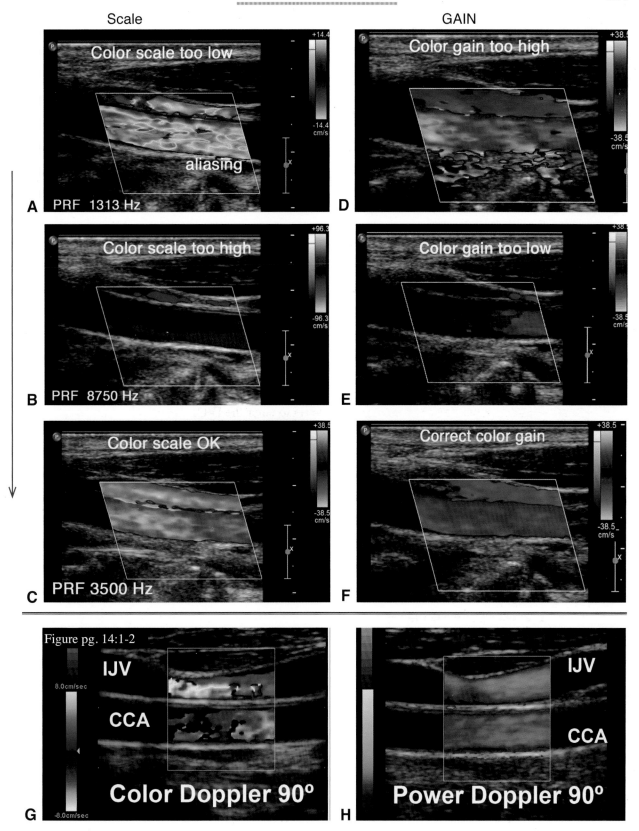

A. Color scale or PRF is set too low = Aliasing. B. Color scale is too high = poor filling in diastole. C. Color scale is optimized. D. Color gain is too high. E. Color gain is too low = poor filling.
F. Color gain is optimized. G & H. Comparison of vessel filling with color Doppler and Power Doppler at 90°.

Color Doppler Color Coding:

Figure pg.12:1-4

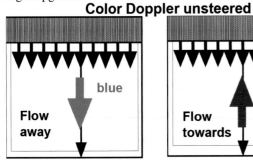

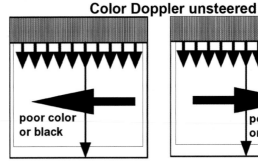

A Flow away from the color Doppler beams is encoded blue; Flow towards is red.

B Flow at 90° to Doppler, flow is neither towards nor away, poor color coding.

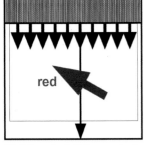
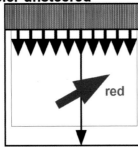

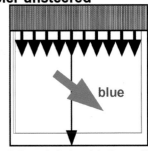

C Flow in left image is from right to left, but it's "towards". Flow in the right image is from left to right, but it's also "towards". Both are encoded red.

D Flow in left image is from right to left, but it's "away". Flow in the right image is from left to right, but it's also "away". Both are encoded blue.

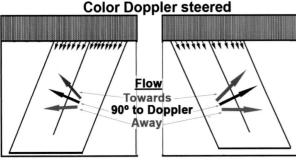

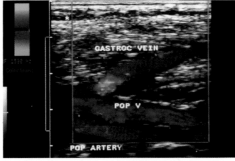

E Color coding depends on whether flow is towards or away from the Doppler beam.

F Gastrocnemius vein flow is encoded red because it's flowing away from the Doppler beam (and into the popliteal vein).

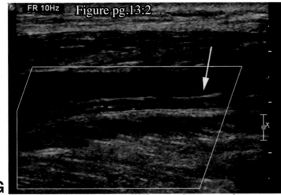

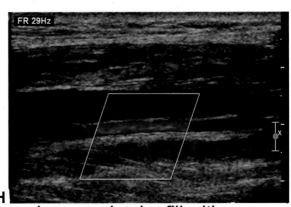

Figure pg.13:2

G Poor color filling due to low frame rate (10 Hz)

H Improved color fill with higher frame rate (29 Hz)

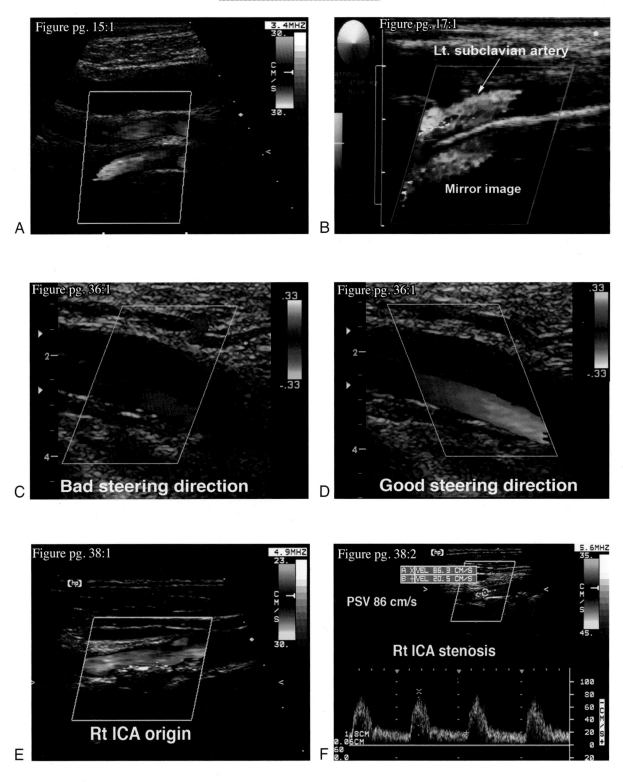

A. Mirror image artifact of the CCA; the upper vessel is the real deal. **B**. Mirror image of the left subclavian artery. The adjacent apex of the lung is the hard reflective surface contributing to the phenomenon.
C. Inappropriate color box steering direction in a popliteal artery with resulting poor fill. **D**. Correct steering direction for this vessel. **E - F**. An ICA stenosis that is less than 50% diameter reduction. Color and spectral Doppler show no increase in velocity over the stenosis. PSV over stenosis is 85 cm/sec.

"Mapping" a > 70% ICA stenosis.

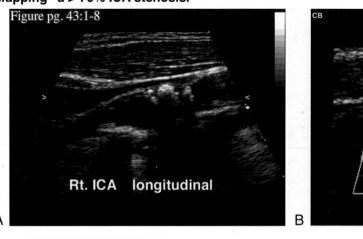

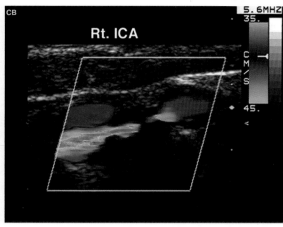

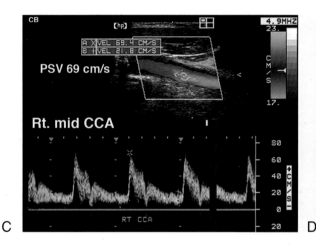

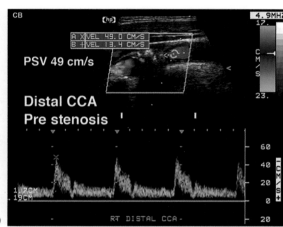

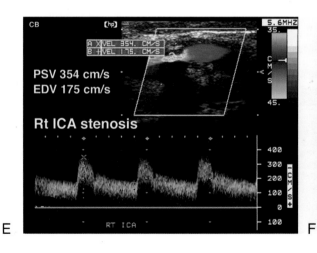

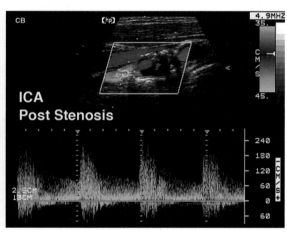

A. Longitudinal image of the ICA with calcified plaque. **B**. ICA imaged from a slightly different scan plane; color Doppler demonstrates frequency increase and aliasing. **C**. Velocity (PSV) in the mid CCA is 69 cm/s. **D**. PSV just before the stenosis is 49 cm/s. **E**. At maximum stenosis velocities are: PSV 351 cm/s, EDV 175 cm/s. Note the lack of spectral broadening in the Doppler waveform; in some stenotic "jets" flow is laminar. **F**. The expected post-stenotic turbulence.

continued next page

> 70% ICA stenosis continued.

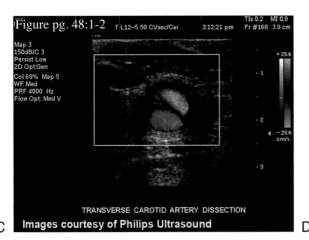

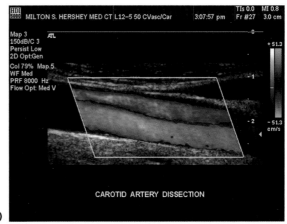

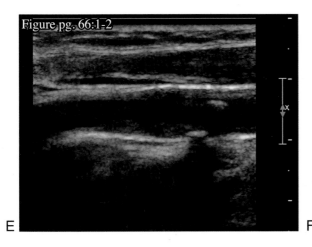

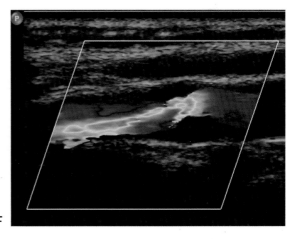

A. >70% continued: Severely disturbed, turbulent flow in the distal ICA. **B**. Unremarkable ECA flow and velocity. **C**. CCA dissection in transverse view. The blue area is retrograde flow within the dissection. **D**. Longitudinal view of the same CCA dissection. Red flow in the main channel flow. **E**. This plaque has mixed echogenicity with hypoechoic areas and some echogenic regions. The plaque appears minor, however, color Doppler outlines a more significant plaque. **F**. Color Doppler defines the contour of this same plaque, and shows frequency increase. Velocity measurements from spectral Doppler waveforms were PSV 218 cm/s, EDV 69 cm/s for a 50-69% stenosis category.

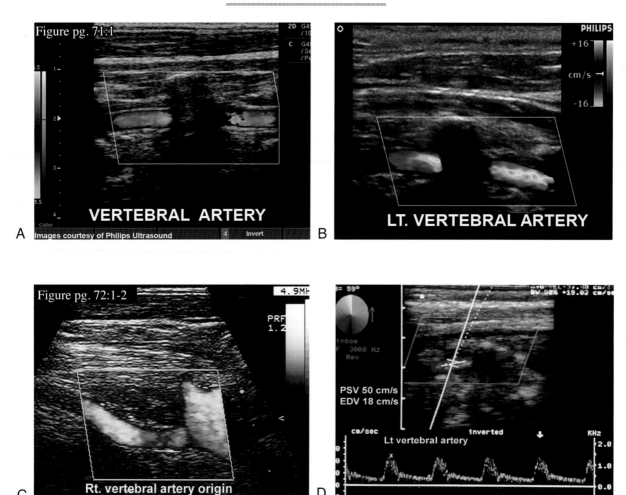

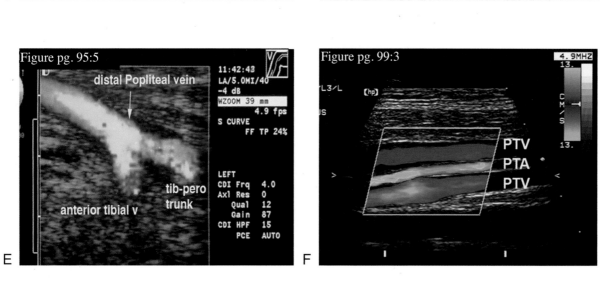

A. Vertebral artery flow is encoded red indicating it's going towards the Doppler beam or scanlines, i.e., normal flow direction. **B**. Vertebral artery flow is encoded blue; color bar is set to "blue away", so flow is away from the Doppler beam, i.e., retrograde flow. **C**. Power Doppler image of the right vertebral artery origin. **D**. Normal left vertebral artery waveform. **E**. Distal popliteal vein courses deep into the proximal calf. Transverse image is often suboptimal due to the oblique "cut" of the beam. **F**. Paired posterior tibial veins with the posterior tibial artery.

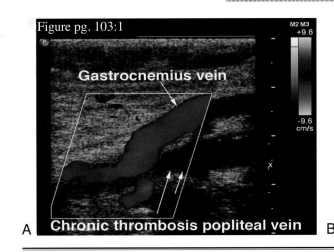

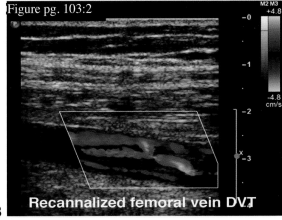

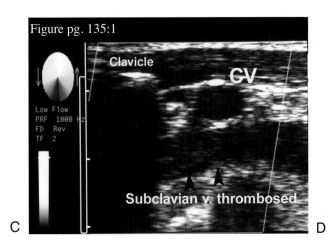

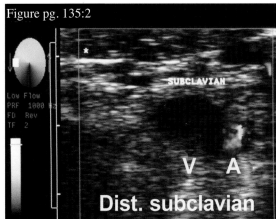

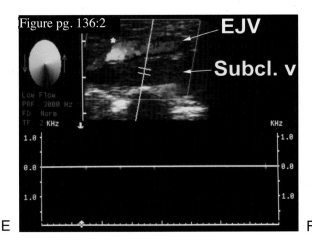

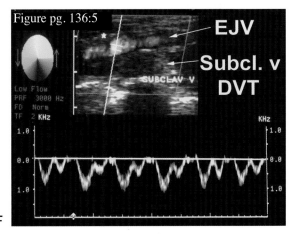

A. Gastrocnemius vein is dilated and functioning as a collateral pathway. The distal popliteal vein is chronically thrombosed. **B**. Different patient: recannalized femoral vein with old thrombosis. **C - F**. Case study #1: Acute upper extremity DVT. **C**. Thrombosed distal subclavian vein in longitudinal. **D**. Same thrombus in transverse planes. **E & F.** No flow in the proximal subclavian vein, but prominent flow in the external jugular vein (EJV). A potential pitfall exists by mistaking the EJV for the subclavian vein.

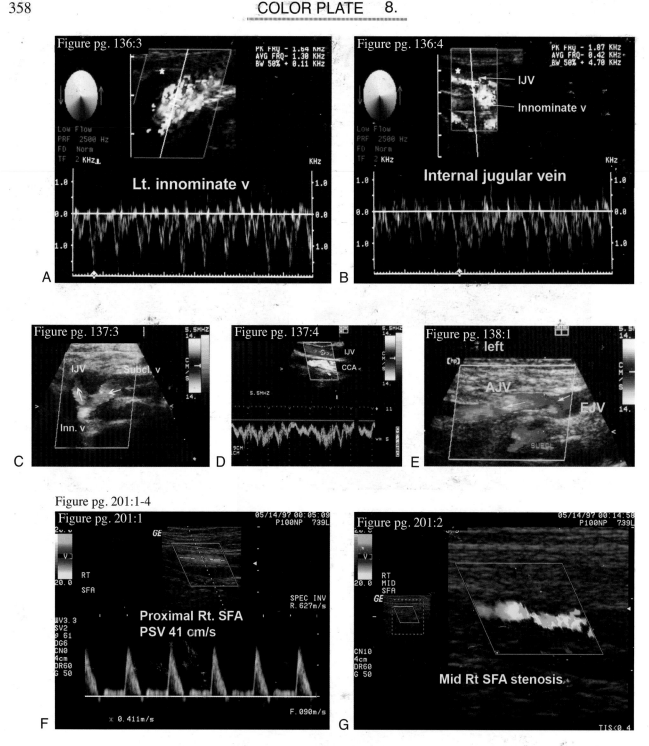

A & B. Case study #1 continued: Normal flow in a patent innominate vein and in the IJV. **C - E**. Case study #2. This patient has a left innominate vein occlusion. **C**. Flow is reversed in the IJV; note it's the same color as the CCA in image D. **E**. Flow in the anterior jugular vein is also retrograde. **F & G**. Series of images "mapping" a superficial femoral artery stenosis. PSV proximal to stenosis is 41 cm/sec. (continued).

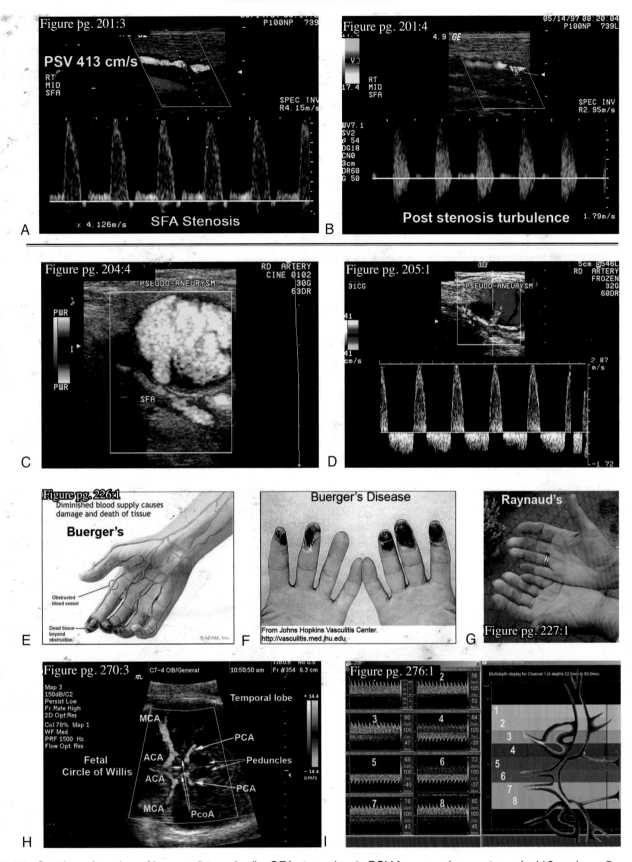

A & B. Continued: series of images "mapping" a SFA stenosis. **A**. PSV from maximum stenosis 413 cm/sec. **B**. post-stenotic turbulence. **C**. Power Doppler image of a pseudoaneurysm originating from an SFA. **D**. Spectral Doppler from the "neck" demonstrating a "to & fro" flow pattern. **E & F**. Illustration and example of Buerger's disease. **G**. Patient with Raynaud's Syndrome. **H**. Transcranial color imaging demonstrating cerebral vascular anatomy. **I**. Transcranial Doppler color "M-mode" with multiple PW sample gates.

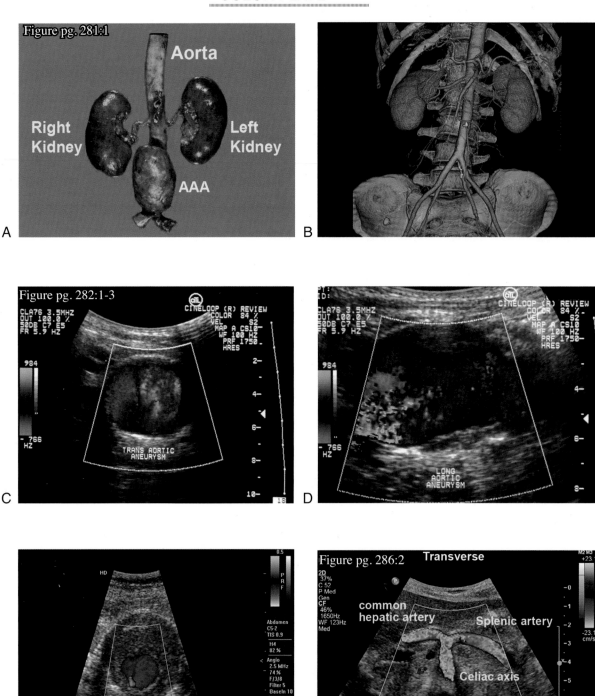

A. Abdominal aortic aneurysm (AAA) from a cadaver. **B.** CTA of normal abdominal vascular anatomy. **C.** Transverse view of a AAA. **D.** Longitudinal view of the same aneurysm. **E.** AAA containing thrombus. **F.** Transverse view of the celiac axis.

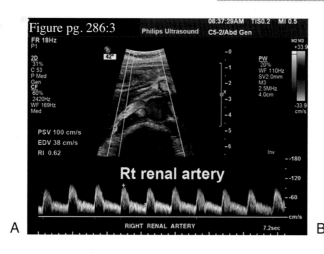

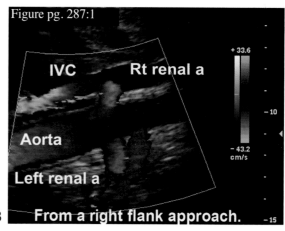

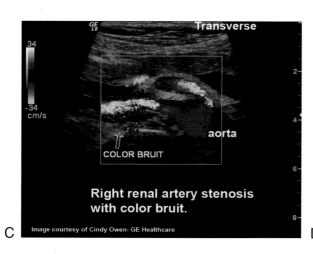

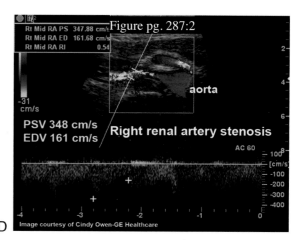

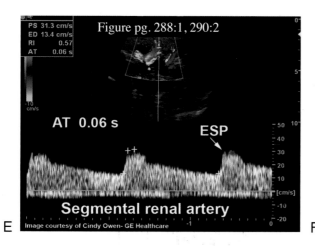

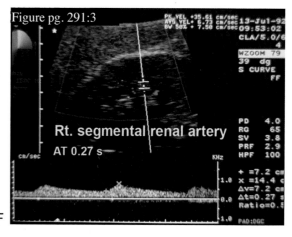

A. Normal right renal artery flow. **B**. Longitudinal view of the renal artery origins from a right flank approach. **C**. Right renal artery stenosis with a color bruit. **D**. Doppler waveforms from within the Rt. renal artery stenosis; PSV 348 cm/s. **E**. Normal segmental renal artery waveform with early systolic peak (ESP), and a fast rise time, 0.06 seconds. **F**. Abnormal segmental renal artery waveform with delayed rise time (0.27 sec.) and tardus-parvus waveform shape. Also noted was reduced color fill in the renal vessels (due to reduced flow). The main renal artery had a > 80% stenosis.

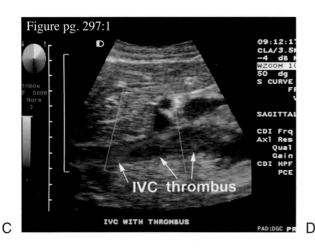

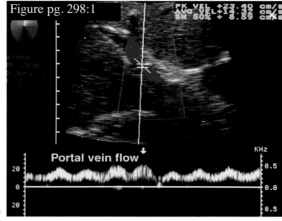

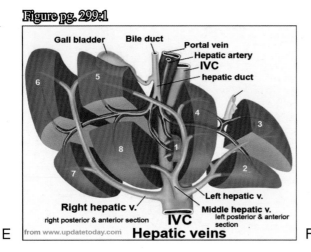

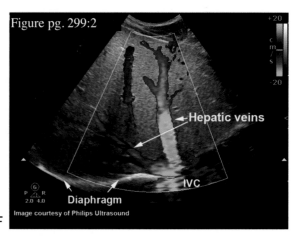

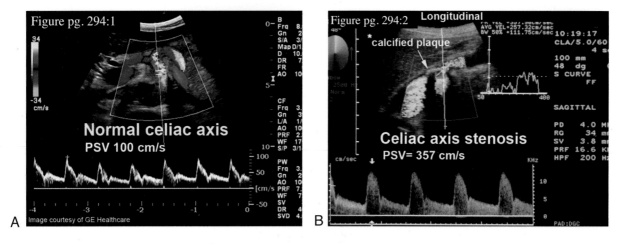

A. Normal, low resistance celiac artery flow. **B**. Spectral waveform from maximum stenosis in a celiac artery. PSV 357 cm/s. **C**. Partially thrombosed IVC; this can cause portal hypertension. **D**. Normal hepatopetal (into the liver) portal vein flow. **E**. Diagram (inverted to resemble an ultrasound image) of hepatic vein anatomy. **F**. Color Doppler image of normal hepatic vein anatomy and flow direction.